MEDICINE WAYS

CONTEMPORARY NATIVE AMERICAN COMMUNITIES
STEPPING STONES TO THE SEVENTH GENERATION

Despite the strength and vibrancy of Native American people and nations today, the majority of publications on Native peoples still reflect a public perception that these peoples largely disappeared after 1890. This series is meant to correct that misconception and to fill the void that has been created by examining contemporary Native American life from the point of view of Native concerns and values. Books in the series cover topics that are of cultural and political importance to tribal and urban Native peoples and affect their possibilities for survival.

Series Editors

Troy Johnson
American Indian Studies
California State University, Long Beach
Long Beach, CA 90840
trj@csulb.edu

Duane Champagne
American Indian Studies Center
3220 Campbell Hall, Box 951548
University of California, Los Angeles
Los Angeles, CA 90095
champagn@ucla.edu

Books in the Series

1. *Inuit, Whaling, and Sustainability*, Milton M. R. Freeman, Ingmar Egede, Lyudmila Bogoslovskaya, Igor G. Krupnik, Richard A. Caulfield and Marc G. Stevenson (1999)
2. *Contemporary Native American Political Issues*, edited by Troy Johnson (1999)
3. *Contemporary Native American Cultural Issues*, edited by Duane Champagne (1999)
4. *Modern Tribal Development: Paths to Self Sufficiency and Cultural Integrity in Indian Country*, Dean Howard Smith (2000)
5. *American Indians and the Urban Experience*, edited by Susan Lobo and Kurt Peters (2000)
6. *Medicine Ways: Disease, Health, and Survival among Native Americans*, edited by Clifford E. Trafzer and Diane Weiner (2001)

Editorial Board

Jose Barreiro (Taino Nation Antilles), Cornell University
Russell Barsh, University of Lethbridge
Brian Dippie, University of Victoria
Lee Francis (Pueblo), University of New Mexico
Carole Goldberg, University of California, Los Angeles
Lorie Graham (Blackfeet), Harvard Law School
Jennie Joe (Navajo), University of Arizona
Steven Leuthold, Syracuse University
Nancy Marie Mithlo (Chiricahua Apache), Institute of American Indian Arts
J. Anthony Paredes, Florida State University
Dennis Peck, University of Alabama
Luana Ross (Confederated Salish and Kootenai), University of California, Davis

Medicine Ways

DISEASE, HEALTH, AND SURVIVAL AMONG NATIVE AMERICANS

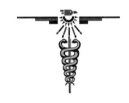

edited by

CLIFFORD E. TRAFZER and DIANE WEINER

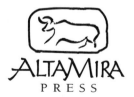

ALTAMIRA
PRESS

A Division of
ROWMAN & LITTLEFIELD PUBLISHERS, INC.
Walnut Creek • Lanham • New York • Oxford

ALTAMIRA PRESS
A Division of Rowman & Littlefield Publishers, Inc.
1630 North Main Street, Suite 367
Walnut Creek, CA 94596
http://www.altamirapress.com

Rowman & Littlefield Publishers, Inc.
4720 Boston Way
Lanham, Maryland 20706

12 Hid's Copse Road
Cumnor Hill, Oxford OX2 9JJ, England

British Library Cataloguing in Publication Information Available

Library of Congress Cataloging-in-Publication Data
Medicine ways : disease, health, and survival among Native Americans / edited by Clifford E. Trafzer and Diane Weiner.
　　p. cm.
　Includes bibliographical references and index.
　ISBN 0-7425-0254-6 (cloth : alk. paper) — ISBN 0-7425-0255-4 (pbk. : alk. paper)
　　1. Indians of North America—Medicine. 2. Indians of North America—Diseases. 3. Indians of North America—Health and hygiene. I. Trafzer, Clifford E. II. Weiner, Diane (Diane E.)
E98.M4 M43 2000
362.1′08997—dc21

00-055867

Printed in the United States of America

CONTENTS

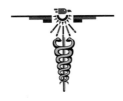

CONTENTS

vi

INTRODUCTION

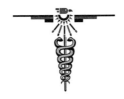

The chapters in this book represent a diversity of academic and practical interests that reflect our varied perspectives on health, illness, disease, and mortality. During a recent interview about their views on common and urgent community health concerns, two American Indian women, Anna and Beth,[1] commenced discussing issues concerning diabetes and obesity. The topic of talk swiftly changed, when, in agreement, the two women began explaining the way local off-reservation politics and economics, framed and mainly controlled by the dominant society, were impinging on community self-sufficiency and thus their communal and individual well-being. These astute young leaders understood that conditions such as diabetes and obesity have physiological, social, emotional, and spiritual symptoms and responses brought on, in part, by aspects of history, politics, economics, psychology, language behaviors, religion, and personal experience. They also asserted that such influences enable groups and individuals alike to become active participants in health, healing, and the prevention of future maladies and predicaments, rather than passive recipients of medical assistance or reactors to health crises.[2] Moreover, health-care decisions and accompanying strategies may be unpredictable, multilayered, and individually and culturally variable.[3] Conditions of health, illness, disease, and even death are socially constructed, based on the perceptions held by members of social and cultural networks.[4]

If all these factors come into play, how might we define health? Medical anthropologists, historians, and sociologists as well as health policy administrators tend to define health as a contrast to or in reference to illness.[5] The World Health Organization declares health to be "a state of complete physical, mental, and social well-being and not merely the absence of disease or infirmity."[6] One American Indian elder from Southern Arizona expanded on this view during an anthropological interview. A retired housekeeper who suffers from chronic knee pain, she explained that "healthy means that you're not sick. You're able to work, to do for yourself—everything." In his chapter in this volume, "The Embodiment of a Working Identity: Power and Process in Rarámuri Ritual Healing," Jerome Levi assures us that this conception of the self as able and productive is not idiosyncratic. Ability and function are multitextual. Critical medical anthropologists[7] and other heirs to Marx, Engels, Virchow, and Parsons may assert that such notions of health reflect issues of economic productivity and reproductive ability; in this vein, health is shaped by ideological and social relations of political and economic structures of production and expropriation.[8] Indeed, chapters by Akers, Castillo, Hassin and Young, Johnson and Tomren, Trafzer, and Weiner give voice to aspects of this stance. Illness and sickness occur *partially* due to non-Indian destruction and manipulation of native sociocultural, economic, and political environments. Illness and sickness are also rooted in personal and collective Native actions; individuals and communities are perceived to be at least somewhat responsible for their own health, a state that also encompasses the complex interactions of social, intellectual, and spiritual essences, symbols, and metaphors of a being and a community.[9]

In Native cultures, health is often expressed as a balance between a body, mind, and spirit or soul.[10] At an abstract philosophical level, health, or, perhaps more appropriately, "wellness," is the possession of moral ways of knowing and enacting this balance.[11] It is obtained, maintained, and experienced through culturally appropriate responses by individuals or groups to actual or perceived events.[12] Raised practicing both his tribal and Catholic religions, a southern California man in his thirties says that health includes "the spiritual, physical, and the mental—you get a good mixture of all those [if you] believe in something higher than yourself." Health is also felt to be influenced by the interactions between people and natural elements, since humans originated from and with the assistance of beings of the natural world. These ideas about health are founded in American Indian oral narratives as well as historical and cosmological teachings that are shaped within sociocultural contexts.

According to oral traditions, during primordial times beings were immortal, and the first "peoples" of earth were in a state of health. Due to jealousy, treachery, or sometimes because of poorly controlled consciousness one or more beings used his/her powers unwisely, resulting in the illness and death of one or more of the first beings. Because of the interdependent scheme of the cosmos, one life effects another. Today, as in centuries past, certain beings give their lives for others; for instance, deer or salmon may offer their lives so that others may be nourished. Although mortality occurs, healing powers also come into existence. Poison plants exist, but so do healing plants, representing positive and negative power. These ideas form the foundation of American Indian cultural perceptions of health, illness, and mortality throughout the continent.

As in the past, contemporary states of health among American Indians may be placed in jeopardy as a result of a disruption of the integration of the body with either secular or sacred social connections. When secular and sacred ties are disturbed,[13] ill health may then ensue. Reactions to disharmony may occur days, weeks, months, years, or generations after the event. What may be considered a health problem or illness among certain individuals or groups might be ignored or be viewed as an observable physical or behavioral distinction. Certain people may consider sadness, disrespect, a cough, or tooth loss as impairments or dysfunctions, while others may perceive these conditions as nothing more than distinguishing markers.[14]

Inherently linked to biomedicine, disease is usually described by health professionals as a purportedly objective, decontextualized,[15] and measured physical change in the structure or functioning of the body.[16] Certain American Indian lay individuals and communities recognize disease as a condition diagnosed by a clinical health professional. For example, among members of certain southern California tribes, lupus and diabetes, defined, diagnosed, and legitimized solely by medical technologies and personnel, are called diseases.[17] Clearly, disease, like health, is a social construct.[18]

Death also may be defined in a variety of ways. Clinicians, biogeneticists, religious leaders, and members of different ethnic groups may all consider death to occur at distinct stages and under different circumstances.[19] In this volume, Donna Akers, Edward Castillo, Troy Johnson, and Holly Tomren eloquently describe and assess the ways extreme spiritual anguish accompanies and aggravates bodily death. Indeed, among the Choctaw during the period after forced migration to Indian Territory, spiritual death may take place even as physiological life holds. Perceptions of the afterworld are also varied. Death of the body does not necessarily bring extermination of the soul.[20] Having passed from this secular world, the soul may still retain power. For this reason, the dead continue to influence the health of their ancestors and others. They are still part of the spiritual world and are honored through memorial services, meals, and stories. According to many Native people, spirits can cause disease and death, or they may contribute to health and well-being.

As revealed in this book, major health concerns of the past centered on medically identified infectious conditions such as respiratory ailments, typhoid, diphtheria, measles, smallpox, syphilis, trachoma, and tuberculosis. The authors also assess Native-identified problems including fevers and sickness of mysterious origins, sorcery, and forced migration from ancestral homelands and spiritual beings. Emotional torment, hunger, and the deterioration of tribal environmental, economic, social, and political resources all contributed to these dilemmas. As Linda Green writes in her analysis of ethnographies of violence, the authors in this collection analyze and pay homage to "the extraordinary and subtle means by which people subvert, contest, and appropriate violence"[21]—both symbolic and physical modes. The writers explicate histories of suffering that influence contemporary constructions of, beliefs about, and strategies to prevent, detect, and treat health problems.

Current health concerns are alarming and may be traced to local and national histories and policies. Clinical typologies include Type 2 diabetes, cancer, depression, suicide, stress, violence, and substance abuse—all of which plague the Native peoples of North America. The only contemporary indigenously defined illness in this collection, detailed by Jerome Levi, is described in English as a "loss of power" accompanied by pain and weakness. It may not surprise readers that these symptoms are often associated with the preceding list of clinical conditions. And even though a single individual may exhibit symptoms associated with a "loss of power," not only may that individual be affected, but friends, family, and community members may be at risk for this problem as well.

The strength of Native peoples in some regions may be in jeopardy because the loss of numerous community healers and shamans throughout the past century has decreased the ability to protect people. Fortunately, American Indian individuals and groups are not passive and fatalistic. They tend to take action and try to rectify ailments. Solutions, both grandiose and minor, are available. Sometimes people are demonstrably proactive, at other times they may appear to be reactionary. Many people tend to be decision-makers, although they may engage different health beliefs and systems at distinct moments in time.[22] As many elders will tell, it is not possible to return to the "Old Ways." However, as Jerome Levi clearly delineates, it is possible and helpful to incorporate tribal and traditional healing processes to treat contemporary woes. These therapies may not resemble all facets of those that took place 20, 50, or 200 years ago, but like the Tongva who attacked an epidemic through the destruction of the sand painting as described by Castillo, or those leaders who initiate social-service and health-care programs in their communities as discussed by Hassin and Young, American Indians are taking actions for positive purposes.

Clinical, native, and popular therapeutic systems are all described herein. Under particular circumstances, certain people utilize one health system: biomedical, native, Christian, or others. A person with a fever may take ibuprofen to assuage this malady. Some individuals have developed syncretic systems, mixing health beliefs and behaviors much as they might combine elements of different religions into one ritual. For instance, someone who has a fever may assert that it was caused by "germs" and must be treated through the joint use of rest, prayer, and aspirin. Other individuals may combine treatments from more than one tribal group, blending herbal treatments from two distinct regions, for instance.

Many people make use of multiple systems of health care, utilizing two or more parallel and seemingly distinct structures of health. Like the person who separately practices both Catholicism and her Native religion, this individual may declare that her fever was possibly caused by germs and by the evil intent of another person. Sometimes the etiologies and associated prevention and treatment methods of a condition form cognitively separate domains.[23] When a multiplicity of health systems exists, there are numerous points at which an individual and/or caregivers have the opportunity to make a usage choice and the health-care decision-making process becomes quite complex.

The health-seeking process is not always sequential; a person may forego care, then seek preventive measures, and later use two or three systems of care.[24] As Nancy Reifel, Diane Weiner, and Brooke Olson write, overall choice seems to be inextricably linked to cultural acceptability, economic and infrastructural access, and efficacy. Todd Benson, Clifford Trafzer, Jerome Levi, and Linda Burhansstipanov, James Hampton, and Martha Tenney keenly observe that political structures greatly impact the utilization of health care as well as health status. These phenomenon are not unique to Natives of North America—such situations are common throughout the world.[25] However, they are particularly acute in American Indian health strategies because of the pervasive domination of Euro-American governments upon American Indian communities. For instance, Burhansstipanov, Hampton, and Tenney describe the limited documentation of cancer statistics about Native peoples. This situation may be interpreted by policy makers to mean that cancer detection and care programs are unnecessary for a particular group of Natives—the underlying perception becomes that if cancer statistics do not exist, the condition itself must be rare. In turn, comprehensive research into the matter and associated means of cancer detection and quality life-saving treatment is often deferred.

The contributors to this volume examine the ways people from a multitude of indigenous communities think about and practice health care within historical and sociocultural contexts on the micro and macro levels. The writers also assess the impact of a variety of social, health, and political systems upon the health of Native peoples. Conditions of health, illness, disease, and death must be analyzed and addressed in this manner. As so eloquently expressed by Eric Henderson, Stephen Kunitz, and Jerrold Levy in their analysis of Navajo youth-gang behaviors, the histories of social maladies must be examined in order to deter these problems in the future.

With the exceptions of Akers, Castillo, and Levi, the writers in this collection analyze clinical categories of illness. As academics we might ask ourselves why there is currently a fascination with and focus on clinically defined health categories. Is it because we are doing our research and writing in English, the language of clinical health in the United States? Is it because American Indians and Alaska Natives currently have a greater tendency to be diagnosed by and cared for by clinical practitioners rather than by Native providers? Is Type 2 diabetes more prevalent than "loss of power"? Are health professionals and lay people more apt to request a study of diabetes than of "loss of power," asserting that the former is more damaging than the latter? Is it because after decades of investigating so-called cultural illnesses, we as academicians prefer not to reveal the perceived sacred, ritual, and private health beliefs and practices of American Indians? Or, in a more cynical vein, are there more sources of funding to examine suicide and cancer than there are to investigate soul loss? These may be unanswerable questions. We must ponder these inquiries and ask ourselves whether these predicaments have value.

All of the authors in this work strive to shed light on information that has been ignored, underreported, misclassified, and obfuscated. The works contribute significantly to the developing body of research by and among contemporary Native peoples of North America. In his chapter, "The Embodiment of a Working Identity: Power and Process in Rarámuri Ritual Healing," Jerome Levi deals with a curing ceremony that a leader underwent in 1989 among his people, the Rarámuri (Tarahumara) of northern Mexico. Levi argues that his research demonstrates that the body is a "house of the souls" as well as an active agent of Rarámuri personhood. The body, he argues, requires serious scholarly study in terms of ritual healing. Levi shows that through the physical body, the people empower themselves and bring forth strength, vitality, energy, and health. He provides a comparative study of healing ritual, and a first-hand, detailed description and analysis of one such ritual.

In his provocative chapter, "Blood Came from Their Mouths: Tongva and Chumash Responses to the Pandemic of 1801," Edward Castillo links the spiritual beliefs of two California Indian peoples to disease, death, and cultural resistance. He examines the Tongva and Chumash Indians of the Los Angeles Basin and adjoining northern coastal region. During the era of the Spanish Mission system, Native Americans often interpreted epidemics as manifestations of their own culture, finding causes and solutions within their own cultural frameworks. During an epidemic in 1801 at Mission San Gabriel, Tongva viewed the sickness and death as an internal, Native phenomenon created by two *Ta.xkw.a* (Indian doctors or medicine men). The disease may have been diphtheria, but Tongva leaders learned that a local *Tumia.R* (or principal chief) had hired two Indian doctors to create a sandpainting on Catalina Island to kill his opponents. After the people killed the two medicine men and their assistant, the epidemic ended among the Tongva. Diphtheria also ravaged the Chumash at Mission Santa Barbara, Santa Ynez, and La Purisima Concepcion.

During the height of an epidemic in 1805, a Chumash woman dreamed of a Native deity named Chupu (Earth Mother) who instructed the people to save themselves from sickness by refusing or renouncing Christian baptism. Castillo links the armed resistance of the Chumash against the Franciscans and presidio soldiers with Native spiritual beliefs that significantly influenced the course of events between the two peoples. He maintains that Native religion played a significant role in response to European diseases and that Native spiritual beliefs tied many people together as a natural cultural response to biological threats brought by the Spanish.

The correlation between Native spiritual beliefs and health is also a theme found in Donna Akers's chapter, "Removing the Heart of the Choctaw People: Indian Removal from a Native Perspective." Akers argues that the forced dispossession of Choctaws from Mississippi was far more than political and economic. Rather, the Choctaws saw their forced exile from their homes as a spiritual uprooting to a place they called, "The Land of Death," that is, the direction or place where the dead lived after ending their lives in Mississippi. Like many Native Americans, Choctaws considered their homelands to be sacred and marked by *Nanih Waiya*, a sacred mound that took generations to build, constructed after the people had completed their migration to Mississippi. The Bookbearer enjoined the people never to surrender their homelands and left a legacy of beliefs and rituals that bound the people together and with plants, animals, water, and places of the south. Furthermore, the government forced most Choctaws into present-day Oklahoma, a dangerous place where spirits of the dead traveled low to the ground or resided permanently. As a result of forced relocation, the Choctaws suffered disease, starvation, suicides, murders, and a general anomie that dislocated the people for generations.

A similar situation is analyzed by Clifford Trafzer in "Infant Mortality on the Yakama Indian Reservation, 1914–1964." Trafzer describes how the government relocated fourteen distinct tribes and bands onto a small land base known as the Yakama Reservation in central Washington State where people died of many diseases. During the 50-year period from 1914 to 1964, the modal age of death on the reservation was infants under one year. He shows that the infant mortality rate on the Yakama Reservation from the 1920s into the 1940s was many times higher than that of whites and nonwhites in the United States as well as that of people in Washington. Infants died primarily of pneumonia, gastrointestinal disorders, tuberculosis, heart disease, and syphilis. Trafzer maintains that bacteria and viruses cause most infant deaths, but that conditions on the reservation—poor housing, lack of traditional food, depression, inadequate public health and medical care, and powerlessness—contributed significantly to high infant mortality. And though it is possible to quantify the numbers of deaths, it is not possible to measure the degree to which housing, food, depression, medicine, public-health education, and so forth contributed to these deaths. On the Yakama Reservation, nearly a third of all deaths during the era from 1914 to 1964 were those of children under six years of age. This is not uncommon among populations throughout the world, but it is disturbing nevertheless.

In her work "In the fall of the year we were troubled with some sickness," Jean Keller also deals with childhood deaths. She traces the deaths of individual students in 1904 who suffered and died from a typhoid epidemic at Sherman Indian Institute located in Riverside, California. Keller details the case histories of each student and discusses the circumstances surrounding the epidemic that took their lives. She offers a critical analysis of Harwood Hall, the school superintendent who failed to report the deaths or epidemic in his correspondence to the Office of Indian Affairs, referring euphemistically to the epidemic as "some sickness." Keller's chapter is one of the first scholarly examinations of Sherman Indian Institute and inaugurates a larger research plan to examine medicine, health, disease, and death at the government boarding school.

Todd Benson also deals with Indian health during the era of the 1920s when the Office of Indian Affairs launched a dangerous campaign to eradicate trachoma among Native American populations. In his chapter "Blinded with Science: American Indians, the Office of Indian Affairs, and the Federal Campaign against Trachoma, 1924–1927," Benson addresses the problem of trachoma, a debilitating eye disease in which tiny red blood vessels form in the conjunctiva or lining of the eyelid and surface of the white of the eye. Trachoma spread through tears, infecting hundreds of Indians. Unable to control the disease, the medical division of the Office of Indian Affairs chose a radical surgical procedure known as "grattage" to eradicate the disease. When this procedure failed, medical doctors working for the government began performing tarsectomies, the removal of the tarsal plate underlying the conjunctiva. Even when administrative and medical officials realized that the radical procedures did not work, they continued to operate on American Indian patients in order to curb the tide of trachoma.

Not all health professionals working on reservations were as callused as policy makers for the Office of Indian Affairs or the surgeons performing tarsectomies. Nancy Reifel provides insightful research into reservation field nurses and their fight against poverty, ill health, smallpox, and tuberculosis. In her chapter "American Indian Views of Public-Health Nursing, 1930–1950," she focuses on two Sioux reservations, Pine Ridge and Rosebud, discussing the role of field nurses and the responses of various Lakota people to white field nurses. The oral histories provided in this path-breaking essay will be of use to anyone interested in health among Native Americans during the early twentieth century. They provide an American Indian voice seldom heard with regard to the efforts of field nurses to stem the tide of disease and death on reservations during the early twentieth century. The use of oral interviews with Native peoples is a hallmark of Reifel's chapter.

Diane Weiner is innovative in her use of oral interviews in her contribution, "Interpreting Ideas about Diabetes, Genetics, and Inheritance." Weiner's work combines original field research with interpretations. She deconstructs the terms "genetics" and "inherited" with regard to cross-cultural discourse between Native American patients and health providers. In a very real sense she deals with four "bodies," including the body of Native people with diabetes, the body of medical-health providers, the body of Native communication, and the body of communication of the medical-health providers. Weiner points out that data regarding perceptions about inheritance helps researchers understand the causes and nature of diabetes as well as illustrate the cultural misunderstandings that arise between and among health-providers and Native patients when discussing diabetes.

In her chapter "Meeting the Challenges of American Indian Diabetes: Anthropological Perspectives on Prevention and Treatment," Brooke Olson offers practical advice to tribal leaders, health providers, and policy-makers about dealing with diabetes. After providing brief overviews of diabetes and genetic considerations regarding the disease among Native American populations, Olson suggests specific strategies by which to deal with diabetes education and prevention among Native cultures. She argues that effective programs depend on understanding the cultures being served, since there is a vast difference between diverse tribes. Traditional health beliefs, concepts of the body, Native exercise and games, storytelling, and Native foods are all topics discussed and analyzed by Olson. These are powerful components of an effective diabetes education and prevention program among Native peoples.

Felicia Schanche Hodge and John Casken describe "Pathways to Health: An American Indian Breast-Cancer Education Project," a practical and culturally sensitive project by which health-care providers developed a breast-cancer educational program with Native American women in California. Using a community-based approach, the scholars worked with six focus groups of Indian women to produce educational materials, including an informational video for native women, breast-cancer treatment guide, resource directory, workshop curriculum, and video for health-care providers. Among the many findings in this work is the fact that these Indian women regard early detection of breast cancer as a low priority in their lives in comparison to the needs of their families. The authors also point out that one of the problems associated with breast cancer and other forms of cancer among American Indians is the lack of accurate data regarding cancer among Native populations.

This situation is the major theme of another chapter found in this book. In "Cancer among American Indians and Alaska Natives: Trouble with Numbers," Linda Burhansstipanov, James Hampton, and Martha Tenney assert that there is a great need to develop cancer programs among Native Americans, but there is a problem obtaining reliable data in order to assess epidemiological trends among Native populations with reference to cancer. Overall, there is a general underreporting of cancer incidences, deaths, and survivals for Native Americans, and the result has been the inability of health professions and Native peoples to recognize increased cancer rates throughout Indian country. The authors argue that while a few states (New Mexico, South Dakota, and Alaska) have access to better databases, there are major problems with databases found in other states.

Most scholars would agree that in order to provide effective health-education and -prevention programs, communities and professions must have a baseline of accurate data on the health problem. This is certainly true with regard to diabetes, cancer, and suicide as demonstrated in works featured in this text, but it is also important in dealing with another health problem that has emerged among Native Americans: the rise of youth gangs on Indian reservations. Eric Henderson, Stephen Kunitz, and Jerrold Levy combine their research to offer "The Origins of Navajo Youth Gangs." The authors argue that youth gangs among *Diné* emerged out of the nineteenth century, after the United States forced thousands of people on a "Long Walk" to the Bosque Redondo for a four-year exile in eastern New Mexico. The Navajo War and forced removal in the nineteenth century were catastrophic to *Diné* men who had previously proven their ascendancy to adulthood through raiding ranchos for horses, cattle, and sheep. This component of Navajo culture largely ended after 1868 when the people returned to their homelands, but some males continued to organize into adolescent male peer groups. Today, officials of the Navajo Nation estimate that sixty youth gangs exist on the reservation, groups that originated in the 1970s. The authors argue that although these gangs have antecedents in the last century, changing demographic, economic, and social conditions on the reservation during the 1970s contributed to the rise of modern Navajo gangs. They maintain that membership in a gang is one way in which Navajo youths may make the transition from childhood to adulthood. Using a theoretical framework advanced by Terrie Moffitt, the authors examine the emergence of modern gangs that are intimately connected with alcohol and drug abuse as well as other antisocial health-related behavior.

One of the themes developed by the authors is that gangs provide young people with a vehicle through which to feel mature, powerful, and in control of their lives. This is also a theme fully developed in "Self-Sufficiency and Community Revitalization among American Indians in the Southwest: American Indian Leadership Training." In this research, Jeanette Hassin and Robert Young argue that Native dependency on the dominant society has created destructive anomie among Native peoples and alienation from non-Indians. In order to correct this trend, the two scholars have launched a vigorous self-empowerment program to encourage Native American self-sufficiency through community involvement. Hassin and Young maintain that permanent change can occur within communities through self-determination and self-sufficiency, a two-tiered process involving one's own personal health, direction, and action as well as a community level of revitalization. The authors provide primary interviews that inform us about views of the body, mind, pain, health, spirit, and many other topics. This is a revealing piece of research that offers suggestions for personal and communal action that will lead to empowerment and better health.

Certainly one's view of body, mind, spirit, pain, and empowerment have a great deal to do with reversing trends among Native Americans that can lead to suicide. This is a main idea found in "Helplessness, Hopelessness, and Despair: Identifying the Precursors to Indian Youth Suicide" by Troy Johnson and Holly Tomren, which is a detailed analysis of suicide, suicide stereotyping, and suicide prevention among Native Americans, particularly young males. Their research is at once contextual and theoretical, drawing on the works of James Shore, Philip May, Teresa LaFramboise, Beth Howard-Pitney, and other scholars who have studied suicide among Native Americans. Johnson and Tomren argue that among American Indian youths ages 15 to 24, suicide is the second most-frequent cause of death in the United States—nearly two-and-a-half times greater than that of other youths from all races in the country. Suicide has been an ever-increasing problem among Native American populations on and off reservations since the 1950s, and it is considered epidemic on some reservations. After deconstructing and analyzing suicide among Native American youths, the authors offer recommendations to families, health-care providers, human-services professionals, and others interested in curbing the tide of youth suicides. Among others, these recommendations include a team approach to combat suicide, incorporating volunteers from among tribal elders, teachers, parents, and spiritual leaders.

Health issues have always been an important element of American Indian culture, and the topic is a continual theme in the traditional oral narratives of all tribes. Since the time of creation, there have always been destructive forces afoot, doing harm to the people depicted in ancient tribal stories. There has never been a time when negative, destructive, and dangerous forces did not exist or threaten Native communities or individuals with annihilation. Traditionally, oral narratives metaphorically depicted disease and death as monsters that consumed plant and animal people, destroying the natural environment and creating confusion among communities. Within the stories, evil monsters continually challenged the people, but through the heroic efforts of individuals and communities, the people always fought back against the forces of destruction. This is an underlying theme of the research presented in this book.

At the beginning of the twenty-first century, Native Americans are taking an ever greater role in fighting disease, death, depression, and destruction among their people. For instance, Anna and Beth and individuals throughout Native nations are developing community economic programs to enhance self-sufficiency and improve their financial, physical, social, spiritual, emotional, and nutritional well-being. Leaders—old and young—are engaging in this struggle with increasing knowledge, although many Native Americans would agree that knowledge is unevenly distributed and access to knowledge is based on one's unique abilities to comprehend.[26] Much of the work in this book explores the ways powerlessness (social, physical, emotional, and spiritual) impacts the body and bodies of Natives and the manners by which it may be replaced by power. An understanding of past and current health dilemmas enables us to engage not only in theoretical conversations about problems, but also offer possible solutions from academics who cross the fence between the walls of the university and the indigenous communities and lives of people whom we describe and analyze. We hope that these investigations of health inspire others to develop means to ensure the health and welfare of future generations of all First Nations people.

Notes

1. These names are pseudonyms.
2. See Robert A. Hahn, *Sickness and Healing: An Anthropological Perspective* (New Haven, CT: Yale University Press, 1995), 7.
3. Linda C. Garro, "On the Rationality of Decision-Making Studies: Part 2: Divergent Realities," *Medical Anthropology Quarterly* 12 (1998): 341–55.
4. Arthur Kleinman, *Patients and Healers in the Context of Culture* (Berkeley: University of California Press, 1980); *The Illness Narratives: Suffering, Healing, and the Human Condition* (New York: Basic Books, 1988); Jennie Joe and Dorothy Miller, *American Indian Cultural Perspectives on Disability* (Tucson: Native American Research and Training Center, 1987); Veronica Evaneshko, "Presenting Complaints in a Navajo Diabetic Population," in Jennie R. Joe and Robert Young, eds., *Diabetes as a Disease of Civilization: The Impact of Culture Change on Indigenous Peoples* (Berlin: Mouton de Gruyter, 1994).
5. See Lesley Doyal with Imogen Pennell, *The Political Economy of Health* (Boston: South End Press, 1979); Hahn, *Sickness and Healing*.
6. World Health Organization. WHO Definition of Health from the Internet, 1997–1998 <http://www.who.int.aboutwho/en/definition.html>.
7. Merrill Singer, "Developing a Critical Perspective in Medical Anthropology," *Medical Anthropology Quarterly* 17 (1986): 128–29; Merrill Singer, "Keep the Label and the Perspective: A Response to 'Emic' Critiques of Medical Anthropology," *Anthropology Newsletter* (March 1989): 15–19; Ronald Frankenberg, "Medical Anthropology and Development: A Theoretical Perspective," *Social Science and Medicine* 14B (1980): 197–207; Ronald Frankenberg, "Gramsci, Culture, and Medical Anthropology: Kundry and Parsifal? Or Rat's Tail to Sea Serpent?" *Medical Anthropology Quarterly*

(1988): 324–37; Hans Baer, Merrill Singer, and John H. Johnson, "Toward a Critical Medical Anthropology," *Social Science and Medicine* 23 (1986): 95–98.

8. See Vicente Navarro, "U.S. Marxists' Scholarship in the Analysis of Health and Medicine," *International Journal of Health Services* 15 (1985): 525–45; Howard Waitzkin, "Micropolitics of Medicine: Theoretical Issues," *Medical Anthropology Quarterly* 17 (1986): 134–35.

9. See Nancy Scheper-Hughes and Margaret Lock, "The Mindful Body: A Prolegomenon to Future Work in Medical Anthropology," *Medical Anthropology Quarterly* 18 (1987): 6–41; Gay Becker, *Disrupted Lives: How People Create Meaning in a Chaotic World* (Berkeley: University of California Press, 1997).

10. For an excellent presentation of this description of health and wellness, see John Molina, "Cultural Medicine," *Journal of Minority Medical Students* (Spring 1997): 28–32.

11. See Jean-Guy A. Goulet, *Ways of Knowing: Experience, Knowledge, and Power among the Dene Tha* (Lincoln: University of Nebraska, 1998).

12. See Robert Lake, Jr., "Shamanism in Northwestern California: A Female Perspective on Sickness, Healing, and Health," *White Cloud Journal* 3 (1983); Carol Locust, *American Indian Beliefs Concerning Health and Unwellness* (Tucson: Native American Research and Training Center 1986).

13. For instance, the majority of accidents and injuries have observable secular causes. Nonetheless, some acts that befall a person may also be traced to social and/or religious violations. A person may state that a child broke her arm while jumping from a rock. This event may be analyzed as a circumstance of visible causal relations. Yet it may also be attributed to the improper social behavior of the child or her kin.

14. Joe and Miller, *American Indian Cultural Perspectives on Disability*; see also, Cecil Helman, *Culture, Health and Illness: An Introduction for Health Professionals* (Boston: Wright Publishers, 1990).

15. See Laura Nader, *Naked Science: Anthropological Inquiry into Boundaries, Power, and Knowledge* (New York: Routledge Press, 1996), for an analysis of scientific knowledge.

16. Helman, *Culture, Health and Illness*, 86–89; see also, Horatio Fabrega and Peter Manning, "Illness Episodes, Illness Severity and Treatment Options in a Pluralistic Society," *Social Science and Medicine* 13B (1979): 44.

17. For more information on this subject, see Diane Weiner, "Luiseño Theory and Practice of Chronic Illness Causation, Avoidance, and Treatment." Doctoral dissertation, University of California, Los Angeles, 1993.

18. J. N. Hays, Introduction, in *The Burdens of Disease: Epidemics and Human Response in Western History* (New Brunswick, NJ: Rutgers University Press, 1998), 1–7.

19. See Robert L. Rubinstein, "Narratives of Elder Parental Death: A Structural and Cultural Analysis," *Medical Anthropology Quarterly* (1995): 257–76; Margaret Lock, "Death in Technological Time: Locating the End of Meaningful Life," *Medical Anthropology Quarterly* (1996): 575–600.

20. Richard Applegate, *Atishwin: The Dream Helper in South-Central California* (Socorro, NM: Ballena Press, 1977).

21. Linda Green, "Lived Lives and Social Suffering: Problems and Concerns in Medical Anthropology," *Medical Anthropology Quarterly* (1998): 3.

22. Diane Weiner and John Molina, Concluding Remarks, in Diane Weiner, ed., *Preventing and Controlling Cancer in North America: A Cross-Cultural Perspective* (Westport, CT: Praeger, 1999), 225; Hays, *The Burdens of Disease.*

23. See also Leo Chavez et al., "Understanding Knowledge and Attitudes about Breast Cancer: A Cultural Analysis," *Archives of Family Medicine* 4 (February 1995): 145–52.

24. Noel Chrisman, "The Health Seeking Process," *Culture, Medicine, and Psychiatry* 1 (1977): 351–78.

25. Susan C. M. Scrimshaw, "Adaptation of Anthropological Methodologies to Rapid Assessment of Nutrition and Primary Health Care," in Nevin S. Scrimshaw and Gary R. Gleason, eds., *Rapid Assessment Procedures: Qualitative Methodologies for Planning and Evaluation of Health-Related Programmes* (Boston: International Nutrition Foundation for Developing Countries, 1992).

26. See Lowell John Bean, "Power and Its Applications," in Lowell John Bean and Thomas C. Blackburn, eds., *Native Californians: A Theoretical Perspective* (Berkeley: California Indian Library Collections, 1976).

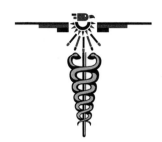

Removing the Heart of the Choctaw People

INDIAN REMOVAL FROM A NATIVE PERSPECTIVE

In 1830, the U.S. Congress passed the Indian Removal Act, effectively authorizing President Andrew Jackson to dispossess and forcibly remove thousands of Native people from their homelands in the American Southeast to lands west of the Mississippi River. The Removal Era has been explored by American historians over the years using classic historical methods and sources. They have recorded and analyzed the usual political and economic happenings and the prominent men with which these events are associated. White America's philosophical and cultural beliefs have been examined in an effort to understand the underpinnings of Manifest Destiny and America's insatiable drive for land and dominance. Various racial and political attitudes have been studied, along with economic factors such as the price of cotton on the world market. What has rarely been examined, however, is what Removal meant to Native people, from a Native point of view.[1]

The archives and other written sources that are often mined by modern scholars are almost exclusively written by non-Native people. Government and military records and accounts, even personal journals and diaries, reflect white authorship. Some of these sources include transcriptions of the speeches and other oral communications made by Native people. But these are, almost without exception, orations that were crafted and intended for white audiences—

1

usually government personnel or national legislatures—and therefore conform to the Native perception of what would be important or meaningful to the larger American culture.

Sources that Native people trust to relate their experiences sometimes differ markedly from those considered valid or reliable by mainstream white historians. Most Native groups passed cultural and historical knowledge from generation to generation, not through written records but through oral accounts. Some mainstream scholars distrust oral sources, so often the information available from these records is omitted from the historical record, leaving a one-sided version of American history. Oral narratives contain an illimitable opportunity for Native cultural understanding and knowledge. Although they may evolve over the years, this makes them not less reliable than written records, but more so—if one is seeking information regarding the Native perception of events within their cultural context. To understand the historical experience of Native Americans it is essential to enter their world to the greatest extent possible. Without an understanding of the Native American experience, historians only relate the experience of white America.

Sources written in Native languages also are largely excluded from the historical record—usually because of pedestrian difficulties inherent in translation. In addition, however, this is due to the racialist/colonialist thinking of the dominant majority, which discounts the value of Native sources. It would be unthinkable for a French historian not to have a working knowledge of the French language. Why is it acceptable for students of Native people not to be familiar with, or knowledgeable about, the language(s) of the people they are researching? To get at the historical experiences and perspectives of all participants during the Removal Era, therefore, it is necessary to consult the oral as well as the written record—and to examine records written in Native languages as well as in European languages.

In 1830 the Choctaw Nation occupied some of the most fertile lands in North America. In the heart of what would become the Cotton Kingdom, the Choctaws' lands encompassed most of the Mississippi Delta, as well as regions of Alabama and Louisiana. According to Choctaw traditions, these lands had been Choctaw lands forever, given to them by the Great Spirit, Chitokaka. The Choctaws resided in villages along rivers and streams, where they followed a primarily agricultural and sedentary lifestyle.

Choctaw society was based on matrilineal kinship. Clans provided the fundamental Choctaw identity, and heritage was reckoned through the mother's line. During the late eighteenth century, a few white men moved among the Choctaws as traders, adventurers, or outcasts of their own European or American homelands. Some married Choctaw women and spent their lives enveloped in Choctaw society. Since matrilineal kinship provided Choctaw identity, their offspring were fully accepted and reared as Choctaws. The children's first language was Choctaw, and their social training and identity was that of Choctaw children. Their paternal heritage sometimes contributed a rudimentary knowledge of the English language. Their father's occasional Euro-American visitors, as well as the tribe's participation in commerce among the white traders, brought exposure to the distant world of Americans on the east coast. But for the most part these influences were limited, and most of the so-called mixed-blood families lived lives dominated, on a day-to-day basis, by the Choctaw world.

In the early nineteenth century the Choctaws sought to appease U.S. demands by ceding sections of land that, at first, seemed of negligible necessity to the Choctaws. However, the demands for land cessions continued and escalated until about 1815, when Choctaws leaders saw that they must halt further cessions altogether. Choctaw participation in the world market was limited primarily to trading deer hides in exchange for guns, ammunition, metal tools, and utensils. A few among the Choctaw had begun to sell crops and cattle to nearby Native or white communities, but as their land base shrank from cessions to the United States, so did the game supply within Choctaw territories. The Choctaw economy had incorporated the fur trade and the resulting acquisition of European manufactured goods into the core of Choctaw life. The sudden contraction of this market and the increased difficulty in obtaining European trade goods created a violent disruption and rapid disintegration of Choctaw society. Simultaneously, white traders smuggled enormous quantities of illegal liquor into the Choctaw Nation, promoting its consumption and hence the erosion of Choctaw lifeways. Real deprivation and economic hardship struck with a vengeance, as a whirlwind of change battered the Choctaws from every direction.

In order to understand the enormous psychological impact the Removal Era had on the Choctaws, one must examine the range of relationships between themselves and non-Choctaws. Relations with outsiders were a fundamental facet of Choctaw being. Reciprocity was at the heart of all relations, including those formed by kinship or clan. Relations with outsiders followed the precepts of kinship, and to Choctaws, these relations were not a parody of kinship relations, but were, in fact, actual kinship realized. White Americans and Europeans had long observed these facets of diplomacy and ritual friendship among the Choctaws and other Native peoples. However, they understood only vaguely that these rituals encompassed a fundamental concept central to Native belief systems.

To the Choctaw, fictive kinship relations with outsiders were essential to human coexistence and could not be avoided. The Choctaw Nation defined outsiders as either kin or foe. They believed that everything in life—the physical, mental, abstract, and concrete—was of one functional whole, one system that tied every being together in permanent yet ever-dynamic relationships. If

3

all were partners in an interconnected system, one could not act without affecting all others. Therefore, harmonious relationships with animal spirits, inanimate objects, and other human beings were essential. In this world view, balance and harmony were fundamental to the community's and the individual's existence and well-being. If balance or harmonic relations were disturbed, dire consequences would follow, causing all to suffer.

In their earliest relations with the United States, the Choctaw Nation came from a powerful position. Allied with the United States during the War of 1812, they provided essential assistance during the Battle of New Orleans, fighting under Andrew Jackson. Subsequently, they assisted Jackson in his assault on the Red Sticks, tipping the balance to the United States during the Battle of Horseshoe Bend. Intense loyalty and fidelity to one's allies and kin permeated these relations. In the second decade of the nineteenth century, even as the relative balance of power shifted and Choctaws became weaker than the ever-strengthening Americans, the Choctaws believed that their relationship with the United States would continue unchanged. Since, in the Choctaw world view, all were part of a non-hierarchical system, each group would continue to recognize and act upon the bonds of kinship, even though their relative power or strength might change.

However, the U.S. government conceptualized its relationship with the Choctaw within a hierarchical framework based on relative power. To Americans, it was natural for Choctaws to assume an inferior role. All their dealings with the Choctaws reflect an arrogance founded on the United States's unquestioning belief in their own cultural superiority. Prior to 1800, and perhaps in the first decade of that century, the United States recognized the strength and military prowess of the Choctaws and sought to engage in a diplomatic relationship between equals. In the next two decades, however, Choctaw power declined precipitously, relative to that of the United States. As a result, Americans began to view their relations with the Choctaws as one of superior to inferior—in both the military and political sense. Having always had a persistent belief in their unquestionable moral and cultural superiority, Americans married the changing relationship of power to their philosophical belief in their inherent superiority, creating a monster that, without compunction, consumed the lands and lives of thousands of Native people.

The 1820s saw the rise of Andrew Jackson to national prominence. He was extremely popular among whites in the backwoods areas of the South, where he consistently called for the expulsion of the resident Native nations. The momentum of expansionism escalated exponentially during this decade, as whites poured into the western reaches of the South hungering for cheap land, and the constituents of U.S. politicians demanded the expulsion, by force if necessary, of the Indians occupying lands they coveted. Whites began invading and squatting on Choctaw soil. The Choctaws thought that surely their

"Father" in Washington would evict these interlopers, as promised in the treaties. The reciprocal relationships long recognized between the Choctaws and the U.S. government demanded this much. The Choctaws were confident, because of their traditional expectations of the behavior of allies and friends, that the U.S. government would stem the incursions into their lands, and would guarantee, as promised, their continued sovereignty and territorial integrity. Despite Jackson's long personal history with the Choctaws, however, he now lead the cry of those calling for their dispossession and exile. This betrayal was met with disbelief and shock. As a traditional people, the Choctaws could not comprehend the pace of events and the sudden shift in U.S. policy from assimilation to dispossession. Even the most biculturally adapted Choctaws never believed that betrayal on such a scale actually would occur. The treachery of their old ally, Jackson, and his sponsorship of their expulsion and exile created a tremendous reaction among the Choctaws. But before we explore their reaction to this betrayal, one must examine what dispossession and exile meant to the Choctaw people.

"Indian removal," as the whites termed it, created moral and spiritual crises intimately linked to fundamental Choctaw beliefs about place, origin, and identity. Choctaws had a deep spiritual and physical attachment to the earth. The earth was the source of all power, a "numinous presence of the divine, the sacred, the truly real by reference to which everything else found its orientation." Most Native people, including Choctaws, vested the earth with an overriding maternal quality: the earth mother gave life and sustained all living things. As siblings, all humans and animals intimately were connected, kindred in a literal sense. All had spirits and destinies irrevocably intertwined with the destiny of humankind.[2]

Many traditional Choctaws believed that humans sprang from the earth from many primeval pairs scattered over the regions of the earth. They were each created separately from the different natural features and substances found in the region of the earth in which each people lived. For example, in a land of forests, the original humans came from the trees; in rugged, mountainous areas, they came from the rocks; on the plains, people emerged from the soil. "Mother earth" gave birth literally as well as spiritually to the Choctaw people.[3]

After their arrival in the American Southeast, sometime back in the ancient mists of time, the Choctaws began to inter their dead in a great mound, built to honor the spirits of the dead. Taking three generations to construct, this sacred mound was called *Nanih Waiya*, known also as *Ishki Chito*, "the Great Mother." This pyramidal mound was located in the southern part of what is now Winston County, Mississippi. Years passed in peace, and then a devastating epidemic struck the people. Everyone died but the headman, who was immortal. When all but this one had perished, the great mound opened and swallowed him.

5

After the passage of many years, the Great Spirit created four infants, two of each sex, out of the ashes of the dead at the foot of *Nanih Waiya*. They were suckled by a panther, and when they were older and strong enough to leave, the prophet emerged from the Mother and gave them bows, arrows, and an earthen pot. Stretching out his arms, he said, "I give you these hunting grounds for your homes. When you leave them, you die." With these words, he stamped his foot; *Nanih Waiya* opened, and, holding his arms above his head, he disappeared forever.[4]

All Choctaw children learned these stories in childhood. The stories were taught as moral and historical lessons, intertwining the spiritual and literal as did the Choctaws in all areas of their lives. Through the oral traditions, Choctaws learned that they not only were part of the Earth, but also part of a specific region of the earth. The gift of the Great Spirit was this land. They were never to leave it, or the nation would die.

The original migration tradition of the Choctaw people emphasizes their attachment to this particular spot of earth (a sacred reciprocal agreement with the dead also is tied to this specific place). This tradition relates how the Choctaw people traveled for forty-three years, everyone carrying the bones of their ancestors. Many of the people carried so many bones that they were unable to carry anything else. Some were so overloaded that they would carry one load forward a half day's journey, deposit it, and then return for the remainder, which they then would carry forward the next day. This task was considered a sacred duty. According to the spiritual teachers, the spirits of the dead "hovered around their bones to see that they were respectfully cared for, and that they would be offended and punished with bad luck, sickness, or even death for indignities, or neglect of their bones."[5]

Each day, at the end of their travels, the people's leader—the *Isht Ahullo*— would plant the Sacred Pole in the ground. At dawn, the leader would rise and see the direction in which the Sacred Pole was leaning—the direction in which the people were to travel that day. One morning at dawn, the leader observed that the Pole "danced and punched itself deeper into the ground; and after some time settled in a perpendicular position, without having nodded or bowed in any direction." The Choctaws' long journey was at last at an end. The Choctaws arrived at the leaning hill—known to the people later as *Nanih Waiya*—in a "plentiful, fruitful land of tall trees and running waters" envisioned by the great Choctaw chiefs in a vision forty-three years before.[6]

At the end of this journey, some of the younger Choctaws did not understand their sacred duty to the dead bones of their deceased kinsmen. The *Isht Ahullo* explained that the people must always take care of "the precious remains of the fathers and mothers," for the Choctaw people were charged by the spirits, who are hovering thick around us now, to take care of them; and carry them whithersoever the nation moves. And this we must not, we dare not fail to do. Were we to cast away the bones of our fathers, mothers, brothers, sisters, for the wild dogs to gnaw in the wilderness, our hunters could kill no more meat; hunger and disease would follow; then confusion and death would come; and the wild dogs would become fat on the unscaffolded carcasses of this unfeeling nation of forgetful people. The vengeance of the offended spirits would be poured out upon this foolish nation.[7]

In historical times, the Choctaws continued to take their responsibility to the spirits of the dead very seriously. Every time they moved their villages, they transported the remains of those who had died. This duty was considered a sacred pact with the dead. In return for honoring the remains of the dead, living Choctaws would be watched over by the spirits of their ancestors. The spirits spoke to the living through dreams and visions, guiding and assisting the Choctaws in all things.

Traditional Choctaws literally believed that they emerged from the Great Mother Mound. In the mid-nineteenth century, the elderly Choctaws, when asked their place of birth, insisted that they emerged from *Nanih Waiya*. Thus, the forced exile from Mississippi separated the Choctaw people from their own mother. They had been warned by the prophets that the people would all die if they ever left their lands.

The Choctaws tried to convey the imperative reasons that they remain in the lands of their ancestors to the U.S. agents and government. They could not understand the whites' assertion that they took the Choctaws' well-being to heart as they forced them away from that which gave them life. One old man haltingly attempted to impart some understanding of their dilemma to an U.S. agent. He said, "We wish to remain here where we have grown up as the herbs of the woods, and do not wish to be transplanted into another soil." The Choctaws saw themselves as part of the soil, an integral element of the ecosystem, tied inextricably to this specific part of the earth. Their world was a vast, complex system of life and spirits, all comprising an indivisible whole. Like the old man's herbs, the Choctaws believed they could not be separated from their mother, the land of which they were a part. The Choctaws could no more be separated from these lands and survive than could the pine forests of the Southeast be uprooted and transplanted hundreds of miles to the West. The Choctaws were part of their homelands. Separation from it meant their death.[8]

Compounding the enormity of the thought of separation from their homelands was the Choctaw understanding of the west as the direction of death. West, both a direction and a place, held special meaning in Choctaw cosmology. The Choctaw afterworld was located on earth, somewhere in the west. According to Choctaw traditions, the *shilup*, or inside shadow, one of the two spirits that every person has, left the body after death and traveled low over the earth to the west, the Land of Death. Choctaw mortuary rituals had to be performed properly or the *shilup* could not make the journey to the afterworld and instead would hover about the place of death, punishing the living kin who had failed him.

Once the *shilup* arrived in the west, it went to a place of happiness and delight, *shilup i yokni*. However, murderers were excluded from this happy ending. They were unable to find the path leading to the land of happiness and instead remained in view of, but unable to reach, that destination. This place of the murderous spirits was called *atuklant illi*, the Second Death. The horror this place conjured up in the minds of Choctaws cannot be overestimated. It was the land of the living dead, the place where the most horrible spirits roamed in unending despair and hopelessness. It was said that in this place, "the trees are all dead, and the waters are full of toads and lizards, and snakes—where the dead are always hungry, and have nothing to eat—are always sick and never die—where the sun never shines, and where the spirits climb up by the thousands on the sides of a high rock from which they can overlook the beautiful country of the good hunting-grounds . . . but never can reach it." This was the destination the United States reserved for the Choctaw people.[9]

To the Choctaw, the west, then, was the Land of the Dead; it was the location of the Second Death, where spirits unable to reach the afterworld roamed forever. The west was the direction from which their ancestors fled in ancient times out of dire necessity. Leaving their homelands in the east meant breaking the covenant with the spirits of the ancestors. In the Choctaw world view, the act of leaving would mean the nation's death. If they left behind the remains of the dead and abandoned their sacred duty, they would commit the most heinous crime in Choctaw cosmology.

The United States's arrangements for their physical removal left the Choctaws no choice. They had to abandon the bones of the dead. Under the best of circumstances, there was no way for them physically to disinter all the remains and transport them. In fact, the Choctaws had to abandon most of their material possessions, since the U.S. government provided few conveyances for people, much less baggage. Most necessities remained behind, such as the hominy mortars that the women considered their most essential tool for food preparation.[10]

Abandoning the bones of the dead was unthinkable to most Choctaws. Even the more acculturated Choctaws of mixed Native and white heritage found themselves unable to reconcile themselves to such an act. Many Choctaws, therefore, refused to leave. The Choctaws believed that every human had two souls. The *shilup* left the body and traveled west to the Land of Death. The *shilombish*, however, remained at the site of death, guarding the remains of the body and its treatment by living Choctaws.[11] One elderly Choctaw man explained this to the U.S. agents: "In those pines you hear the ghosts of the departed. Their ashes are here, and we have been left to protect them. Our warriors are nearly all gone to the far country west, but here are our dead. Shall we go, too, and give their bones to the wolves?"[12] Women, especially, were reluctant to leave. Many families were split apart, as mothers and grandmothers adamantly refused to abandon the bones of their dead children and their *shilombish*, the outside shadow.[13]

The Treaty of Dancing Rabbit Creek was the instrument used by the United States government to force the Choctaws from their homes. Under the guise of legality, this treaty was procured in 1830 by fraud and deception, against the consent of almost the entire Choctaw Nation. Over the subsequent protests of thousands of Native people and white missionaries, the U.S. Senate ratified the treaty, and the government informed the Choctaws that they had three years in which to leave.

This news produced the most profound reactions among the Choctaw. Chaos was the immediate result. The people quit planting crops; many simply gave up. The months of summer passed without a harvest, and when the winter came, the people began to starve. Alcoholic bingeing became the norm, and the children suffered. Drinking led to violence, as hopelessness engulfed the nation. Thirteen Choctaws died from alcohol poisoning in one month. One missionary reported that the entire nation was in utter disarray. The men stopped hunting, the women stopped planting, starvation and disease followed. Children wailed all night from hunger and inattention. Missionary Cyrus Kingsbury reported that the consequences of the treaty "almost beggars description. Loud exclamations are heard against the treaty in almost every part of the nation. . . . The nation is literally in mourning. . . . Multitudes are so distressed with their prospects as to sit down in a kind of sullen despair. They know not what to do."[14]

In 1831 the first parties were assembled to leave at certain appointed gathering places throughout the nation. The night before one party departed, the women covered their heads with their skirts, keening the death songs all night long. The warriors sat stoically, facing away from the fires, into the woods. In the morning, as the soldiers stirred the reluctant Choctaws, men and women lovingly touched the leaves and branches of the trees as they departed. They left in autumn, as one of the worst winters in memory struck throughout the South. When they reached the Mississippi River, they were stopped indefinitely by ice floes obstructing passage. The ferries and steamboats stopped running, forcing parties of Choctaws to camp out night after night in freezing rain. The Choctaws seemed unsurprised by the suffering; they were forewarned by the oral prophecies.[15]

The journey to the west was characterized by American ineptitude, incompetence, and fraud. Many Choctaws died or became seriously ill due to exposure, disease, and inhumane arrangements for their journey. Most of the nation was forced to walk the entire journey, which was more than five hundred miles.

They traveled in kinship groups. Stories are still related of the suffering and death inflicted on the Choctaw people. One large group of emigrants was lost in a Mississippi swamp. The men, women, children, and elderly walked in chest-deep swamp water for thirty miles. They went without food for nearly six days, and many began dying from exposure and starvation. They had given up and were singing their death songs when a rescue party reached them. One witness reported that among the bodies of the dead Choctaws were one hundred horses standing up in the mud, stiff from death. The survivors were so disoriented that their rescuers had to lead them out of the swamp by their hands, like little children.[16]

A Memphis citizen observed a group of exiled Choctaws on the road, completely unprepared for the harsh winter weather. They had no tents—nothing with which to shelter themselves. Not one in ten had even a moccasin on their feet and the great majority of them walked. This same man witnessed the travails of another Choctaw party that camped in the woods near his home. One night a hail storm began, followed by two days of heavy snowfall. The Choctaw party was stranded in the coldest winter weather the region had ever experienced. He reported that they lay in their camp for more than two weeks without shelter of any kind and with very few supplies. The second week, the weather averaged twelve degrees Fahrenheit. The abrupt departure had left many with little or no time to prepare or pack necessities, which they were told would be supplied by the U.S. government. The government failed to do so. Only one blanket was issued per family—and most families averaged six members.

Yet another party traveled through sleet and snow for twenty-four hours, most barefoot and nearly naked, in order to reach Vicksburg without exhausting their inadequate supplies. The disgusted U.S. Army captain who was their official escort reported that "If I could have done it with propriety I would have given them shoes. I distributed all the tents and this party are entirely without." He complained about the inadequate provisions made for the Choctaws, and said that the sight of these people and their suffering would convince anyone of the need for an additional allowance for transportation.[17]

As if the weather were not enough, the Choctaws were dogged by sickness on their exile west. Cholera, the most dreaded scourge of the times, struck again and again. A report of its presence in Memphis caused all the wagon drivers hired by the U.S. government to abandon their teams, leaving 150 wagons for the sick and aged standing with full teams of horses. Agent William Armstrong reported that these Choctaws had suffered dreadfully from cholera, stating, "The woods are filled with the graves of the victims. . . . Death was hourly among us and road lined with the sick."[18]

The Choctaws were forced to abandon traditional mourning rituals on the journey west. The bodies of the dead were not scaffolded. Typically lasting more than three months, the rituals were viewed as superstitious and heathen by the U.S. agents. The Choctaws sought to take their dead with them to the new lands, but the U.S. agents did not allow them to do so. One group's U.S. agent forced the Choctaws to bury their dead the morning after their death, according to Euro-American tradition. He expressed his satisfaction in his report to his superiors in Washington that the dead had been "decently interred." The Choctaws, of course, understood that the *shilup* of these people were unable to travel to the land of death without the proper ritual of scaffolding and funeral cries. They would be forced to wander the earth, and would punish those who had thus abandoned their sacred duty.[19]

Nearly one-third of the Choctaw Nation died on the march west. Many of these were young children and elderly tribespeople, who disproportionately suffered from exposure, hunger, and disease. The enormous death toll produced social and political chaos. The council of elders that governed each town no longer existed when the Choctaws tried to rebuild in the west. The clans could not survive the death of so many of the elders. The elders were the leaders of each clan—they made the important clan decisions, and all those affecting the smaller kinship units. Since clans traveled together, some suffered death disproportionately, thus upsetting the checks and balances of power so carefully constructed over the centuries by the Choctaw. Their deaths also severely impacted the transmission and survival of cultural knowledge and ritual.[20]

Place always had played an important part in the identity of the Choctaw people. Red and white towns informed the martial or civil responsibilities and emphases of the townspeople. The dispersion of representatives of all clans throughout towns in the nation formed an essential network of unity and cohesiveness, and mitigated conflict among men. The deaths of so many of their people prevented the Choctaws from replicating the physical organization essential to their identity in the new lands of the west. This severe blow to kinship and identity rent the Nation and exacerbated the confusion and depression they suffered after their arrival.[21]

The Choctaws always have been survivors, and have shown themselves adept at meeting the challenges of a changing environment. Within a few years the majority had found kinsmen, erected shelters, and cleared fields. As early as 1833, several hundred Choctaw families had settled on the banks of the Arkansas River, planting crops in anticipation of the arrival later of many more emigrants, for whom they planned to provide corn. Perhaps these folks thought they had escaped the worst, for the spring planting had gone well and most of the people who survived the march were recovering. However, some saw the anger of the spirits raining down on the nation when in June 1833 the Arkansas River overflowed its banks in the greatest flood in its history. In astonishment at the damage done by the raging waters, the U.S. agent wrote that the Choctaw houses and fields were completely washed away, as though they had never existed. The cattle and horses some Choctaws had managed to bring with them drowned. Incessant rains continued all spring, flooding the entire river network in the new Choctaw Nation. Since the agrarian Choctaws always lived near rivers and streams, many new farms, if not most, were ruined that year. Some families were completely stranded by the high waters, and many began to starve.

Terrible sickness followed the floods. Carcasses of dead animals lined the riverbanks and floated in the waters, making it unfit for human consumption. The U.S. agent wrote that many were starving: "more than they ever suffered before from hunger." He reported many came to him begging for food, having had nothing to eat "for 10, 12, 15 days." The children cried continuously from hunger, and many died. "Within the hearing of a gun from this spot," he wrote, "100 Choctaws had died within the past week."[22] He reported that of the entire number of emigrants, one-fifth died from the floods, disease, and starvation. Many Choctaws were "even reduced to eating the flesh of animals found dead in the woods and on the wayside," reported the agent. He appealed to a nearby army unit for food for the Choctaws. The provisioning officer sent them fifty barrels of pork that had putrefied and spoiled. Earlier in the year, the Choctaws had refused to accept his proffer of these provisions, but now, the officer reported to his superior, "he was happy to inform General Gibson that since they were reduced to starvation, they would doubtless be glad to get it."[23]

In fulfillment of the prophecies, the nation was dying. As soon as they departed from their beloved homelands in the east, the Choctaws succumbed to exposure, illness, accidents, depression, misery, and death. No one was left unscathed. Even the U.S. agents were appalled at the suffering of the Choctaw people. The official U.S. government reports indicated that some 20 percent of the Choctaw people had died on the journey, and a great number more—perhaps another 20 percent—died soon after their arrival. The elders died disproportionately, making reestablishment of social and political institutions problematic. Old living patterns, important to the cohesion of the nation, proved impossible to duplicate in the west. Many survivors of the journey did not move from their point of entry into the new lands. According to U.S. observers, they were so depressed, they simply stayed put where they landed and did nothing. Some did not even build shelters or make any effort at all to clear fields or plant crops. Suicide became commonplace, whereas it was almost unknown in prior times.[24]

After removal of most Choctaws to Indian Territory, those Choctaws remaining in Mississippi kept a correspondence and relationship with those living in the new Choctaw nation. Choctaw families in the west reported the great tragedy befalling the nation. Some of the newly arrived émigrés turned around and started back. Others wrote kin that they should not come west. Those who stayed behind in Mississippi, intending to come later, now decided not to make the journey at all. These people became the prey of invading whites, many of whom were unscrupulous and had no compassion for Native people in distress. The thousands of Choctaws still in Mississippi were forced off their lands and into the remote and worthless swamplands. From there they sometimes would return to look upon their former bountiful homes and farms, all in the hands of white men.[25]

The new lands of the Choctaws in the west became known among Choctaw as the Land of Death. The misfortunes continued. On November 13, 1833, Choctaws experienced a terrible omen. That night, an extraordinary meteor shower lit up the night sky as bright as day "with myriads of meteors darting about in the sky." Some of the women and children screamed and cried in terror, while others hid. All night long the showers continued. The terror was not limited to the Choctaws. The Kiowas recorded this event, too, finding it so important that they named the season "the Winter that the Stars Fell." The Choctaws knew that the Great Spirit spoke through natural events such as this and that the unnatural event portended great misfortune. This celestial event coincided with the U.S. announcement that no more provisions would be provided for the people. The period covered by the treaty for their emigration had expired. And despite the terrible floods and illness and death suffered in the past two years, the United States intended to do nothing more to assist the exiles.[26]

The suffering of the Choctaw people intensified with the horror of a smallpox pandemic that struck Native people throughout the west from 1836 to 1840. More than ten thousand Native people died in the northern plains alone. Newly arrived emigrants in the Choctaw Nation brought the disease with them. More than a thousand Choctaws died, including their renowned and beloved leader, Mingo Mushulatubbee. Some families were destroyed completely, all members succumbing within days of each other. Whooping cough decimated the population of babies and toddlers among the Choctaws. One observer reported that all of the small children for miles were killed by one whooping-cough epidemic in the old and new Choctaw nations.[27]

As the decade of the 1840s began, the Choctaw people struggled to survive and rebuild in their new lands. The nation had been decimated by Indian Removal. Some estimate that more than one-third of the nation died as a result of their forced exile west and as many as four thousand Choctaws remained behind in the Southeast, to be dispossessed from their homes and relegated to wandering in the swamplands, working occasionally as stoop laborers on lands that had been their own. The social and political organization of the nation was in shambles. The clans so central to Choctaw identity and community barely survived the exile. Despite the terrors of the 1830s, however, the nation refused to die. The Choctaws began to rebuild, and in an uneven fashion social and political institutions began once again to function.

The story of the U.S. policy of Indian Removal must be reexamined and retold. It was not merely an official, dry, legal instrument as it often is portrayed. Removal, as experienced by Native people, was an official U.S. policy of death and destruction that created untold human pain and misery. It was unjust, inhuman, and a product of the worst impulses of Western society. Indian Removal cannot be separated from the human suffering it evoked— from the toll on the human spirit of the Native people. It cannot be remembered by Americans as merely an official U.S. policy, but must be understood in terms of the human suffering it caused, and the thousands of deaths and lives it destroyed.

Notes

1. Regarding Indian Removal, see Arthur H. DeRosier, Jr., *The Removal of the Choctaw Indians* (Knoxville: University of Tennessee Press, 1970); Grant Foreman, ed., *Indian Removal: The Emigration of the Five Civilized Tribes of Indians* (Norman: University of Oklahoma Press, 1932); Michael Paul Rogin, *Fathers and Children: Andrew Jackson and the Subjugation of the American Indian* (New Brunswick, NJ: Transaction Publishers, 1991). For an eyewitness account of the departing Choctaws, see Horatio B. Cushman, ed., *History of the Choctaws, Chickasaws, and Natchez Indians* (New York: Russell & Russell, 1962), 114–16.

2. Cushman, *History*, 94–95; and Denise Lardner Carmody and John Tully Carmody, *Native American Religions: An Introduction* (New York: Paulist Press, 1993), 19.

3. John R. Swanton, *Source Material for the Social and Ceremonial Life of the Choctaw Indians* (Washington, DC: Government Printing Office, 1931; reprint, Birmingham, AL: Birmingham Public Library Press, 1993), 202.

4. J.F.H. Claiborne, *Mississippi as a Province, Territory, and State with Biographical Notes of Eminent Citizens* (Jackson, MS: Power and Barksdale; reprint, Baton Rouge: Louisiana State University Press, 1964), 518–19.

5. Swanton, *Source Material,* 13–14.

6. Charley Jones, address to Choctaws, Choctaw Labor Day Festival, September 1997; and Annie Haley, interview, September 1991. Notes in possession of author.

7. Cushman, *History*, 15.

8. Claiborne, *Mississippi as a Province, Territory, and State*, 512; "Mingo Pushmataha," *American State Papers, Indian Affairs*, II, (Washington, DC: Gales and Seaton, 1832–1861), 230; and Simpson Tubby, quoted in Swanton, 100.

9. George Catlin, *North American Indians*, ed. Peter Matthiessen (New York: Penguin Books, 1989), 404; *The Missionary Herald* 24(6): 182–83; and Ruth Fowler Dodd, interview, August 1992. Notes in possession of author.

10. Jesse O. McKee and Jon Al Schlenker, *The Choctaws: Cultural Evolution of a Native American Tribe* (Jackson: University of Mississippi Press, 1980), 19; and Foreman, ed., *Indian Removal*, 79.

11. Swanton, 216–17; and *The Missionary Herald*, 182–83.

12. Claiborne, *Mississippi as a Province, Territory, and State*, 512–14.

13. John Pitchlynn to Peter P. Pitchlynn, June 13, 1834, Box 1, Number 41, Peter P. Pitchlynn Collection, University of Oklahoma.

14. Cyrus Kingsbury to Jeremiah Evarts, October 16, 1830, File 6, Number 24, Cyrus Kingsbury Collection, Western History Collection, University of Oklahoma, Norman.

15. Cyrus Kingsbury to Jeremiah Evarts, October 16, 1830, File 6, Number 22, Cyrus Kingsbury Collection, Western History Collection, University of Oklahoma, Norman; Greenfield Leflore to Eaton, November 19, 1830, Office of Indian Affairs, "1830 Choctaw Emigration," in ed. Foreman, *Indian Removal*, 39; Colquhoun to Gibson, July 1, 1832, Senate Document 512, I, 719; Annie Herchel Hanie, interview, May 1987.

16. Senate Document 512, I, 719; Harriet B. Wright to David Greene, "Missionary Letters," Andover-Harvard Theological Library, LXXII, no. 138, 1832.

17. Foreman, ed., *Indian Removal*, 53, 60.

18. Langham to Commissary General of Subsistence, November 8, 1832, Office of Indian Affairs, "Choctaw Emigration," 387, 737.

19. Letter from George S. Gaines, *Mobile Commercial Register* (November 12, 1831): 1.

20. Cushman, *History*, 95, 148, 176.

21. John Edwards, "The Choctaw Indians in the Middle of the 19th Century," in *Chronicles of Oklahoma*, ed. John R. Swanton (Oklahoma Historical Society, 1932), 10, 395, 400, 401.

22. Armstrong to Herring, September 17, 1833, Office of Indian Affairs, "Choctaw Agency," quoted in Foreman, *Indian Removal*, 97.

23. U.S. Senate Document 512, Twenty-third Congress, first session, "Indian Removal," I, 324.

24. William H. Goode, *Outposts of Zion, With Limnings of Mission Life* (Cincinnati: Poe and Hitchcock, 1863), 53; *Report of the Commissioner of Indian Affairs*, 1833 (Washington, DC: Government Printing Office, 1833), 254; and Annie Haney, personal communication, August 1991. Notes in possession of author.

25. John Pitchlynn to Peter P. Pitchlynn, November 23, 1832, Box 1, File 31; John Pitchlynn to Peter P. Pitchlynn, February 21, 1833, Box 1, File 35; John Pitchlynn to Peter P. Pitchlynn, January 30, 1834, Box 1, File 40; John Pitchlynn to Peter P. Pitchlynn, June 13, 1834, Box 1, File 41; and John Pitchlynn to Peter P. Pitchlynn, September 30, 1834, Box 1, File 43, Peter P. Pitchlynn Collection, University of Oklahoma, Norman.

26. James Mooney, *Calendar History of the Kiowa Indians* (Washington, DC: Smithsonian Institution Press, 1979), 260–61; Cushman, *History*, 195–97; and John Pitchlynn to Peter P. Pitchlynn, October 7, 1834, Box 1, File 44, Peter P. Pitchlynn Collection, University of Oklahoma, Norman.

27. Lavinia Pitchlynn to Peter P. Pitchlynn, December 14, 1841, Box 1, File 72; Rhoda Pitchlynn to Peter P. Pitchlynn, December 29, 1841, Box 1, File 73; Rhoda Pitchlynn to Peter P. Pitchlynn, January 5, 1842, Box 1, File 74, and January 15, 1842, Box 1, File 75, Peter P. Pitchlynn Collection, University of Oklahoma, Norman; and Cyrus Kingsbury to Jeremiah Evarts, November 24, 1830, Cyrus Kingsbury Collection, University of Oklahoma, Norman.

TWO

EDWARD D. CASTILLO

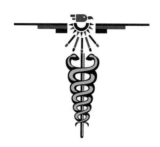

Blood Came from Their Mouths

TONGVA AND CHUMASH RESPONSES TO THE PANDEMIC OF 1801

The arrival of Spanish invaders on the shores of Alta California in 1769 spawned a biological holocaust among Southern California Indians.[1] The epidemics that swept across the coast, mountains, valleys, and deserts of California were catastrophic, causing Native Californians to attempt to comprehend the sickness and death stalking their various communities. European diseases significantly affected the lives of many Indians of California, including the Tongva of the Los Angeles basin and the Chumash north of them along the Santa Barbara coast. Tongva and Chumash people responded to epidemics brought to their homelands by the Spanish in a manner consistent with their spiritual and practical world view. In one sense they internalized the diseases, attempting to comprehend the massive suffering and death in a way that made sense to them. Traditional Native views of death and sicknesses shaped their response to them. This was clearly the case of the Tongva people living near Mission San Gabriel.

The Tongva of the Los Angeles basin spoke a dialect of the Takic family of languages derived from the larger Uto-Aztecan linguistic stock. The mainland Tongva were divided into two groups, one associated with the San Fernando Valley, and the other embracing the watershed of the Los Angeles and Santa Ana river basin. Ninety percent of their territory was within the rich Sonoran life zone whose ecological resources included vast quantities of acorn, pine nut, small game, and deer. On the coast, shellfish, sea mammals, and fish were taken. They followed an economy of hunting, collecting, and fishing that supported a population of approximately five thousand just prior to the Spanish invasion. The religious beliefs, practices, and mores of the Tongva centered on the cosmological belief that humankind was not the apex of creation but simply a strand in the web of life. Humans, like plants, animals, and even the landscape, shared reciprocal obligations to one another. According to creation stories, each provided something for the other and required a display of mutual respect and care. Careful stewardship of food resources and sacred places was proscribed.[2]

Indian doctors or shamans, called *Ta.xkw.a*, provided curing services, distributed foods from communal hunts, and sometimes practiced witchcraft. The diagnosis of illness was broadly divided into two categories: "loss of soul," and the intrusion of foreign objects in the patient's body due to taboo violations or sorcery. The *Ta.xkw.a* were important members of the elite class of citizens and leaders in the Toloache ritual complex,[3] which was based on the ingestion of the highly narcotic properties of datura, or jimsonweed, as it is commonly known. This dangerous and sometimes toxic substance was used both ritually as well as pharmacologically in male puberty ceremonies and medicinal contexts. In coastal California, two major religious subsystems developed out of the Toloache movement of southern California. Among the Tongva there emerged the Chingichnigish religion, and among the Chumash, the *?Antap* practices developed.[4]

Modern demographic studies have shown that American Indian populations in California were perhaps the highest in America (north of the valley of Mexico) and that just prior to the arrival of permanent colonization the "birth and death rates were substantially equal, and the total number of persons was more or less constant. With the arrival of the Spaniards the equilibrium in the coastal areas was profoundly disturbed."[5] According to the beliefs of these people, they enjoyed an abundance of food and good health, due in large measure to a careful observation of their religious mandates and faith in the Indian doctors. That faith would be seriously challenged by events that followed the arrival of Spanish colonial forces.

The Tongva were first reported by explorer Juan Rodriguez Cabrillo in 1542. However, permanent colonization forces did not arrive in Tongva territory until the late summer of 1771. Near the Los Angeles River, two Franciscan missionaries accompanied by ten soldiers staked their claim to the territory of the people of Porciuncula village by founding a mission called San Gabriel on September 8, 1771. Sporadic Tongva resistance ensued until October 2 when the *Tumia.r* (principal chief) of Porciuncula organized a large force of warriors to attack the Spanish compound in an attempt to kill a soldier who had raped his wife. The *Tumia.r* was killed by the soldiers, and two of his followers were wounded. The soldiers promptly decapitated the chief and displayed his severed head on a stake at the entrance to the mission.[6] There followed an ugly pattern of sexual assaults by the soldiers that did not spare even young children. A Scotsman married to a Tongva woman of high lineage reported on the typical soldier's sexual assault upon Tongva women:

> [A] large party [of soldiers], who commenced tying the hands of the adult males behind their backs; and making signs of their wish to procure women— these having fled again to the thicket, at the first appearance of their coming. Harsh measures obtained for them what they sought, but the women were considered contaminated, and put through a long course of sweating and drinking herbs, etc. They necessarily become accustomed to these things, but their disgust and abhorrence never left them till many years after. In fact every white child born among them for a long period was secretly strangled and buried![7]

Such depraved behavior by the colonists did little to enamor the Spanish to the bewildered Tongva.

As a result of the military violence and wholesale sexual assaults reported by early chroniclers of Mission San Gabriel, recruitment into mission society was slow. However, the Franciscan missionaries were well trained in methods of recruitment, gained from more than two centuries of missionary activities among Indians of New Spain.[8] Perhaps the greatest ally aiding in the recruitment process was the sudden appearance of a glut of horrible new diseases, virtually unknown to the Tongva and indeed all Native peoples of North America. Children's diseases such as measles, mumps, and chicken pox killed thousands of Tongva; while smallpox, diphtheria, typhoid, and other unidentified "fevers" killed more. Syphilis, introduced by the Spanish, while not fatal by itself, often accompanied other ailments, adding to the suffering and pain of a population that lacked immunities to these maladies.[9] Through a careful study of mission baptismal, marriage, and death registers, historian Robert Jackson has analyzed the Tongva population at San Gabriel and reported the rate of decline of the population to be a staggering 78 percent. Forced separation of female children from their parents, beginning at about the age of six, locked up in filthy and disease-ridden female barracks called *monjerios*, occurred at all missions. According to Jackson's study, "gross imbalance in the age structure developed with children under the age of ten making up a small percentage of the total population, and a growing gender imbalance, with few women surviving." Children's life expectancy averaged 6.4 years.[10] Worse still, everything Tongva shamans tried could not stem the tide of death and misery that overwhelmed their people. Experienced missionaries knew, and others soon learned, that the appearance of such deadly diseases would provide an opportunity for evangelization. Baptismal records at San Gabriel reveal that the earliest baptisms occurred among dying children and elders (those most vulnerable to epidemic diseases).[11] Under church law and Franciscan policy, such baptisms can occur without the permission of the dying individual. Consequently, when children occasionally survived, the grateful parents believed they owed it to the missionaries' efforts, and in gratitude often allowed themselves to be baptized. It is likely that they believed the spiritual power of the padres to be a good insurance policy against the periodic and terrifying waves of epidemic diseases that washed over the Tongva peoples.[12]

Colonists' medical efforts on behalf of the growing flood of sick and dying mission Indian laborers were uncoordinated and haphazard at best. Spanish, and later, Mexican medical doctors were stationed in the Monterey Royal Presidio and seldom were available to the neophyte population. During the great diphtheria epidemic of 1801 in southern California, the official surgeon was Juan de Dios Morelos. Apparently there was some doubt as to the professional credentials of Morelos, and he did not receive full pay as such. Nevertheless, there is no evidence that Morelos or any visiting naval surgeon was present to assist the Indian victims of that epidemic. During a study of Spanish surgeons in Alta California, physiologist Sherburne F. Cook of the University of California's medical school concluded that "these physicians actually accomplished relatively little, aside from local practice in the region of Monterey and San Francisco."

Consequently, most Western medicine available to sick Indians was through the padres themselves. It is known that some of the possible remedies offered by the attending Franciscans were raw potatoes; their leaves were applied to the head to stop pain. Fever was treated with verbena leaves boiled in water and swallowed. In an attempt to stop the bleeding, Yerba de Pollo (*Commelyna tuberosa*) was applied internally and externally. After a study of Spanish medical practices in Alta California, one medical historian concluded: "The Franciscan Padres came to Alta California with the avowed purpose of proselytizing; to cure the souls of the Indians not their bodies."[13]

Alarming accounts of the decimation of California Mission Indians by disease eventually prompted the viceroy of New Spain to order a medical survey of both *gente de razon* (the empire's Christian citizens) and Indian populations to determine their cause. In response, José Benites, the surgeon general at Monterey, undertook a journey as far south as Mission San Luis Obispo in the winter of 1804–1805. His report found dangerous public-health practices in general, and general poor health, especially among the Indians. This report further confirmed earlier official reports that the filthy and disease-ridden missions were the principal cause for the decline of the Indian population, especially among females. Tragically, little effective reform was undertaken, which took a steady toll on Indian lives.[14]

Serious disruption of the Native wildlife and flora and fauna resulted from the introduction of non-Native domesticated animals; horses, cattle, hogs, and sheep began to gobble up native food supplies. Within a few years, these grazing animals, allowed to wander unfenced, soon overran surrounding village territories. Serious disruption in neighboring village food supplies resulted. If local Tongva killed offending animals, the soldiers would launch punitive expeditions, whip and humiliate suspected village chiefs, and take hostages back to the mission. It is clear that many neighboring villages soon succumbed to mission recruitment activities as they faced the real possibility of hunger and starvation because of the depletion of native foods caused by introduced animals.[15]

The mission's goal was to transform the hunting and collecting California Indians into a well-disciplined and docile medieval-style labor force, ruled by a small class of Spanish male elites. The missions would train them in ranching and farming skills and convert them to Spanish Catholicism. Native peoples were expected to surrender their lands, resources, independence, and culture for the dubious status of inferior peons of the empire.[16] The advantage for the Franciscans was the opportunity to convert "pagans" to Christianity and demonstrate to their critics that God's empire on earth could be accomplished by the padres (with a little help from the army). The missionaries were supposed to complete this task in ten years, a goal never achieved; in fact, the Franciscans clung to their vast California empire for nearly seven decades. They blamed their failure to meet that deadline on the "stupidity" of the Indians. The imperial crown, on the other hand, would gain the advantage of an unpaid labor force that could be expected to support the colonial forces economically and secure Spanish territorial claims to this part of the New World.[17]

Prior to 1776, there developed a messianic movement known as "Chingichnigish" among the Tongva that soon spread to nearby tribes. The highly secretive sect is reported to have first appeared at the village of Puvugna in the person of an evangelizing messiah-shaman who introduced a new body of beliefs that became syncretized with the older beliefs and practices of the Toloache complex.[18] Revealing its connection with cosmotheism, the name Chingichnigish itself means "all dangerous, all seeing and present in all places."[19] New rules of behavior and numerous moral injunctions and taboos were required of followers. To enforce this strict new class of rules, avenger spirits (rattlesnakes, spiders, tarantulas, bears, stingrays, and ravens) would enforce compliance. Violations of the rules resulted in the admonition, "To him, I will send black bears to bite him, Pacific rattlesnakes to bite him, bad luck, sickness and sicknesses that he will die of."[20] The early-nineteenth-century Franciscan Padre Geronimo Boscana reported that the Tongva prophet explained, "the laws and establishing the ceremonies necessary to the preservation of life."[21] Because the prophet and his doctrines emphasized survival, the movement has been characterized as a crisis religion that developed in response to the biological holocaust enveloping the Tongva people.[22]

An extremely rare Native American account of how one group of Tongva at Mission San Gabriel perceived a mysterious sickness that was destroying them was collected from Native consultant José de los Santos Juncos by the

Smithsonian Institution's linguist John P. Harrington. About 1801, a serious "contagious fever" ravaged the Indians at San Gabriel. According to Juncos,

> the people at San Gabriel were dying. They had headaches, and blood came out of the mouth, and so on. The priests at San Gabriel were concerned. At first only single graves were dug, but they could not keep up, so they later made big pits and would throw the bodies of dead people in. When these were full they would cover it with earth and dig another pit.[23]

Just prior to these events, according to Juncos, a local *Tumia.r* (or captain) had paid two Catalina Island *Ta.xkw.a* brothers to kill his enemies with sorcery. The captain warned the shaman that none of his family was to be injured. They pursued their witchcraft in a remote canyon on the island, by use of a sand painting. However, this description of its use in sorcery illustrates the role that sickness and avenger spirits played in providing a culturally relevant explanation for the unhappy events they could not otherwise understand. Juncos reported: "When they were finished painting the world, they began to paint infirmities and blood, all over the world, as well as such dangerous animals that cause pain by biting, clawing and so on, to occupy places in the world—all of these things for sickness."[24]

The fever that erupted in 1801 caused considerable fear, as all the Indians sought to comprehend the source of the sickness. According to this Native account, "Only the Captain knew who was doing it—no one else knew."[25] Unfortunately, the captain's daughter grew sick and died along with the others. Believing himself betrayed, the captain journeyed to the coast and hired some *ti'ats* (ocean-going plank canoes) to take him and his followers to Catalina Island for revenge. Upon arrival they approached the local captain and explained the nature of their expedition. It would appear that the local captain also feared the *Ta.xkw.a* and agreed to help kill them. Without hesitation the two war parties located the isolated canyon where the sorcerers lived and surrounded their house. The Tongva captain challenged the brothers to come out and fight. As each emerged, they met a swift death. A young male apprentice was discovered within the house and showed the San Gabriel party the sand painting used to cause the sickness and death on the mainland. The boy was compelled to destroy the painting. Fearing that he too might be able to replicate the epidemic for revenge on the mainland people, the apprentice was likewise shot with arrows and killed. The house and bodies of all three were burned to prevent their resurrection. Juncos concludes his account by declaring, "The plague was over at San Gabriel."[26]

Just north of the Tongva lived the Chumash peoples. They spoke six dialects of the Hokan language stock. Their territory started from above Malibu and extended along the coast and adjacent to San Luis Obispo. About 3,200 Chumash populated the northern Channel Islands: Anacapa, Santa Cruz,

Santa Rosa, and San Miguel. The hunting, fishing, and collecting economy was based on the intensive exploitation of sea mammals, fish, and other marine foods. Females collected acorn, tubers, and grass seeds, while males hunted deer, small game, and waterfowl. The rich natural resources of the mainland coast supported an extraordinarily large population, which reached 12,000 or more before contact.[27]

The Chumash shared many cosmological aspects of their hunting and collecting neighbors, the Tongva. Nevertheless, their Toloache traditions were somewhat different. The precontact datura-based ?Antap religion was restricted to the elite classes and focused its ritual and cosmological attention on the sun, the earth, and her three aspects: wind, rain, and fire. ?Antap also functioned to control professions, displaying characteristics of craft or guild associations by restricting access to some trades and rights to certain property.[28] Following missionization, a significant messianic revitalization movement evolved from ?Antap traditions.

As among the Tongva, the arrival of permanent Spanish colonists set in motion a deadly vortex of invasion by a foreign army, relocation, forced labor, physical coercion, sexual assaults, destruction of the natural habitat through ranching and agricultural practices, and terrifying plagues that brought these robust peoples to the very edge of extinction.[29] Northern Chumash territory was occupied by the Spanish beginning in 1772 with the establishment of Mission San Luis Obispo. Santa Barbara followed in 1786 and La Purisima Concepcion the next year. San Buenaventura was founded in 1782, and finally Santa Ynez in 1804.[30] Although no epidemics were reported between 1772 and 1788, a thorough study of mission registers demonstrates a significant underrepresentation of children surviving in the early contact period. A pronounced gender imbalance rapidly became apparent.[31] As many as seven epidemics swept over the Chumash mission populations in their forty-nine years of occupation by Spanish and Mexican authorities. An overall average Chumash mission Indian mortality rate was sixty-six deaths per thousand people. According to anthropologists Phillip Walker and John Johnson: "This is extremely high; for instance, the average death rate in Sweden for the period 1751–1800 was 27.4 per 1,000 population. In the United States, the age-adjusted mortality rate is now 5.4 per 1,000."[32] For nearly half a century, typhoid, pneumonia, consumption (tuberculosis), measles, influenza, and smallpox epidemics cut a murderous swath through the Chumash population. Like elsewhere, the population rapidly became saturated with syphilis, weakening the already staggering population and creating an alarming number of sterility cases.[33] Chumash religious leaders' failure to control these epidemics worked further to disillusion loyalty to a system that seemed to have lost its authority and power.

One of the most devastating epidemics occurred between 1800 and 1802. It has been identified as diphtheria (*cerramiento de garganta*) and is believed to have originated at San Gabriel and spread to the Chumash. Hit especially hard were the Chumash at Mission Santa Barbara, where they suffered a rate of 14.68 deaths per 100; in other words, it resulted in the death of 15 percent of the population.[34]

In a letter written March 1, 1805 to Governor Jose Joaquin Arrillaga, Padre Estevan Tapis reported what he characterized as a "revelation" of a "deception" by a female neophyte that led the padre to distrust his flock and fear for his life.[35] According to Tapis, amidst the chaos, suffering, and death of the epidemic an unnamed female neophyte entered a trance state at midnight and awoke to report that the Chumash deity *Chupu* (Earth Mother Deity)[36] had appeared to her with the threat that death would befall the non-Christian Chumash who became baptized and that the only hope for survival of the neophytes was to make offerings to Chupu and undo their baptisms by washing their hair with a special water called "tears of the sun." The deity further threatened to kill immediately any who would inform the missionaries. Word of the vision spread quickly throughout the neophyte housing at the mission. Desperate Chumash, including trusted alcaldes, anxiously made offerings of seeds and beads and performed the symbolic act of renouncing their Christianity. Tapis lamented that the movement had gone unchecked for three days and was sweeping distant Chumash communities on the coast as well as the interior. Finally, an unnamed male informant revealed the movement to the astounded missionaries. Tapis's letter ends with the speculation that had the visionary prescribed a revolt against the Spanish,

> [w]ho would have escaped death, and who would have warned the presidio, although it is only half a league away? This did not happen thanks to god, but it is enough that such a thing might have happened, and that the neophytes know how to scheme their plots at night with such secrecy and reserve so that the custody of the missions with a thousand neophytes altogether should not be entrusted to two, three, or a few more soldiers who might compose their guard.[37]

Unfortunately, the nature of the Spanish response is not revealed in this letter, and further related documentation has yet to materialize. However, we do know that the good padre was correct in assuming that Indians would secretly continue to worship Chupu, for the movement resurfaced again in 1810 among the Chumash neophytes at La Purisima Concepcion.[38] Fourteen years later the Chumash revolt erupted, and among the most militant were the La Purisima rebels.

The extent to which the Chumash continued to adhere to traditional belief patterns is dramatically evident in the great Chumash uprising of 1824. A series of events pitting aboriginal beliefs against pressures to conform to missionary and military authority led to widespread Chumash participation in the revolt.

About the time of the winter solstice (December 1823), a twin-tailed comet appeared and was visible until March 1824. According to Chumash cosmology, such an astronomical anomaly foretold a sudden change and new beginning.[39] Furthermore, the annual pre-Easter confessions cajoled from the neophytes were increasingly becoming a sophisticated device with which to probe the extent of the neophyte population's abandonment of ?Antap beliefs.[40] Tensions mounted and finally exploded into violent resistance when the routine beating of a La Purisima neophyte at Mission Santa Ynez occurred February 21, 1824. Chumash informant Maria Solares provided linguist John P. Harrington with a rare Native account of the decidedly non-Christian perceptions of participants:

> The Indians began to prepare themselves and they did not go to bed that night. Some of the Indians said, "The priests can not hurt me—I am a medicine man. . . . If they shoot at me water will come out of the cannon; if they shoot at me, the bullet will not enter my flesh."[41]

Other supernatural elements are reported in Maria's account, including an Indian who could not be killed because he wore an amulet of woven human hair, a Chumash vaquero who mounted a horse in front of the soldiers and disappeared to a nearby hilltop, and a man who entered a prison cell through a keyhole.[42]

Colonial records report that the Santa Ynez mission guards were attacked and a building was torched. Two Indians from that mission were killed in this initial skirmish. Trapped soldiers and padres barricaded themselves in a building until the rebels fled to nearby La Purisima the next day.

At La Purisima, neophytes under the leadership of Pacoimo revolted simultaneously with their Santa Ynez neighbors. Four colonists were killed, while the soldiers and padres were driven into a storeroom. Seven neophytes died in this brief but violent action. The soldiers fled to Santa Ynez and the bewildered padre observed the La Purisima rebels' astounding display of military preparation to defend their newly acquired fortress. The rebels erected palisade fortifications, cut weapon slits in the mission buildings, and positioned two small cannons in anticipation of a punitive military response.

Messages of warning to the trusted Santa Barbara alcalde Andres Sagiomomatsse resulted in his demand that the soldiers withdraw from Mission Santa Barbara. Breaking into the weapons locker, the neophytes armed themselves, wounded and disarmed several soldiers, and eventually fought a pitched battle against presidio troops within the mission compound. The rebels drove Mexican soldiers from the mission, wounding an additional four. Indian casualties were three dead and two wounded. Sagiomomatsse and his followers soon fled across the San Marcos Mountains, seeking refuge in the lower ?San Joaquin Valley. Presidio troops promptly looted both the neophytes' and the padres' quarters, killing five helpless Chumash neophytes either too old or sick to join their kinsmen.

During the next few weeks, Sagiomomatsse and his Santa Barbara followers could not be persuaded to return, nor would Pacomio's La Purisima rebels surrender the mission at La Purisima. In mid-March, Mexican cavalry, infantry, and artillery troops surrounded La Purisima and began an attack. As the soldiers came into range, they were met with a volley of musket shot, the blast of the neophytes' cannon, and a shower of arrows. Eventually the more experienced Mexican artillery crews shattered the rebels' defenses. Following a failed attempt to break out of the siege, a surrender was negotiated with the aid of a padre.[43]

It is worth noting that Andres and the Santa Barbara Chumash were celebrating their newfound freedom. Captured rebels reported baptized Christians and non-Christians marrying and divorcing each other, gambling, and failing to pray to the Christian god. The defiant rebels issued this message to the authorities attempting to recoup their unpaid laborers, "We shall maintain ourselves with what god will provide us in the open country. Moreover we are soldiers, stonemasons, carpenters, etc., and we will provide for ourselves by our work."[44] Several subsequent expeditions eventually persuaded a significant number of rebels to return to Santa Barbara. A decision to remain outside of one's aboriginal territory was not an easy decision to make. After all, individuals had to choose between a life among Yokut peoples far away from all the sacred places and the graves of one's Chumash ancestors or a return to the totalitarian labor regime of the Franciscans. Nevertheless, several hundred Chumash choose freedom. A decade later it was reported they were living prosperously in northeast Kern County, raising corn, pumpkins, melons, and other crops and engaged in a lively horse trade. It is a tragic irony that these defiant and exiled Chumash were virtually wiped out in the great Central Valley malaria epidemic of 1833.[45]

About 1940, demographer Sherburne F. Cook began the first scientific investigation into the question of what caused the California Indian population to suffer a gut-wrenching dive that reduced the once-healthy population of over 310,000 prior to contact to a shattered 17,000 survivors by the year 1900.[46] In 1976, historian William H. McNeill wrote in *Plagues and Peoples*:

> It is worth considering the psychological implications of a disease that killed only Indians and left the Spaniards unharmed. Such partiality could only be explained supernaturally and there could be no doubt about which side of the struggle enjoyed divine favor. The religions, the priesthoods, and way of life built around the old Indian gods could not survive such a demonstration of the superior power of the god the Spaniards worshiped. Little wonder then the Indians accepted Christianity and submitted to Spanish control so meekly. God had shown himself on their side, and each new outbreak of infectious disease imported from Europe renewed the lesson.[47]

With the development of more recent ethnohistoric methodologies utilizing historical, ethnographic, archeological, and linguistic data, a fuller and more balanced understanding of these events can be achieved that moves beyond McNeill's simplistic supposition. Perhaps of equal importance is this new approach's focus on comprehending events as they were understood by nonliterate groups undergoing the stress of colonization and dispossession while enduring a series of frightening plagues.

This chapter provides an examination of the religious, demographic, and cultural response of two southern California Indian tribes to introduced Spanish diseases and colonization. I have attempted to describe the aboriginal pre-contact religious cosmology of both groups and to show how subsequent diseases and colonial policies triggered profound changes in the aboriginal belief system. In the first case, some Tongva blamed the plague on Native sorcery and destroyed the two shamans they deemed responsible. This reaction illuminates the growing suspicion aimed at aboriginal Native religious leaders whose failure to control the diseases undermined their authority. The reactions of the Chumash appears to be consistent with classic messianic movements among Native Americans, of which the best known was the 1870 wave of the Ghost Dance.[48] And like the second wave of the Ghost Dance of 1889, its suppression ultimately resulted in violent resistance.[49]

Tongva and Chumash are simply two examples among hundreds in which Native people turned inward to explain, interpret, and contend with foreign invaders who introduced deadly diseases, ill health, and social anomie. Native California Indians did not simply abandon their ancient belief systems and become Christians. They held strongly to their Native religious beliefs, as illustrated in the examples provided here. The coercive Christianization that so characterized Spanish colonial policy resulted in new forms of religious beliefs built upon ancient dogma that offered Native explanations and responses to the new frightening diseases. In this way, Indians maintained some control of their world. To be sure, some mission Indians adopted Christianity and synchronized compatible elements of the old and new religions. But some Tongva and Chumash responded to Spanish colonization and European-borne pathogens in a Native manner, offering responses understood only through an examination of California Indian cultures and religions as well as the voices of Native people.[50]

Notes

1. Sherburne F. Cook, *Population Trends among the California Mission Indians* (Berkeley and Los Angeles: University of California Press, 1940), 23–28. For an analysis of Cook's contribution to historiography, see Albert L. Hurtado, "California Indian Demography, Sherburne F. Cook, and the Revision of American History," *Pacific Historical Review* 57:3 (August 1989): 323–43.

2. Lowell J. Bean and Charles R. Smith, "Gabrielino," and Robert F. Heizer, "Natural Forces and Native World View," in *Handbook of North American Indians*, vol. 8, *California*, ed. Robert F. Heizer (Washington, DC: Smithsonian Institution Press, 1978), 538–49 and 649–53. See also Alfred L. Kroeber's "The Nature of Landholding Groups in Aboriginal California," in *Two Papers on Aboriginal Ethnography of California*, eds. Hynes and Heizer, *University of California Archaeological Survey Reports* 56 (1962): 19–58.

3. Bean and Smith, "Gabrielino," 544. The aboriginal people of Los Angeles called themselves Tongva and I have followed suit. Few Indians want to be known only on the basis of a colonial experience. The term "Gabrielino" was used by colonists to describe Tongva peoples associated with Mission San Gabriel.

4. Lowell J. Bean and Sylvia Brakke Vane, "Cults and Their Transformations," in *Handbook of North American Indians*, vol. 8, *California*, 662–72.

5. Sherburne F. Cook, *The Population of the California Indians 1769–1970* (Berkeley: University of California Press, 1976), 24.

6. Zephyrin Engelhardt, *San Gabriel Mission and the Beginnings of Los Angeles* (San Gabriel: Mission San Gabriel Press, 1927), 12–14; Maynard Geiger, *The Life and Times of Fray Junipero Serra O.F.M. or the Man Who Never Turned Back*, vol. 1 (Washington, DC: Academy of Franciscan History, 1959), 304–8; Hubert Howe Bancroft, *History of California*, vol. I, *1542–1800* (Santa Barbara: Wallace Hebberd, 1963), 180–81.

7. Robert F. Heizer, ed., *The Indians of Los Angeles County: Hugo Reid's Letters of 1852* (Los Angeles: Southwest Museum, 1968), 70. For a detailed analysis of Tongva females in Mission San Gabriel, see Edward D. Castillo's "Gender Status Decline, Resistance and Accommodation in the Missions of California: A San Gabriel Case Study," *American Indian Culture and Research Journal* 18:1 (1994): 67–93. See also Albert Hurtado, "Sexuality in California's Franciscan Missions: Cultural Perceptions and Sad Realities," *California History* 71:3 (fall 1992): 371–85.

8. Daniel McGarry, "Educational Methods of the Franciscans in Spanish California," *The Americas*, vol. 6 (Washington, DC, 1950), 335–58; Daniel Matson and Bernard Fontana, eds., *Friar Bringas Reports to the King: Methods of Indoctrination on the Frontier of New Spain 1796–1797* (Tucson: University of Arizona Press, 1977); for a critical analysis of recruitment techniques, see, Edward D. Castillo's "Neophyte Resistance and Accommodation in the Missions of California," in *The Spanish Missionary Heritage of the United States: Selected Papers and Commentaries from the November 1990 Quincentenary Symposium*, ed. Howard Benoist (San Antonio, TX: United States National Park Service, 1992), 62–64.

9. Sherburne F. Cook, *The Conflict between the California Indians and White Civilization* (Berkeley: University of California Press, 1976), 13–55. Syphilis generally weakened neophyte populations and made them more susceptible to other diseases. Among females, it caused sterility.

10. Robert Jackson, "The Economy and Demography of San Gabriel Mission 1771–1834: A Structural Analysis." Paper presented at an international symposium, *The Spanish Beginnings in California 1542–1822* (University of California, Santa Barbara, July 15–19, 1991), 13–18. Paper is in author's possession.

11. Ibid., 16.

12. Castillo, "Neophyte Resistance and Accommodation," 62. There is no evidence

to suggest that baptized individuals understood the relocation, family dismemberment, and unpaid labor obligations of their new status. Florence Shipek, "California Indian Reaction to the Franciscans," *The Americas* 41:4 (April 1985): 480–91. Shipek's oral histories of San Diego Mission Indians concluded that the Kumeyaay viewed the padres as the most dangerous thieving witches they ever encountered.

13. William Shuman, "Historical Medicine, California Medicine, Part II: Spanish Medicine," *Medical Journal and Record* 131 (1930): 374.

14. Sherburne F. Cook, "Monterey Surgeons during the Spanish Period in California," *Bulletin of the Institute of the History of Medicine* 5 (1937): 67–68; and Sherburne F. Cook, "California's First Medical Survey: Report of Surgeon General Jose Benites," *California and Western Medicine* 145 (1936): 352–54. See also Shuman, "Historical Medicine," 373–77.

15. G. James West, "Early Historic Vegetation Change in Alta California: The Fossil Evidence," in *Columbian Consequences: Archaeological and Historical Perspectives on the Spanish Borderlands West*, vol. 1, ed. David H. Thomas (Washington, DC: Smithsonian Institution Press, 1989), 333–48; see also Thomas Blackburn and Kat Anderson, eds., *Before the Wilderness, Environmental Management by Native Californians* (Menlo Park, CA: Ballena Press, 1993); for a thoughtful analysis of the coercive nature of Spanish colonial policy, see Cook, *The Conflict between the California Indians*, 113–34. See also, Robert F. Heizer's "Impact of Colonization on the Native California Societies," *Journal of San Diego History* 24:1 (1978): 121–39. The classic Franciscan defense of such policies can be read in Francis F. Guest's, "An Inquiry into the Role of the Discipline in California Mission Life," *Southern California Quarterly* 71 (spring 1989): 1–68. Guest argues that flogged, incarcerated, and chained Indians were criminals who deserved punishment under Spanish–Mexican and church laws. Cook, on the other hand, analyzed a sample of disciplinary actions by Franciscan and army authorities from 1775 to 1831 and concluded that punishment for political crimes against the colonial authorities constituted a whopping 90 percent of the cases. See Cook, *The Conflict between the California Indians*, 122. A Catholic French explorer visiting Alta California in 1786, shocked by the harsh punishments he witnessed, wrote, "Corporal punishment is inflicted on the Indians of both sexes who neglect the exercises of piety, and many sins, which in Europe are left to Divine justice are here punished by irons and stocks." Malcolm Margolin, ed., *Monterey in 1786: The Journals of Jean Francois de La Perouse* (Berkeley, CA: Heyday Books, 1989), 82.

16. Alan Hutchinson, *Frontier Settlements in Mexican California: The Hijar-Padres Colony and its Origins, 1769–1835* (New Haven, CT: Yale University Press, 1971).

17. Robert H. Jackson and Edward D. Castillo, *Indians, Franciscans, and Spanish Colonization: The Impact of the Mission System on California Indians* (Albuquerque: University of New Mexico Press, 1995).

18. Bean and Vane, "Cults and Their Transformations," 669. The only undisturbed section of Puvugna that remains today is located on the California State University, Long Beach campus. Despite the fact that it is a protected historic site and registered as such with the State Office of Historic Preservation, the university's administration is attempting to disturb the site to build a mini-mall. A lawsuit is currently pending.

19. Geronimo Boscana, Chinichnigish, *A Revised and Annotated Version of Alfred*

Robinson's Translation of Father Geronimo Boscana's Historical Account of the Beliefs, Usages, Customs and Extravagancies of the Indians of Mission San Juan Capistrano Called the Acagchemem Tribe, annotations by John P. Harrington (Morongo Indian Reservation: Malki Museum Press, 1978), 138–39.

20. Ibid., 129.

21. Ibid., 33.

22. Bean and Vane, "Cults and Their Transformations," 669.

23. Travis Hudson, ed. and trans., "A Rare Account of Gabrielino Shamanism from the Notes of John P. Harrington," *Journal of California and Great Basin Anthropology* 1:2 (1979): 357.

24. Ibid. Such sand paintings were also used by the Tongva sorcerers to cause earthquakes; see Alfred L. Kroeber's, "A Southern California Ceremony," *Journal of American Folklore* 21:80 (1908): 40.

25. Hudson, "A Rare Account of Gabrielino . . .," 357.

26. Ibid., 359.

27. Cambell Grant, "Chumash: Introduction," "Eastern Coastal Chumash," and "Interior Chumash," in *Handbook of North American Indians*, vol. 8, *California*, 505–19, 530–34. Reliable population figures can be found in Alan K. Brown's "The Aboriginal Population of the Santa Barbara Channel," *University of California Los Angeles, Archaeological Survey, Annual Report*, vol. 69 (1967), 79.

28. Lowell Bean and Thomas King, eds., *?Antap: California Indian Political and Economic Organization* (Ramona, CA: Ballena Press, 1974), 93–110; and Bean and Vane, "Cults and Their Transformations," 669. See also Richard Applegate, "The Dantura Cult among the Chumash," *Journal of California Anthropology* 2 (summer 1975): 7–17.

29. Edward D. Castillo, *Native American Perspectives on the Hispanic Colonization of Alta California* (New York: Garland Publishing, 1991). Spanish colonization practices are analyzed in the introduction, xvii–xxxvi. For a Chumash view of missionization, see Travis Hudson, ed., *Breath of the Sun: Life in Early California as Told by a Chumash Indian, Fernando Librado to John P. Harrington* (Morongo Indian Reservation: Malki Museum Press, 1979); Daniel Larson, John Johnson, and Joel Michaelson, "Missionization among the Coastal Chumash of Central California: A Study of Risk Minimization Strategies," *American Anthropologist* 96:2 (June 1994): 263–99. These authors have built a convincing argument that a combination of droughts and a warming of the coastal waters for half a century during missionization may have caused starvation among the Chumash, thus making the acceptance of missionization a lesser of two evils. The authors use both baptismal records and high-resolution dendrochronological and marine sedimentary records to reconstruct paleoenvironmental conditions. Anthropologist John Johnson nevertheless reported "only a remnant population had survived when the Mission period came to a close"; see John Johnson, "The Chumash and the Missions," in *Columbian Consequences*, vol. 1, ed. David H. Thomas (Washington, DC: Smithsonian Institution Press, 1989), 373.

30. Ibid., 365.

31. Phillip L. Walker and John Johnson, "The Effects of Contact on the Chumash Indians," in *Disease and Demography in the Americas*, eds. John Verano and Douglas Ubelaker (Washington, DC: Smithsonian Institution Press, 1992), 129–32.

32. Ibid., 133.

33. Ibid., 133 and 136. A padre at Mission Santa Barbara made this report on the extent of syphilis among the Chumash there: "All are infected with it for they see no objection to marrying another infected with it. As a result, births are few and deaths many so that their number of deaths exceed births by three to one." In Maynard Geiger and Clement Meighan, eds., *As the Padres Saw Them* (Santa Barbara: Santa Barbara Mission Archive Library, 1976), 74. For a general discussion of the effect of venereal diseases on mission Indian birthrates and survivability, see Cook, *The Conflict between the California Indians*, 23–30. Cook writes, "Perhaps there were some [Mission Indians] who were able to avoid the infection, but this must have been rare," 27.

34. Walker and Johnson, "The Effects of Contact on the Chumash Indians," 135.

35. Robert F. Heizer, "A Californian Messianic Movement of 1801 among the Chumash," *American Anthropologist* 43 (1941): 128–29. Heizer's article provides a translated version of the Tapis letter.

36. Richard Applegate, "Ineseno Chumash Dictionary," Manuscript on file at Santa Barbara Museum of Natural History, n.d.

37. The Tapis letter can be found in Archivo de la Mision de Santa Babara, *Papeles Miscelaneos* 6, 33–34, the Bancroft Library, University of California, Berkeley. Travis Hudson and Ernest Underhay, *Crystals in the Sky: An Intellectual Odyssey Involving Chumash Astronomy, Cosmology and Rock Art*, in Ballena Press Anthropological Papers Number 10 (Socorro, NM, and Santa Barbara, CA: Ballena Press/Santa Barbara Museum of Natural History, 1978), 21–22, 72. This groundbreaking study identified the visionary as an 'Alchuklash or a Chumash astrologer and member of the elite ?Antap society.

38. Alfred L. Kroeber, *Handbook of the Indians of California* (Washington, DC: Smithsonian Institution, *Bureau of American Ethnology Bulletin* 78, 1925), 567.

39. James D. Sandos, "Levantamiento!: The 1824 Chumash Uprising Reconsidered," *Southern California Quarterly* (summer 1985): 128. This article provides the best account of that much-reported rebellion. It utilizes interdisciplinary data and is a good example of the balance that can be achieved by ethnohistoric methodologies. See also James Sandos, "Christianization among the Chumash: An Ethnohistoric Perspective," *American Indian Quarterly* 21:4 (1991).

40. Ibid., 115–19. See also Madison Beeler, ed., "The Ventureño Confesionario of Jose Senan, OFM," in *University of California Publications in Linguistics* 47 (Berkeley and Los Angeles: University of California Press, 1967); and Harry Kelsey, ed., *The Doctrina and Confesionario of Juan Cortes* (Altadena, CA: Howling Coyote Press, 1979).

41. Thomas Blackburn, ed., "The Chumash Revolt of 1824: A Native Account," *Journal of California Anthropology* 2:2 (1975): 224. This account is taken from the field notes of linguist John P. Harrington's interview with Ineseno Chumash consultant Maria Solares. For an additional Chumash account, see Travis Hudson, ed. and trans., "The Chumash Revolt of 1824: Another Native Account from the Notes of John P. Harrington," *Journal of California and Great Basin Anthropology* 2:1 (1980): 123–26.

42. Ibid., 224–25.

43. Scholarly published accounts of the Chumash revolt can be found among the following: Maynard Geiger, OFM, ed. and trans., "Fray Antonio Ripoll's Description of the Chumash Revolt at Santa Barbara in 1824," *Southern California Quarterly* 52

(1970): 345–64; Hubert H. Bancroft, *History of California*, vol. II, 527–37; Gary B. Coombs, "With What God Will Provide: A Reexamination of the Chumash Revolt of 1824," *Noticias Santa Barbara Historical Society* 26:2 (summer 1980): 21–29; and Gary Stickel and Adrienne Cooper, "The Chumash Revolt of 1824: A Case for an Archaeological Application of Feedback Theory," *Annual Report Archaeological Survey*, University of California Los Angeles (1969): 5–21. For a comparison and analysis of the Chumash revolt with other mission Indian resistance movements in California, see Edward D. Castillo, "The Native Response to the Colonization of Alta California," *Columbian Consequences*, 377–94. Mexican authorities tried and executed seven Chumash rebels; four leaders of the revolt got ten years of presidio labor and perpetual exile. Eight others received eight years of presidio labor.

44. Unnamed Chumash rebel to Padre Ripoll, quoted in Maynard Geiger, "Fray Antonio Ripoll's Description of the Chumash Revolt . . .," *Southern California Quarterly* 52 (1970): 352.

45. Sherburne F. Cook, "Expeditions to the Interior of California, Central Valley, 1820–1840," *Anthropological Records* 20:5 (1962); see section, "The Purisima Rebellion," 152–57. For a report on the Chumash exiles in Kern County, see John C. Ewers, ed., *Adventures of Zaenas Leonard Fur Trader* (Norman: University of Oklahoma Press, 1959), xi, 121–23. For an account of the epidemic, see Sherburne F. Cook, "The Epidemic of 1830–1833 in California and Oregon," *University of California Publications in American Archaeology and Ethnology* 43:3 (1955): 303–26.

46. Cook, *The Conflict between the California Indians.*

47. William H. McNeill, *Plagues and Peoples* (Garden City, NY: Anchor Press, 1976), 2.

48. Anna Gayton, "The Ghost Dance of 1870 in South Central California," *University of California Publications in American Archaeology and Ethnology* 28:3 (1930): 57–82; and Cora DuBois, "The 1870 Ghost Dance," *Anthropological Records* 3:1 (1939): 1–151.

49. Alice B. Kehoe, *The Ghost Dance, Ethnohistory and Revitalization* (Fort Worth: Holt Rinehart and Winston, 1989).

50. For a comparison, see the fascinating essay by Helen Jaskoski "Andrew Blackbird's Smallpox Story" (*Genre* 25 [spring 1992]: 1–11), which analyzes a nineteenth-century Ottawa Indian writer, Andrew Blackbird, and his Native account of a smallpox plague that ravaged his people in 1763.

THREE

JEAN A. KELLER

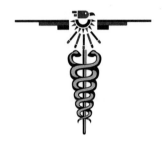

"In the fall of the year we were troubled with some sickness"

TYPHOID FEVER DEATHS AT SHERMAN INSTITUTE, 1904

On July 1, 1904, the new school year began at Sherman Institute, a nonreservation Indian boarding school in Riverside, California, with an enrollment of 722 students. By November 14, 1904, nine of these students were dead. Seven of the children died from an epidemic of typhoid fever between October 29 and November 14, and at least 35 other students were stricken with the disease.[1] Yet in his annual report to the Commissioner of Indian Affairs, Sherman Institute Superintendent Harwood Hall did not mention the deaths of these students. Instead, he stated only that in the fall of the year they had been "troubled with some sickness."[2]

By most accounts, Hall was a man dedicated to the health and well-being of his young Indian charges, yet he chose not only to dismiss the deaths of the seven children killed by typhoid fever in the fall of 1904, but the deaths of four children earlier in the year as well. This exclusion was particularly relevant because the 1904 mortality rate at Sherman Institute exceeded that of all previous years combined, including those of its predecessor, the Perris Indian School.[3] The death of eleven children, seven of which were from typhoid fever, was clearly an uncommon occurrence. In his official report, however, Hall did not acknowledge that anything out of the ordinary had transpired, apparently deciding that the deaths of these children were irrelevant to his report.

Prior to becoming superintendent of Sherman Institute, Hall had been superintendent of the Phoenix Industrial Boarding School (hereafter, the Phoenix Indian School) near Phoenix, Arizona. The school had been established in September 1891 for the specific purpose of preparing Native American children for assimilation.[4] By the time Hall arrived at the Phoenix Indian School in 1893, the school had already experienced considerable growth and was on its way to becoming a major component in the federal assimilation program. During his tenure at the school, Hall fostered this growth, equating it with progress and accomplishment.[5]

Hall was an experienced educator who wanted the Phoenix Indian School to be the quintessential Indian boarding school of the western United States, and he lobbied relentlessly for additional funding to expand and improve the school.[6] His efforts had a significant impact. Between 1893 and 1895, he succeeded in obtaining sufficient funding to build a boys' dormitory, hospital, employees' quarters, and a small office, enabling the school to accommodate three hundred students.[7] By the end of the 1895–1896 school year, almost 350 students attended and the school continued to grow, primarily due to Hall's efforts.

In addition to his fund-raising skills, Hall recognized the value of public relations and succeeded in creating strong community ties between the Phoenix Indian School and the citizens of Phoenix.[8] The Phoenicians supported the school in large part because it contributed to their financial well-being through Hall's outing and apprentice programs, as well as through the federal expenditures that resulted from Hall's lobbying. However, perhaps of equal importance was the fact that the Phoenix Indian School, through Hall's instigation and promotion, became a center of community social life.[9]

Under the direction of Harwood Hall, the Phoenix Indian School also became integral to the promotion of tourism, which was beginning to assume importance in Arizona. Prominent civic leaders in Phoenix staged a multitude of special events at the school, all of which were designed to attract visitors and bring in tourist dollars.[10] Superintendent Harwood Hall was a popular schoolmaster, reportedly respected by Phoenix Indian School students, their parents, and the community. The only problem was that Harwood Hall simply could not stand the hot weather of Arizona. Therefore, despite having to take leave of his successful work-in-progress, Hall commenced a quest to be transferred from Phoenix to another Indian boarding school. After several requests to the Commissioner of Indian Affairs, he was placed in charge of the industrial boarding school at Perris, California.[11]

The Perris Indian School had formally opened on January 9, 1893, with only eight enrolled students. By the first of March, 113 students were enrolled and by the end of 1893, 118 students were boarding at the school. By 1897, the physical plant of Perris Indian School included boys' quarters, girls' quarters, a hospital, and several miscellaneous buildings such as a laundry, barn, boys' wash house, and a shop building equipped with a carpenter shop, paint shop, shoe and harness shop, engineering shop, and storeroom.[12] Despite an almost continuous building program, the enrollment was always larger than the available living space.

In addition to problems in the physical plant, it became apparent within the first year of operation that there existed inherent problems in the geographical location of the Perris Indian School. The school was situated on the path that Indians traveled going to and from the Indian Agency in Colton. In addition, it was also in an area that Indians traveled through on their way to more settled areas to find work. Clearly this was not an environment considered healthy for the assimilation of Indian youth; there were simply too many Indians around.

> It is to be regretted that a site was not secured in the vicinity of one of the
> many thriving cultural communities with which southern California abounds,
> where the highest type of civilization would be a constant example to inspire
> these Indian youths with lofty ambitions to become intelligent industrious
> men and women assimilating with this progressive age.[13]

Despite these problems, the school continued to be productive and to grow. An academic program coincident with that of public-school programs was instituted and later expanded to include an extensive music program. Religious instruction was provided when possible and social gatherings between students and employees were frequent. Both Superintendent Savage and his successor, Edgar A. Allen, recognized the spatial and locational problems of Perris Indian School, but felt that they were not insolvable and strove to improve conditions at the site throughout their respective tenures.

When Harwood Hall arrived at Perris Indian School in 1897, the school's isolation, inadequate facilities, and the poor quality of its employees shocked him. In his first annual report as superintendent, he deplored the school's inadequacies, going so far as to state that, ". . . a poorer place for an Indian school, it seems to me could not have been found in southern California." It may be that compared to the established and relatively cosmopolitan Phoenix Indian School, from which Hall had only recently arrived, almost anything would look bad.[14]

Much of Hall's first year at Perris had been spent essentially laying the groundwork for what he considered to be the very obvious and necessary next step in the development of the school—moving it to a better location. During the fiscal year 1898–1899, Hall formally suggested that a new site be found for the Perris Indian School due to the inadequacy of available water.[15]

On November 13, 1899, Reel wrote to Hall,[16] reassuring him that she would do everything possible to acquire a large appropriation from the Senate.

She enclosed a copy of her report on the Perris School and said she hoped it met with his approval. Also included in Reel's letter were two very important pieces of information. First, she congratulated Hall on the fact that both Los Angeles and Riverside have taken so much interest in the location of the school. This indicates that Hall was confident enough his request for a new school would be granted that he had discussed its new location with two competing cities. It also suggests that Hall recognized the potential value his new school would have to a community, as well as the benefits to the school that such value could reap. The second piece of information found in Reel's letter was that there already existed considerable opposition to the school's move from Perris. It seems that not everyone concurred with Hall's assessment of the current site's inadequacies, especially concerning the water and soil.

According to further correspondence between Hall and Reel,[17] the influential people of Riverside had begun taking an active interest in the location of the large Indian school by November 1899. One of these individuals was Frank Miller, owner of the Glenwood Mission Inn and Riverside's streetcar company.[18] At the same time, opposition to the move was apparently increasing, with letters from landowners and residents of the Perris area being sent to the Commissioner of Indian Affairs. The most scathing indictments of Hall's reasons for moving came in letters from Mr. T. Gibbon of the Los Angeles Terminal Railway Company[19] and from Horatio Rust, Indian Agent of Colton, California.[20] Both accused Hall of misrepresenting the facts, that independent investigations had shown that there was abundant water available for use by the school, and that there existed no logical reason for moving the school to another location.

During the May 22, 1900 session of the United States Senate, discussion of these letters in relation to Hall's request resulted in an argument regarding "conflicting testimony."[21] Hall countered Gibbon's and Rust's letters by collecting support letters.[22]

Despite considerable Senate and local opposition, the Indian Appropriation Act for a new school in Riverside, California, was passed in the United States Senate on May 31, 1900. The Secretary of the Interior subsequently approved $75,000 for the purchase of land and erection of new buildings. In June of 1900, the U.S. Supervisor of Schools, Mr. Frank Conser, was instructed to investigate a site located on Magnolia Avenue, five-and-a-half miles from the center of the City of Riverside and three-quarters of a mile from Arlington Station on the Santa Fe Railroad.[23] It is interesting that the site was adjacent to Frank Miller's streetcar company in Chemawa Park, owned by Miller's sister and brother-in-law, and that apparently no other sites were offered for consideration. On July 31, 1900, the Department of the Interior granted permission to negotiate with Frank and Alice Richardson for the purchase of the land, and on August 18, 1900, a deed was executed conveying the land to the United States for $8,400.

The move to Riverside involved far more complex issues than simply the improvement of student health. Superintendent Hall saw the move as a necessary step in realizing his dream of establishing the ideal Indian boarding school. Hall's school required the elements that had been present in Phoenix, but with a more favorable environment. In Riverside, he found such a place and the potential was recognized by others. As such, local businessmen and other influential citizens were instrumental in procuring the new Indian school for Riverside and they were diligent in their efforts to expedite its foundation. They saw the school as representing a significant financial benefit to the city and were anxious to get things going. As an exuberant commentary in the *Riverside Enterprise* stated shortly after the purchase of the school property had been completed,

> [t]he securing of this government institution is one of the great strides in the
> progress of Riverside. It will provide for large number of Indian children and
> must in a very few years grow to proportions and importance that few people
> can imagine. It will be a feature to attract tourists and secure their money in
> permanent investments. It will enhance values of taxable real estate in the
> vicinity and thereby proportionally increase public revenues. And in addition,
> the Indian school will bring to the city for the benefit of merchants no
> insignificant amount of trade.[24]

Superintendent Hall played an important part in the design of the new school. In a letter to the Commissioner of Indian Affairs, dated August 1, 1900, Hall submitted a detailed explanation of his plans for the school.[25] This plan showed a genuine concern for the physical and mental health of his young charges and it is clear that a great deal of thought went into his plan. Realistically, many of Hall's ideas were not born of compassion as much as they were born of a desire to maximize assimilation and expedite the "civilization" of his Indian board students. His attitude was paternalistic, as was common in Indian school administration during most of its history. However, if viewed in the context of the time, Hall's plans for the new school were somewhat revolutionary because they took into consideration the individuality and vulnerability of the students. Two particular passages are illustrative of Hall's rather ambitious plans:

> It is very unwise, I find, to have a mixed set of employees to room in children's quarters, outside of matrons and disciplinarians, as the children cannot
> feel free and are always subject to the whims and idiosyncrasies of tired, sick,
> and nervous employees. The herding of larger children in dormitories simply
> breeds disease and immorality, and lessons a larger boy or girl's self respect.
> They can have no individuality or privacy in dormitories, as everything of a
> necessity held in common and no privacy for any one. Boys and girls both
> will take great interest in their rooms, manufacturing various little room dec-

orations, making them attractive and homelike; will advance them in my opinion along lines of general civilization greater and faster, than in any other way, as it will give them an idea of the possibilities in arranging a home of their own.[26]

In his plans for the new school, Hall not only took into consideration the mental and physical health of his young Indian students, but the needs of the community and school, as well. He clearly acknowledged the important symbiotic relationship between a successful Indian school and the community in which it exists.

The cornerstone of the Sherman Institute, named after James Schoolcraft Sherman, chairman of the Committee on Indian Affairs of the House of Representatives and considered a true friend of the school, was laid on July 18, 1901. Another friend of the school, Frank Miller, had apparently decided to take on the planning of the cornerstone ceremony because he assumed full responsibility for sending the invitations out and responses were sent not to the attention of Harwood Hall, but to Frank Miller.[27] Miller also had commemorative volumes of Helen Hunt Jackson's *Ramona* printed for select guests of the ceremony, his way of thanking them for their support of the school and the improved living conditions the Indian students were soon to enjoy.[28] The local newspapers were filled with detailed accounts of the festivities, which proved to be the major social event of the year:

> Riverside was in gala attire today, the occasion being the laying of the cornerstone of Sherman Institute, the new United States Indian Industrial School. And more than 7,000 persons were present at the ceremony. This was the most significant event in its history as a city since the water, which has transformed the arid plains into a fertile garden, was first turned on thirty years ago. The town was prettily decorated.[29]

Harwood Hall had obviously been correct in his vision of Sherman Institute being a prime attraction for people in the City of Riverside. He had also been correct in his recognition of the benefits resulting from strong community support, particularly by a businessman as influential as Frank Miller.

Sherman Institute formally opened on September 8, 1902, with an enrollment of 350 students. This population was comprised of students transferred from the Perris Indian School, as well as eight students from the Pima Reservation in Arizona. Unfortunately, problems obtaining furnishings and supplies in a timely manner necessitated sending forty-three of the younger children back to the Perris school location. Presumably the unhealthful conditions cited by Hall in his quest to have the Perris school closed were not so great as to preclude the housing of this small number of children.

The formal dedication of Sherman Institute was postponed until February 10,

1903.[30] Sherman faced serious financial problems from the beginning, which at one point led to the dismissal of all but the most essential employees and the students themselves taking over the day-to-day operation of the school. Conditions improved during the 1903–1904 fiscal year and Hall's annual report presents a glowing picture of progress being made at the school, especially in terms of the physical-plant expansion.[31] By June 30, 1904 the average enrollment was 583 and average attendance was 501. Fiscal year 1903–1904 had already realized Hall's vision of Sherman Institute's capacity to garner community support and increase tourism in Riverside:

> The residents of southern California take no little interest in the school and are ever ready to lend a helping hand. A fair library has been donated by individuals of Riverside, and the pupils have the privileges of reading standard works, of which they may avail themselves. By reason of location the school is visited by thousands throughout the tourist season; and while it would seem, where so many sightseers are shown through the school, the pupils and employees would be demoralized, such is far from the true facts, for it seems to stimulate all concerned to do their best work and really is a help, as the general routine is not permitted to be affected thereby.[32]

In closing his report, Hall again lamented the conditions at the Perris Indian School, at which some of the younger students were still housed. He proposed that upon completion of the buildings at the Riverside school, all children at Perris should be transferred to Riverside, and the Perris plant should be abandoned, at least for use as a school. Shortly after his annual report had been submitted, there was a complete failure of the water system at Perris and the danger of disease and sickness was so great that Hall felt immediate action should be taken. He telegraphed the Bureau of Indian Affairs in Washington stating the conditions and seeking permission to move the children to Riverside, even if it meant housing them in tents. On October 6, 1904 Hall wired the Commissioner of Indian Affairs that he had received permission from the BIA to close the school and transfer the students to Riverside.[33]

Superintendent Hall's concern for the health of the children at Perris Indian School was commendable. However, there existed health problems at the Riverside school that he apparently chose not to recognize. By the time Hall wrote his annual report on September 1, 1904, four children had already died at the Riverside school.[34] This was particularly significant because the annual mortality at Perris had never exceeded two children. Yet less than a year after the move to Riverside, that number had doubled. In Hall's official annual report, however, he mentioned nothing of these deaths or of student health in general.

On January 1, 1904 a fourteen-year-old Rogue River boy by the name of Chester Moore died at Sherman Institute; and on May 17th eighteen-year-old Lizzie Edwards (Concon) died.[35] The cause of their deaths is unknown. Death certificates were never filed with the County of Riverside Recorder's Office and although the National Archives maintains classified student records from Sherman Institute beginning in 1903, they have no records of either these children or of the others who died in 1904.[36] The deaths of Lizzie and Chester were simply noted in the student registers for the 1903–1904 school year.

The other two children who had died by the time Hall wrote his report were fourteen-year-old Harry Seonia (Pueblo) and six-year-old Nancy Lawrence (Tejon). Death certificates were filed for these children and are currently on microfilm at the County of Riverside Recorder's Office.[37] Harry died on July 20th of pneumonia and Nancy died on July 27th of pneumonia following measles. During their illnesses, Dr. A. S. Parker of Riverside had attended to the children at Sherman Institute, but to no avail. School officials buried both children in Sherman's cemetery: Harry on the day of his death, and Nancy on the day following hers. At the time of the children's illnesses, a hospital had not yet been built at Sherman and it is unclear why they were treated at the school instead of admitted to Riverside General Hospital, which was less than a mile away. It is possible that Dr. Parker did not realize the seriousness of the illnesses. Cost would not have been a factor, since the hospital was established specifically to care for the indigent of the county and it is unlikely that charges would have been incurred for the children's medical care.

Since the deaths of Nancy Lawrence and Harry Seonia occurred shortly after the beginning of fiscal year 1904–1905, which was also considered the beginning of the new school year, it may be that Hall planned to report their deaths in that year's annual report. However, he failed to do so. Perhaps in dealing with the events and problems of 1903 and 1904, the deaths of the children slipped Hall's mind, particularly because there were only four and they had been spread out over the year. In fiscal year 1904–1905, this was not to be the case.

On November 2, 1904, a single line appeared in the "Local News at Arlington" column of the *Riverside Enterprise*: "There are thirty cases of typhoid fever in Sherman Institute." Nothing more appeared until November 9, 1904. In the "Items of News from Arlington" column of the *Riverside Enterprise*, another single sentence stated, "There have been three deaths from typhoid fever at the Indian School within the last few days." Although no further information was forthcoming, action was apparently being taken, for in the November 16, 1904 edition of the *Los Angeles Daily Times* the following news article appeared:

TYPHOID FEVER AMONG INDIANS—SERIOUS CONDITION AT THE SHERMAN INSTITUTE

Riverside Board of Health Trying to Find the Source of the Disease. Three Deaths and Thirty Cases the Present Record—Result of Official Canvas.

Riverside, Nov. 15—The Riverside Board of Health made a trip this morning to the domestic wells of the Riverside Water Company and tested them for evidences of typhoid germ life. The water was entirely pure. This and kindred investigations being made by the Board of Health all over the city is the result of the outbreak of typhoid at the Sherman Institute Indian School. Three deaths have resulted within the last few days from the epidemic, and thirty other cases are reported today. The seriousness of the outbreak has stirred the entire community, and every effort known to medical science is being made to locate the root of the trouble and to try in some manner to remedy it. The Board of Health promises to make a report to the Trustees at their next session, and that report may be something of a nature startling in the extreme.[38]

It is interesting that this article states that the seriousness of the outbreak stirred the entire community, since beyond the two sentences printed in the November 2 and 9 editions of the local newspaper, nothing else was ever written about the epidemic. The *Los Angeles Daily Times* article provided far more comprehensive coverage and the newspaper certainly did not have the circulation enjoyed by the local press. Unless news of the typhoid-fever epidemic spread by word of mouth, it is unlikely that there was widespread knowledge of its existence, let alone concern over the Indian children at Sherman Institute. However, those who were aware of the typhoid-fever epidemic were obviously very concerned, not by the fact that it was at Sherman Institute, but because the possible source of contamination could infect the general population. The wells of the Riverside Water Company provided domestic water not only to Sherman Institute, but also to the residents and businesses of the City of Riverside. Consequently, if the well water were contaminated, typhoid fever could potentially spread throughout the entire city. Of further concern to knowledgeable citizens was that some of the city's most influential citizens were shareholders in the Riverside Water Company. Typhoid contamination of their wells would certainly have proved catastrophic, thus the expeditious, but ill-publicized, investigation by the Board of Health.

Typhoid fever is a bacterial infection caused by *Salmonella typhi*. It is spread via contaminated food and water supplies. Following ingestion, the bacteria spreads from the gastrointestinal tract to the lymphatic system, liver, and spleen, where they multiply. Salmonella can also directly infect the gallbladder and seed other areas of the body via the bloodstream. Common early symptoms include fever, malaise, and abdominal pain. Diarrhea develops, along with weakness, fatigue, delirium, and obtundation. A rose-colored rash consisting of flattened spots about one-quarter inch across appears on the chest and abdomen. Complications include intestinal hemorrhaging, intestinal perforation, kidney failure, and peritonitis. Treatment includes intravenous hydration and antibiotics, with the illness usually being resolved in two to four weeks. Cases in children are usually milder than in adults.[39]

While water is not the only source of typhoid fever, it was the principal one during the nineteenth and early twentieth centuries. The usual mode of transmission was through well water that had been contaminated by "discharges from the bowels" of a carrier—a person with the bacteria already in their system. From the privy, fecal material traveled into a cesspool, soaked into a well through the soil, and infected the drinking water. Milk was also a relatively common mode of typhoid transmission during this period because it was often mixed with contaminated water. Flies could also transmit typhoid fever by carrying germs from a carrier's fecal matter to others, upon whom they landed.[40]

Although the local press did not publicize the tests the Board of Health ran on the Riverside Land Company domestic wells, they quickly printed the full text of the investigation results—even before they were formally presented to the County Board of Trustees. In addition to providing a lengthy, detailed description of the source of water for the wells (flowing artesian wells in San Bernardino County, 400 to 500 feet deep, with iron casings), they concluded that at no time was water in the wells exposed to contamination from any source. The water was pure—absolutely free from all pollution and disease. Once it was known that the general population was not in danger of being exposed to typhoid fever from the domestic water wells, nothing further was written about the epidemic at Sherman Institute; it had become an internal problem. The County Board of Trustees took no action after receiving the report, except, perhaps, to breathe a sigh of relief.

It is interesting that more concern was not shown regarding this issue, since by this time, Sherman Institute and its resident Indian children had become quite a tourist attraction in Riverside. The possibility of tourists contracting typhoid fever while visiting the school or of the school no longer being accessible to tourists because of the epidemic, was apparently not considered, at least publicly.

Whether a source of the Sherman Institute typhoid fever was ever found is not known. Although it may have originated in the school's dairy.[41] According to the report of Dr. A. S. Parker, Sherman Institute's contract physician:

Cause of the epidemic—previous to Oct. 18th there had never been a case of typhoid fever in the school, this enumeration shows that during the first week of the outbreak over half of the total number of cases come down. It was observed also that they were about equally distributed among the four dormitories, this points to the conclusion that either the water or the food supply became infected at that time. That it was not the water would seem to be proven by the fact that there was no outbreak in the town at large other than a scattering case here and there, the school using the same domestic water supply as the town. It is decidedly uncertain as to how the food could have become infected, other than the fact that there were swarms of flies on the premises that could spread an infection once started. The grounds, kitchen, cellars, urinals, every thing that could possibly figure in contagion, were immediately and rigorously cleansed and renovated, and it was ordered that every drop of milk should be boiled.[42]

Newspaper accounts noted that thirty cases of typhoid fever existed as of November 2, and that three deaths had occurred by November 9. According to Dr. Parker's report, the total number of students infected with typhoid between October 18 and November 28 was forty-two. A total of six children died of typhoid fever between October 29 and November 14. However, the information contained within Parker's report frequently contradicts that found on the children's death certificates filed with the Riverside County Recorder, so the figures presented in his report are suspect.

Based on information contained within death certificates of the Indian children who succumbed to typhoid fever, the first student became ill on October 15, 1904. The name of this student was Mateo Couts, a seventeen-year-old Luiseño boy from Rincon who had come to Perris Indian School as a six-year-old. Mateo was attended by Dr. Parker until his death on November 6; he was buried in Temecula. Interestingly, in Parker's report, forwarded to the Commissioner of Indian Affairs, the first five students became ill on October 18th and Mateo Couts was not listed as being ill until October 20th. The reason for the discrepancies in Parker's reports is unknown, although it is apparent that he either had difficulty maintaining consistent records or keeping track of student identities.

Three students, including fourteen-year-old Lilly Edwards (Round Valley), seventeen-year-old Mamie Alpheus (Klamath), and seventeen-year-old John Powers (Wylachi) took ill on October 22. Parker treated them for seven, twenty, and twenty-two days respectively, but unfortunately, all of them died. School officials buried the children in the Sherman cemetery in caskets. Again, Parker's report differs from the death certificates, listing the onset of illness as October 24 for Edwards and Powers, and October 27 for Alpheus. On October 24, two more students became ill. Their names were Dan Edwards (Round Valley) and George Summersell (Pomo). Dan was fourteen years of age and was ill for seventeen days before his death; twenty-two days passed before twelve-year-old George finally succumbed to typhoid fever. The place of burial for each of these boys was listed as U.S.A. Grounds, but it is unclear exactly where this was. Parker's report does not even list Dan Edwards and gives a date of November 1 as the onset of Summersell's illness.

In each case, Parker's report, compiled at the request of the Commissioner of Indian Affairs, indicates that the victims of the typhoid-fever epidemic were ill for significantly shorter periods of time than what was entered on their death certificates. It is possible that Parker's inaccuracies were intended to convey a less critical situation at Sherman than actually existed. Alternately, Parker may have spent so little time actually caring for the children that he was uncertain as to the length and extent of their illnesses and perhaps even who the individual children were.[43]

Whether parents were notified of their children's illnesses and deaths is not known; Hall stated that such was the case, but corroborating correspondence has not been found. None of the children who died during this period were from the local area so it is improbable that their parents would have learned of the epidemic and their children's illnesses unless specifically notified by Hall.

At the time of the typhoid-fever epidemic, a hospital had not yet been built at Sherman Institute. However, two salaried resident nurses, Mrs. Lida Bartlow and Mrs. Lucretta Wrigley, cared for the children.[44] Two additional nurses, Minnie Virtue and Mattie Higgins, also worked at the school and received salaries, but apparently did not live there. The services of local physician Dr. A. S. Parker were contracted for at a rate of $180 per quarter. Since Parker maintained a successful private practice, it is doubtful that Parker spent a great deal of time at Sherman, particularly since it was located across town from his offices.[45]

Despite the fact there was no hospital or infirmary at Sherman Institute in 1904, the Riverside County General Hospital was located on Magnolia Avenue less than one mile from the school. Yet the Indian children at Sherman Institute suffering from typhoid fever were not treated at the hospital.[46] Instead, the children were kept at the school, where Parker and the nurses took care of them, aided by five "irregular nurses." It is apparent that instead of sending the children to the hospital to be cared for, Hall decided to keep them at the school and simply hire extra practitioners to care for them.[47]

According to Hall's correspondence with the Commissioner of Indian Affairs, he had received permission to move the remaining students from Perris and transfer them to Riverside, even if he had to house them in tents until the buildings under construction were finished. On October 27, Hall purchased eight tents for temporary housing for the transferred students; it is probable that at least some of them were used for the sick children, particularly if by November 2, thirty students were ill.[48] Since the living quarters of Sherman Institute students were broken up unto a series of individual rooms, it would have been far more difficult to care for the ill students if they had been left in these rooms instead of being moved into large tents.[49] This would also be in keeping with the prevailing medical opinion that a typhoid-fever patient's sick room should be kept well ventilated day and night. It is doubtful, however, that a tent infirmary such as this would have had sufficient facilities for disinfecting bodily discharges, beds, linens, and toilet facilities, practices critical to controlling the spread of infection.[50] Available records do not specify where the sick students were housed.

Although neither treatment nor medication records have been found, it is known that drugs were only purchased by Sherman Institute on September 30, approximately three weeks before the epidemic began, and on December 31, six weeks after it ended. It is unlikely that sufficient medication was in stock to treat the forty-two children suffering from typhoid fever.[51] The method of treatment utilized by Dr. Parker and the nurses can only be imagined, but obviously it was not terribly effective.

The last student, George Summersell, died of typhoid fever on November 14, 1904 and was buried the same day. Additional deaths did not occur during the year, so the total deaths for 1904 remained at eleven. Considering that the cumulative number of student deaths at both Perris and Riverside schools locations since 1892 had only been six, the mortality rate for 1904 was extraordinarily high. Yet on August 31, 1905, in his annual report to the Commissioner of Indian Affairs for fiscal year 1904–1905, Harwood Hall stated only:

> The general health of the pupils has been good, although in the fall of the year we were troubled with some sickness. We have been handicapped, however, owing to the fact of not having our hospital completed. It is now finished and in use.[52]

The deaths of eleven children in 1904, seven from a typhoid-fever epidemic, did not warrant mention or recognition in Harwood Hall's report, which was the official government statement regarding Sherman Institute for the fiscal year ending June 30, 1905. Further, although the Commissioner of Indian Affair's office had been minimally notified of the typhoid-fever epidemic and resulting deaths, Hall's report was accepted as submitted and no attempt was made to require elucidation or change.[53] In not recognizing the deaths of the children, they were essentially dismissed as irrelevant, and as a result not only was the official report falsified, but the lives of these children were trivialized.

According to available accounts, Hall was reputably a compassionate man who had dedicated his life to the education of Indian children. Of course realistically, this equated to encouraging their assimilation, teaching them to be more white, and hence more "civilized." His letters to the Commissioner of Indian Affairs and others reveal a man who seemed to be trying to do the right thing, a man of good intentions. The Superintendent of Indian Schools for the Department of the Interior, Estelle Reel, admired and respected Harwood Hall. Considering the many Indian School superintendents she had to deal with, it seems plausible that she would be able to recognize traits that were exemplary in a superintendent, and in Hall, she found them. Mary Jamison and her sister, Mary Fish, who were students at Sherman Institute in the early days, expressed their great love for Hall and his wife:

> We loved them. We were so happy because they were so wonderful. They were just like our parents. Mrs. Hall especially. Every Christmas time Mr. Hall would invite all the little girls to his home (located on the grounds). He would have a party on the lawn and have a present for all there. We cried when Superintendent and Mrs. Hall left Sherman.[54]

It is difficult to understand why such a man as Harwood Hall reacted to the deaths of his students as he did. Certainly he felt some sense of grief or sorrow, especially for Mateo Couts, who had literally grown up at the school. However, instead of truthfully reporting what had happened during the year, he chose to deny that children under his care had died. Hall notified the Commissioner of Indian Affairs about the existence of a typhoid-fever epidemic, but his letters provided cursory information at best and were typically only requests for reimbursement of funds. It was in his official report to the Commissioner of Indian Affairs for inclusion in the annual report of the Department of the Interior, presented to the House of Representatives, that Hall neglected to mention the depth of the troubling sickness.

The fact that it was typhoid fever to which the children succumbed should have had no relevance, because in 1904, numerous epidemics of typhoid fever occurred throughout the state of California. However, it is possible that Hall felt he had not provided adequate care for the students by keeping them at the school instead of admitting them to the local hospital. By not reporting the students' deaths, he would not be held accountable for the adequacy of their treatment. This may in fact have played a part in Hall's falsified reporting. According to the California State Board of Health report for October 1904,[55] typhoid fever had increased to a considerable degree and was quite prevalent throughout the state; the cause was usually found to be the water supply. In thirty-two reports covering a population numbering 1,009,500, there were twenty-eight deaths from typhoid fever. The student population at Sherman Institute during the epidemic period was approximately six hundred, and of those, seven children died of typhoid fever. Obviously, the mortality rate was significantly higher at Sherman Institute than throughout the state of California during the same time period.[56] It is quite possible that Hall recognized this and chose to ignore the deaths instead of explain them. This may also be the reason the Commissioner of Indian Affairs requested a report from the school physician. Why the information provided by the school physician was not then required to be included in Hall's report is inexplicable.

In reality, Hall's reason for not reporting the student deaths at Sherman Institute in 1904 probably had far less to do with accountability than with his professional credibility and career aspirations. Harwood Hall was a man who, from his earliest days with the Indian Service, had visions of building the *ideal* vocational school for assimilating young Indians; he sought to create the quintessential Indian school of the West. His dream began with the Phoenix Indian School in Arizona and would have continued there had it not been for his inability to adapt to the hot weather. In Phoenix, Hall was able to put into practice his personal ideas concerning Indian education and assimilation, although his abilities in these areas were somewhat questionable. Of critical importance to his tenure at the school was the institution of outing and apprentice programs he had developed. Primarily through these programs, the community saw Phoenix Indian School as representing a considerable financial benefit to them.

Hall's prolific federal fund-raising efforts contributed to the community's financial interest in the school, as did his efforts to make the school both a tourist destination and community social-cultural center. The school was perceived as being good for the community, thus warranting its support. As the administrator of the school, Hall was in a position of power and he quickly learned to use that power to benefit the Phoenix Indian School and its students. It would be cynical to believe Hall's sole motive in directing the Phoenix School in the manner he did was to attain personal power and glory. Considering the type of man he was purported to be, it is more plausible to believe he acted primarily for the benefit of the children. However, Hall's tenure at the Phoenix Indian School gave him a taste of what could be, provided the climate was better.

Transfer to an Indian vocational boarding school in southern California seemed the ideal solution to Hall's problems. That is, until he arrived at the less-than-ideal school in Perris, California. Even today, much of this area is relatively desolate. Although he diligently tried to improve conditions at the school, it was immediately clear to Hall that his dreams of creating the ideal Indian school would not be realized at Perris. Hall embarked on an ambitious campaign to move his Indian school to a more favorable location, citing the poor water supply at Perris as the primary reason for the move. The proposed move was very controversial and the specter of Hall's alleged falsification of data arose more than once. However, the move was eventually approved, not an instant too soon for Hall.

Moving the Indian school to Riverside was the first concrete step in the realization of Hall's ideal Indian vocational boarding school and he took full advantage of the situation. Preliminary lobbying for his vision of the proper design resulted in the school essentially being built to his specifications. Hall's mastery of public relations resulted in the creation of a strong community support network before construction of the school had even begun. Despite a somewhat rocky financial start, Hall succeeded in obtaining sufficient federal funding to continue his expansion program. Under Superintendent Hall's skillful direction, Sherman Institute was growing nicely and becoming a thriving tourist destination and cultural center for the city. In its very short existence at the new location, the school promised to be everything Phoenix Indian School had been, and more. A thriving Indian school with considerable community support, in a beautiful city, with a perfect climate; Hall's vision of creating the quintessential Indian school in the western United States was seemingly a reality.

In the year 1904, however, Hall was forced to deal with some rather important distractions. During the early part of the year, two children died, but this was not a wholly unusual occurrence and probably did not warrant much concern. In July, two more children died within two days of each other, both from pneumonia. Again, this probably did not cause any alarm on Hall's part, despite the fact that the children were only six and nine years old. Then, there was the problem of finally closing the Perris school. Hall had been very anxious to close the Perris school for some time. It was twenty-two miles distant and running both schools was very difficult. In October, the water system fortuitously suffered complete failure and Hall was finally given permission to transfer the remaining children to Riverside. Unfortunately, just as this was to occur, a typhoid-fever epidemic was visited upon Sherman Institute, and Hall was faced with the very significant, very real problem of many sick and dying children. Hall made choices in the care of these children that may or may not have been wise or responsible, but they were choices he alone had the authority to make as their temporary guardian. It is unlikely that others in his position would have made vastly different choices.

When it was time for Harwood Hall to submit the 1904–1905 fiscal year report to the Commissioner of Indian Affairs, he made one more critical decision that involved the care of the children who had become sick and died during the past year. Quite simply, Hall chose to ignore their deaths, to treat them as if they had not happened. By doing this, the lives of eleven children, who had died far away from their homes and families, were dismissed as irrelevant and unimportant. Not only did Hall consciously disregard his fiduciary duty to accurately report the condition of students in his care at Sherman Institute to the federal government, but by denying the deaths of these students, he denied their short lives. The complicity of the Commissioner of Indian Affair's office in not requiring at least some elucidation regarding the sickness and its victims, even if it was simply a bureaucratic oversight, further negated the lives of Indian children they were required by federal law to protect.

Although Hall must certainly have felt some degree of sorrow for the children at the time they died, nine months had passed by the time he wrote his annual report and the children were then just memories. The Sherman Institute, on the other hand, was rapidly expanding, running smoothly, and becoming ever more successful. Superintendent Hall's vision of the ideal Indian school was finally coming to fruition and there was nothing that he would allow to tarnish that. What had happened in the fall of 1904 was over and done, and except for being a little troublesome, it really had very little to do with the big picture of Sherman Institute's continuing success.

NOTES

1. "Local News at Arlington," *Riverside Enterprise*, November 2, 1904. The single sentence, "There are thirty cases of typhoid fever in Sherman Institute," was the first public acknowledgment of the epidemic. However, according to the report of Sherman Institute's physician A. S. Parker, 42 students contracted typhoid fever between October 18 and November 28, 1904. See A. S. Parker's Report to Commissioner of Indian Affairs, December 7, 1904 (Letter Press Books, 1904), 357–58, National Archives, Pacific Southwest Region, Laguna Niguel, California, Record Group 75. The author wishes to thank Lori Sisquoc, Curator of the Sherman Indian Museum, for her assistance and continued support of my research. Without her help, this project could not have been completed.

2. "Report of School at Riverside, California, August 31, 1905," *Annual Report of the Department of Interior for the Fiscal Year Ended June 30, 1905* (Washington, DC: Government Printing Office, 1906), 416. Hereafter cited as *Annual Report of the Department of Interior, 1905*. Hall stated that "The general health of the pupils has been good, although in the fall of the year we were troubled with some sickness. We have been handicapped, however, owing to the fact of not having our hospital completed. It is now finished and in use." Neither the seven deaths from typhoid fever, nor the additional four deaths that had occurred earlier in the year were noted. Hall also failed to report that at least 35 additional children had contracted typhoid.

3. Pupil Registers, 1892–1904, Sherman Indian High School Museum Collection, Riverside, California. Hereafter cited as Sherman Indian Museum Collection. Deaths recorded between 1892 and 1903 totaled six.

4. Robert A. Trennert, *The Phoenix Indian School* (Norman: University of Oklahoma Press, 1988), xi.

5. Ibid., 32–33.

6. Ibid., 41.

7. Ibid., 45.

8. Ibid., 51.

9. Ibid., 54–55.

10. Ibid., 55.

11. Hall to Commissioner of Indian Affairs, April 3, 1897, NA, PSWR, RG 75, 13036-1897.

12. Hall, "Report of School at Perris, California, August 31, 1897, *Annual Report of the Department of Interior, 1897*, p. 345.

13. M. H. Savage, "Report of the School at Perris, California," August 15, 1893, *House Executive Document*, 53rd Congress, 2nd Sess. (Washington, DC: Government Printing Office, 1895), 408.

14. Hall, "Report of School at Perris, California," August 31, 1897, *Annual Reports of the Department of Interior, 1897*, p. 345.

15. Estelle Reel, Superintendent of Indian Schools, to Commissioner of Indian Affairs, June 3, 1899, Sherman Indian Museum Collection. "The general condition of this school, so far as regards the buildings, management and supervision is excellent. The Perris school could easily be made one of the largest nonreservation schools in the

service were it not for the fact that so far it has been impossible to obtain sufficient water supply. . . . While I was at Perris the Bear Valley Irrigation Company entirely closed off the water supply. . . . The Superintendent stated that the school had been dependent upon this supply of water, both for domestic and irrigation purposes, since the school was first located in 1891. Now that the supply is entirely cut off this condition of affairs involves the question of no water, no sewerage, etc. . . . I earnestly recommend that an appropriation be granted by Congress for the establishment of an Indian Industrial School plant at some suitable location in Southern California where sufficient water facilities can be obtained." Reel supported Hall's request to move the Perris school to a new location.

16. Reel to Hall, November 13, 1899, Sherman Indian Museum Collection.

17. Ibid., December 5, 1899.

18. Tom Patterson, *A Colony for California* (Riverside, CA: Museum Press, 1996), 240. Patterson argues that Frank Miller is generally given the credit for bringing the Indian school to Riverside in 1902. The location of Sherman Indian Institute next to Miller's streetcar company's Chemawa Park was by design, and Sherman's Mission Revival architecture mirrored that of Miller's Mission Inn in Riverside.

19. T. Gibbon, Los Angeles Terminal Railway Company, to the Commissioner of Indian Affairs, May 14, 1900, Sherman Indian Museum Collection.

20. Horatio N. Rust, Indian Agent, Colton, California, to Merrill E. Gates, May 10, 1900, Sherman Indian Museum Collection.

21. *U.S. Congressional Record Proceedings*, May 22, 1900.

22. University of California College of Agriculture, Berkeley, to Sherman Indian Institute, June 12, 1900, Sherman Indian Museum Collection.

23. Kathleen Svani, "The Last Song: History of Sherman Institute, Riverside, California," unpublished manuscript, 1966, Riverside Public Library, pp. 29–30.

24. *Riverside Daily Enterprise*, September 28, 1900.

25. Hall to Commissioner of Indian Affairs, August 1, 1900, Book of Letters, Indian School, Perris, California, September 1, 1898–April 6, 1901, Sherman Indian Museum Collection.

26. Hall to Commissioner of Indian Affairs, August 1, 1900, Sherman Indian Museum Collection.

27. Personal communication, author with Lori Sisquoc, Curator of the Sherman Indian Museum. Copies of invitations and responses are in the Sherman Indian Museum Collection.

28. Personal communication, author with Dr. Vincent Moses, Curator of History, Riverside Municipal Museum. The Frank Miller Collection is housed at the Riverside Museum.

29. *Riverside Daily Enterprise*, July 18, 1901.

30. Svani, "The Last Song," pp. 36–37.

31. Hall, "Report of Riverside School, California," September 1, 1904, *Annual Reports of the Department of Interior, 1904*, pp. 436–38.

32. Ibid., pp. 437–38.

33. Hall to Commissioner of Indian Affairs, October 7, 1904, NA, PSWR, Letter Press Books, p. 288. Hereafter cited as LPB.

34. Pupil records contain information regarding deaths, and these registers are a wealth of information regarding individual students and the student population. Each student register contained these variables: the date of entry into school, enrollment date, name, age, blood quantum, tribe, residence, parents' names, and whether the parents were alive. Student registers also recorded the student's activities, outing program participation, vacations, being dropped from school because of illness, and date of death. Four registers contain vital statistics for students, including height, weight, pulse, forced expiration, forced inspiration, etc.

35. Generally studies such as this do not share the names of individuals, but in consultation with Lori Sisquoc, I have chosen to do so to give greater meaning to their lives, much more so than that accorded by Harwood Hall. The children who perished due to typhoid fever were real humans, not mere statistics, and their deaths indicate that in 1904 Sherman pupils suffered more than a little "sickness."

36. Classified student records for these children do not exist, although the National Archives preserves a letter press book from 1904 containing correspondence to the Commissioner of Indian Affairs regarding the deaths from typhoid fever. See Hall's and Parker's correspondence, November 16 and December 7, 1904, LPB, NA, PSWR, RG 75.

37. Death Certificates, Riverside County, Microfilm 1893–1906, for Harry Seonia (#182) and Nancy Lawrence (#194).

38. *Los Angeles Daily Times*, November 16, 1904.

39. William Budd, *Typhoid Fever* (New York: Arno Press, 1977), 176–77.

40. Ibid.

41. *Nineteenth Biennial Report of the State Board of Health of California, July 1, 1904–June 30, 1906* (Sacramento: State Publishing, 1906), 15.

42. Parker to Hall, December 7, 1904, LPB, 1904, p. 358, NA, PSWR, RG 75. Records prior to 1950 have been discarded at what is now the Public Health Department of Riverside; it is impossible to determine if the investigation included more than just the Riverside Water Company's wells.

43. Ibid.

44. *Riverside City Directory, 1905* (Los Angeles: Riverside Directory Company, 1905), 42, 292. A city directory for 1904 could not be found. The names of these individuals were found in a ledger book filed at the Sherman Indian Museum Collection.

45. The Cash Ledger Book, 1904, listing monetary distributions for the year indicate that Bartlow and Wrigley each received a salary of $50 per month.

46. Riverside General Hospital Book of Admissions, 1904, Riverside General Hospital Files.

47. During the epidemic, the Office of Indian Affairs hired five irregular nurses at $3.60 per day. None of the women listed as serving as nurses appeared in the *Riverside City Directory*. See Cash Ledger Book, 1904, Sherman Indian Museum Collection.

48. Hall to Commissioner of Indian Affairs, LPB, p. 354, NA, PSWR, RG 75. The correspondence does not reveal why Hall and Parker kept the children at Sherman and did not admit them to the hospital.

49. Parker's Report suggests that the students were being housed in four dormitories, when in fact administrators housed them in individual rooms within the four dormitories.

50. Budd, *Typhoid Fever*, p. 177.

51. Cash Vouchers, Hall to Commissioner of Indian Affairs, October 20, 1904, LPB, pp. 299–300, NA, PSWR, RG 75, indicate that in 1904 Sherman had little medicine and purchased some from Boyd Keith, Voucher 49 for $21.45, and from Charles E. Weck, Voucher 63 for $4.10. These purchases do not appear in the Cash Ledger Book, Sherman Indian Museum Collection.

52. Hall to Commission of Indian Affairs, December 5, 1904, LPB, p. 416, NA, PSWR, RG 75.

53. In the late-nineteenth and early twentieth centuries, the Commissioner of Indian Affairs often asked agents, superintendents, doctors, and other employees of the Office of Indian Affairs to clarify issues mentioned in their letters and reports. However, the Commissioner never asked Hall to clarify or illuminate his report of the typhoid fever epidemic.

54. Interview with Mary Jamison, former pupil of Sherman, as found in Svani, "The Last Song," pp. 46–47.

55. "California State Board of Health Report," *Riverside Enterprise*, November 26, 1904.

56. In 1904, the Crude Death Rate for typhoid fever among the general California population was 2.77 per 100,000 population, while the same year, it was 1,166.68 per 100,000 population among the student population at Sherman.

FOUR

TODD BENSON

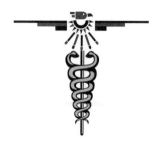

Blinded with Science

AMERICAN INDIANS, THE OFFICE OF INDIAN AFFAIRS, AND THE FEDERAL CAMPAIGN AGAINST TRACHOMA, 1924–1927

In December of 1924, Charles Burke, the Commissioner of Indian Affairs, received a letter from H. J. Hagerman, a former governor of New Mexico Territory who had been appointed by the Office of Indian Affairs (OIA) as "Special Commissioner to the Navajo."[1] Hagerman reported that he had received a troubling piece of correspondence from an OIA physician head-quartered on the Navajo reservation. This physician, Polk Richards, had found some disturbing aftereffects among Navajo patients who had been treated by government doctors for trachoma, a painful, infectious eye disease that produced damaged vision or blindness. Two of these patients could no longer close their eyelids completely, a condition known as "lagophthalmos," and at least two others suffered from entropion, in which the eyelashes had turned inward and were scratching the surface of the eyeball.

All of these patients had been treated as part of a national campaign by the OIA to eradicate trachoma from Indian communities. Their condition, Hagerman told Burke, suggested that perhaps the OIA needed to rethink its strategy. The trachoma campaign was based on the use of a radical surgical technique known as tarsectomy, in which the surgeon treated the disease by cutting out the tarsus, the supportive tissue underneath the eyelids. Unless patients were selected judiciously, Hagerman warned, and unless those who performed the operation were highly skilled surgeons, it was quite possible that the trachoma campaign would produce "very harmful results," potentially causing Indian patients to lose all confidence in OIA doctors.[2]

Burke replied with a letter designed to reassure the Special Commissioner. The OIA would, Burke said, make every effort to ensure that the operation was performed only in carefully selected cases, and only by carefully trained physicians. OIA doctors who showed no aptitude for the surgery would not be provided with money to buy the special instruments necessary to perform the procedure. And while it was true that aftereffects such as entropion and lagophthalmos would sometimes occur, such problems could be treated with additional surgery.[3]

Hagerman was not mollified. He pointed out, in reply, that there was a severe shortage of OIA physicians qualified to perform such a delicate procedure, and noted that if performed improperly a tarsectomy could "result disastrously to the patient."[4] This time Burke failed to reply. Rather than heed Hagerman's warnings, he issued an official circular that made it mandatory for *all* physicians to perform the surgery, or risk losing their jobs. Henceforth, he said, the OIA would "require all our physicians to learn to perform the approved operations for the cure of trachoma, or give place to those who will learn."[5]

With Burke's order, the campaign against trachoma, which had previously been confined solely to the Southwest, began to expand dramatically. But Hagerman's warnings would prove prophetic. It would not be until 1927 that OIA officials would come to accept any evidence that tarsectomy was dangerous. But by then the procedure had been performed on at least three thousand American Indian men, women, and children, with disturbing results.

The Campaign Begins

But how did this disaster come about? Why and how would the OIA be so willing to design their campaign around an untested radical form of surgery? And why would the OIA ignore repeated warnings, such as those by Hagerman, that their campaign was harming Indian patients?

The OIA's use of tarsectomy was driven by factors similar to those that had given rise to a national program of Western-style health care for American Indians in the first place. Between 1908 and 1912, scientific studies financed by the OIA confirmed what many in American Indian communities had known for some time: health and sanitary conditions on reservations and in government boarding schools were deplorable.[6] Two diseases in particular, trachoma and tuberculosis, had reached near-epidemic proportions. The studies revealed that nearly one in four American Indian men, women, and children—on some reservations the figure reached as high as one in two—suffered from trachoma.[7] And American Indians were nearly ten times more likely than the rest of the population to contract pulmonary tuberculosis, and four times as likely to die from the disease.[8]

Anecdotal evidence of such problems had been available to government administrators for several years but had been largely disregarded. In the late-nineteenth century, OIA officials had ignored warnings of possible health risks and recruited and enrolled in boarding schools many Indian students with active tuberculosis.[9] Why, then, did policy-makers suddenly display such concern for investigating Indian health? The answer was twofold. First, American Indians and whites were, in many areas, living closer to each other. In the years following passage of the Dawes Act, the government sold off or leased millions of acres of so-called surplus Indian land to whites, and Congress passed legislation that opened other tribal lands to white settlement.[10] The increasingly close contact between the two groups meant that American Indians afflicted with infectious diseases represented a threat to neighboring whites as well as to members of their own community. As Commissioner Francis Leupp put it in 1908, the OIA was "confronted by the urgent necessity of doing more than has ever been done before in the way of protecting the Indians against the ravages of the disease, not only for their own sakes, but because the infected Indian community becomes a peril to every white community near it."[11]

Policy-makers also argued that poor Indian health threatened the process of assimilation. "[T]he physical welfare of the Indian is, and always must be," Commissioner William Jones said in 1904, "the fundamental consideration in the scheme to educate or civilize him. It is impossible to develop his mental and moral capabilities without healthy material to work on."[12] The results of the OIA-financed health surveys confirmed Jones' views and led several prominent federal health officials to worry that inferior health conditions might threaten Indian peoples' capability to become economically self-sufficient. The high incidence of trachoma, Surgeon General Walter Wyman argued, threatened the "economic usefulness" of individual Indian people, and the "economic efficiency" of the entire race. Other officials in the Public Health Service agreed, noting that trachoma endangered Indian children's potential "power to earn a living," thus increasing the possibility that they would "become permanent charges on the State."[13]

Beginning in 1909, OIA officials used such arguments to win regular congressional appropriations for a national Indian health program. By 1912, Congress appropriated approximately $350,000 annually "to relieve distress among Indians and to provide for their care and for the prevention and treatment of tuberculosis, trachoma, smallpox, and other contagious diseases."

Although the OIA used these funds to implement a major expansion of government health efforts during the 1910s, the onset of World War I led to a retrenchment of the Indian health program, as doctors and nurses in the Indian Service resigned their positions by the dozens to enter military service or seek more lucrative private employment. Inflation caused by the war, meanwhile, forced the OIA to reduce or in some cases even eliminate its purchases of medical equipment and supplies.[14]

The situation did not improve, given the postwar climate of fiscal conservatism that dominated the nation during the early 1920s, even after the war ended. Between 1919 and 1924 Congress failed to increase the OIA's health budget above prewar levels. It was not until 1923 that Hubert Work, the Secretary of the Interior, requested an increased appropriation from Congress for Indian health programs. His request specified that the increased funds would be used "for the purpose of enlarging the present facilities for the treatment of trachoma among Indians."[15] Although the secretary's motive in focusing on trachoma, rather than on tuberculosis or on general health needs, remains unclear, it is likely he was driven by two primary considerations. In 1891, the PHS had begun conducting medical examinations on all immigrants. Those with trachoma (or deemed to be insane or mentally retarded) were denied entry. Two decades later, the PHS initiated a campaign to reduce the incidence of the disease among Appalachian whites. The success of these two programs left American Indians as the last major affected group in which the trachoma epidemic had not been addressed. Second, Work knew that he would need to demonstrate that any new appropriation would produce results. In contrast to a disease such as tuberculosis, which stubbornly resisted all attempts at a cure, trachoma appeared susceptible to control efforts, as the PHS program in Appalachia demonstrated.[16]

Congress responded to Work's request, increasing the OIA's health budget for 1924 by $500,000, and OIA officials made plans to begin an anti-trachoma campaign in the Southwest, with a particular focus on the Navajo reservation.[17] They did not do so blindly, since there existed a significant body of knowledge about how the disease progressed. In trachoma's initial stages, tiny, reddish clumps of blood vessels form in the conjunctiva, the clear layer of tissue lining the inside of the eyelids and the surface of the white of the eye. As time progresses, granular follicles, filled with debris and discharge (and, we now know, with the *chlamydia* microorganism that causes the disease) also develop in the conjunctiva and on the tarsus, a cartilagelike plate of tissue that lies between the conjunctiva and the eye muscle, which gives the eye its shape. Although doctors did not understand the exact cause of the disease, they knew that people could spread it to others through tears. A person can easily catch trachoma simply by wiping his or her face with a towel an infected person has just used.[18]

Trachoma can cause serious damage, as OIA physicians knew. Over time, the blood vessels that initially form on the conjunctiva may expand onto the surface of the eyeball, producing a dark spot that causes impaired sight or blindness. The granular follicles, meanwhile, rupture, causing scarring, which in turn leads to the contraction of the tarsal plate. A condition known as "entropion" may then ensue. In serious cases, this causes the eyelashes to rub against the cornea, causing blurred vision or blindness.[19]

There were three possible approaches that the OIA could have followed separately or in combination in designing the trachoma campaign. The first was utilizing public-health measures such as improving sanitation and providing health education about the spread of the disease. The second possible method, which was widely employed by American ophthalmologists of the period, was to treat the disease with medications such as silver nitrate, copper sulfate, alum, or bichloride of mercury.[20] The Public Health Service used both of these techniques to control trachoma in Appalachia.[21]

But the OIA opted for a third method: surgery. Following the advice of John McMullen, a PHS specialist brought in to plan the trachoma campaign, administrators established several field hospitals at Navajo in the summer of 1924.[22] There, government physicians performed a procedure known as "grattage." Stated crudely, grattage involved scraping away all infected conjunctival tissue. To perform the operation, a practitioner anesthetized patients locally, used a forceps to evert—turn inside out—their eyelids and vigorously scraped the infected tissue with a scalpel or surgical roller, breaking open the conjunctival follicles. The final step in the procedure consisted of rubbing off the diseased material with a brush or cloth. Postoperative care involved applying medicines to the treated area for several days.[23]

The campaign began on July 1, 1924 and received an immediate positive response from the Navajo community. By August 6, five weeks after the campaign began, over 5,100 people had reported to the new field hospitals for trachoma screening. The doctors found 1,174 cases of the disease, 962 of which they treated surgically.[24] In spite of this early success, the physicians in charge of the campaign soon experienced difficulties. In funding the antitrachoma program, OIA officials had followed McMullen's recommendation and budgeted for an average of six days of postoperative care per patient.[25] But the doctors soon found that postsurgical inflammation, which in their view necessitated a hospital stay of anywhere "from two to four weeks," was an inevitable consequence of the surgery. Patients discharged before the inflammation had subsided, they told Commissioner Burke, would not only continue to infect others, but might experience more damage from their inflamed eyes than "if no operation had been performed." One doctor wrote that he would consider himself "derelict in duty and malpracticing" to dismiss cases so soon after surgery.[26]

A Radical Solution

Although Burke reluctantly granted the doctors' request to extend the six-day limit on postoperative care, the campaign's financial difficulties perhaps made it inevitable that OIA officials would seek a magic bullet to cure trachoma. The solution to their problems came in September 1924, when Dr. L. Webster Fox of Philadelphia took a vacation in Montana's Glacier National Park. Fox, a professor at the University of Pennsylvania, was one of the country's leading ophthalmologists and the author of a standard textbook in the field.[27]

On a similar vacation one year earlier, Fox had discovered that 30 percent of the population of the nearby Blackfeet reservation suffered from trachoma and had used Blackfeet trachoma patients to demonstrate his treatment methods to reservation physicians. When Fox returned to the area in 1924, he agreed to repeat his demonstration. This time, though, his audience included Assistant Commissioner Edgar B. Meritt, who was visiting the Blackfeet agency. Impressed, Meritt sent Commissioner Burke a glowing report of Fox's clinic, and on Burke's orders, "a large number" of OIA doctors—including J. S. Perkins, the director of the trachoma campaign at Navajo—subsequently traveled to Blackfeet to observe Fox's procedure firsthand.[28]

Fox's technique included two separate procedures, the first of which was a more extreme version of the method used by the OIA physicians at Navajo, and which Fox labeled "radical" grattage. In this operation, surgeons used sharp three-bladed knives to scrape the inner eyelids "both longitudinally and laterally," which produced "rather free bleeding." Then they dipped a stiff toothbrush in a bichloride of mercury solution and brushed "very vigorously" across the eyelids. Aftercare involved the application of medicinal dressings for four to six days. Fox recommended this operation for the earlier stages of the disease but not before the follicles had formed and slight scarring had occurred.[29] For more advanced cases he advocated a second more radical operation known as "tarsectomy." To perform it, physicians everted a patient's upper eye and used a scalpel to excise both the diseased tarsal plate and most of the underlying conjunctiva. To compensate for the removal of this tissue and provide support for the eyelid, they used a small forceps to grasp the edge of the remaining conjunctiva near the top of the eyelid, pulled it down, and stitched it to the margin of the eyelid. Aftercare consisted of the application of anesthetics in a dressing for eight to ten days.[30]

The advantage of these two surgeries, Fox believed, was that they cured quickly and completely, eliminating the need for any extended form of treatment. With just a few cuts of the knife, the disease could be eliminated. Those who attended Fox's demonstration were suitably impressed. "Judging by the past," wrote Perkins, "a lot of the work we are doing now will have to be repeated because it does not cure, in a large number of cases." Fox's "great ability and wide experience," on the other hand, guaranteed that his methods would be more effective, more efficient, and less costly in the long term. Walter Stevens, a high-level OIA medical supervisor, agreed. "With the elimination of aftertreatment," he wrote, "it can readily . . . be seen that our present methods of treatment will be greatly simplified."[31]

However, Stevens noted that tarsectomy could produce a serious side effect. Stretching the remaining conjunctiva to the lid margin after the excision of the tarsus produced tension, which could cause the lid to turn inward on itself, possibly leading to blindness. This was the same condition found in many advanced cases of trachoma. To prevent this complication, Fox ended a tarsectomy operation by using an electric cautery to puncture a double row of tiny holes along the margin of the lid. "The theory," Stevens wrote, "is that the scar resulting will counter act [sic] the shortening of the conjunctiva."[32]

Stevens himself was skeptical about this procedure. "This is probably the result in many cases," he said, "but I am of the opinion that secondary operations to correct the entropion will be necessary in a number of cases." He also noted that a tarsectomy might not always cure the disease. "We have the possibility, that the granules may again form . . . in which instances a secondary operation will be necessary," he said. It was unclear, however, what those operations would be: one could neither apply medication to the underside of the tarsus nor scrape the granules off it once it had been surgically removed.[33]

It was clear, though, that either a recurrence of trachoma or the development of entropion would require further medical treatment, contradicting Fox's claim about the benefits of a tarsectomy. But Stevens ignored this potential problem, as well as the potential damage that failed tarsectomies could cause. "Presuming we get only 50 percent successful operations," he wrote, "our results will be far more reaching than we could hope to obtain through the prolonged aftertreatment method." The procedure itself was relatively simple to learn, Stevens said, and required neither "any more time nor a more developed technique" than the mild form of grattage then used. He recommended that all OIA traveling ophthalmologists learn tarsectomy, as well as radical grattage, and that both procedures be given a one-year trial.[34]

OIA administrators enthusiastically endorsed Stevens's recommendations, but ignored his suggestion for a trial period. On September 12, Commissioner Burke ordered Stevens to travel to the Southwest and begin teaching the Fox operations to agency doctors. Shortly thereafter, Meritt instructed him to devote "the major part of his time to the trachoma campaign," and, with Perkins's assistance, to organize a clinic where other OIA doctors could learn to perform tarsectomies. The first clinic was held on the Navajo reservation on November 3, 1924. The physicians who attended, some of whom had never before performed surgery, received an abrupt introduction into Fox's methods. After first watching an instructor operate on one eye of a trachoma patient, the new ophthalmological trainees then had to operate on the other eye, with their instructor's assistance.[35]

About the same time, Burke informed a congressional committee that the OIA was striving "to make every physician in the Indian Service a trachoma expert." The OIA had employed a number of ophthalmologists as regional trachoma specialists even before the trachoma campaign had begun. The intent now was to have them learn Fox's operations and then have them demonstrate the procedures to other physicians in their own districts. By January, the program of radical surgery in the Southwest was operating "full blast," and one of the OIA's trachoma specialists had been directed to begin a similar campaign in the Dakotas.[36] Fox then agreed to give another demonstration clinic at Albuquerque. Commissioners Burke and Meritt ordered both Perkins and Robert Newberne, the OIA's chief medical director, to participate in Fox's demonstration, and Newberne authorized OIA ophthalmologists from as far away as South Dakota and Michigan to attend.[37]

Fox's second clinic was held in January 1925 and had what can only be described as a major impact on those who attended. "THIS CONCLUDES ONE OF THE GREATEST TRACHOMA CLINICS EVER HELD," Perkins telegraphed Washington after the clinic had ended. It was "IMPOSSIBLE TO ESTIMATE THE AMOUNT OF GOOD DONE," he added, noting that those attending had been fortunate to learn from "a master."[38] By then all of the OIA's traveling trachoma specialists and medical supervisors ("with," according to Commissioner Burke, "the possible exception of one") had received instruction in Fox's radical approach. During the next five months the OIA held two other formal clinics in the Fox technique, at Phoenix, Arizona, and at Riverside, California, and by September over fifty OIA physicians had "become skilled operators in trachoma." By then the OIA had also initiated new campaigns against the disease in Wisconsin, Oklahoma, and on the Crow agency in Montana. As a report by the Board of Indian Commissioners put it, on "almost all the reservations and in all the schools the agency and school physicians were examining, treating, and operating for trachoma."[39]

It was at this point that the first signs of trouble appeared. Indeed, even before Hagerman had forwarded Polk Richards's troublesome findings to Burke, W. C. Barton, an OIA physician who had attended Fox's initial clinic at Blackfeet, wrote the Commissioner to express his reservations. Although Barton had left the Montana clinic a proponent of the Fox techniques, he wrote the Commissioner cautioning that a tarsectomy was "an operation requiring considerable surgical skill." Moreover, patients who underwent the procedure required approximately two weeks of postoperative care. "For this reason," Barton concluded, "only a comparatively few patients can be handled at one time, and a larger number of helpers and workers is required."[40]

But Barton's concerns, like those of Richards and Hagerman, were ignored in favor of Burke's veiled threat of termination for any physician who did not learn tarsectomy. As the campaign progressed into late 1925 and 1926, these heavy-handed tactics began to achieve results. OIA physicians cut out an ever-growing number of Indian tarsal plates, and Indian Office administrators publicly expressed optimism about the results of their radical experiment. Marshall C. Guthrie, who became the OIA's Chief Medical Director in 1926, told a congressional subcommittee that the campaign "should" produce a decrease in the incidence of Indian trachoma. Assistant Commissioner Meritt, testifying at another subcommittee hearing, noted that while trachoma would likely remain a problem for "some time into the future," since the Fox technique had been adopted, "considerable progress" had been made. And the campaign's chief budget officer wrote a glowing report of the tarsectomy program, which was published in the *Santa Fe New Mexican* and five other Southwestern newspapers. Fox's clinics had, the report stated, allowed "a large number" of OIA physicians to receive "special training which added greatly to their fitness for handling trachoma and treating it by the most improved methods." Thousands of Indians had been treated by government doctors, and in the coming year "many times as much [would] be accomplished."[41]

But even as administrators were heralding what they saw as the OIA's achievements, and even as growing numbers of American Indians were undergoing the surgical removal of their tarsal plates, events were transpiring that would force the end of the trachoma campaign. In October 1924 the American Medical Association, at the request of Interior Secretary Work, had appointed a committee of leading ophthalmologists to advise the OIA and the Secretary on trachoma-control activities. Within five months, the three members of the committee had submitted a report to the Commissioner that stressed the need for public-health education as a means of controlling the disease. The committee concluded that both grattage and tarsectomy were "severe" forms of treatment to be used only in carefully selected cases.[42]

Assistant Commissioner Meritt penned what appears to have been a disingenuous official response to this recommendation. The OIA was, he told the members of the advisory committee, relying on milder forms of surgery (including a mild form of grattage) as its principal weapons in the trachoma campaign.[43] But Meritt knew this to be false. His reply came several months after he himself had attended Fox's initial clinic at Blackfeet. Meritt's attempt to mislead members of the advisory committee suggests that he (and presumably other top OIA officials as well) knew that tarsectomy was a controversial procedure. Had Meritt told the truth, the AMA consultants would likely have recommended abandoning the tarsectomy campaign immediately. But because he did not, the campaign of radical tarsectomy continued another eighteen months, until the advisory committee members began a firsthand investigation of the OIA's trachoma program. Only then did the truth about the trachoma campaign began to emerge.

In November 1926 a member of the committee wrote an apparently innocent letter to Polk Richards, the physician whose reports had led Hagerman to warn Commissioner Burke two years earlier, requesting Richards's opinion on how best to treat trachoma. Richards replied by cautioning against the use of radical surgery, which in his experience could cause damage to the patient even while failing to cure the disease. He noted that he was treating two patients "tarsectomized two years ago" who suffered from severe cases of the disease.[44] Richards repeated these conclusions a few months later in a letter published in a professional ophthalmological journal. Radical grattage, he reported, had caused "much unnecessary damage" to Indian trachoma patients, including extensive scarring to the conjunctiva and a condition called "symblepharon," in which the eyelid became stuck to the eyeball. Tarsectomy also had caused significant damage. "We have had and seen others have," Richards said, "some bad results following these operations, varying degrees of lagophthalmos being the most common." Tarsectomy also often failed to cure the disease: "[a]cute flareups in the so-called cured cases," Richards said, "are common." He himself was treating three tarsectomized patients suffering from a reoccurrence of trachoma.[45]

By then, members of the advisory committee had finished firsthand visits to the field. (Two of them had traveled to Oklahoma the previous spring, and one more had visited the Southwest just a few months earlier.) The committee published the results of these investigations in the *Journal of the American Medical Association* on April 9, 1927. It concluded that OIA boarding schools, because they admitted both healthy and infected students, were a major source of trachoma infection, and recommended as a way to correct this problem the establishment of segregated schools that would exclusively enroll trachomatous pupils. The committee also recommended that health education and the use of trained field workers to conduct home visits represented the best way to control the disease. "We doubt the efficacy" of a tarsectomy campaign, the committee members noted, "for trachoma is a disease that demands continuous after treatment and cannot be cured by one radical treatment, operative or otherwise." In a second article published one month later, one committee member noted that he and a colleague had observed cases where the tarsectomy operation had produced horrible disfigurement, and had heard of another where it had caused blindness.[46]

In spite of the committee's recommendations and Richards's descriptions of tarsectomy's destructive consequences, Medical Director Guthrie waited more than three more months before taking any action to limit use of the procedure. Even then his predominant concern, rather than simply protecting Indian eyesight, seems to have been assuaging potentially hurt professional feelings among OIA physicians. Before issuing an official pronouncement on trachoma treat-

TABLE 4.1

NUMBER OF TRACHOMA OPERATIONS PERFORMED BY OIA PHYSICIANS,
FISCAL YEARS 1925–1927

Year	Operations Performed
1925	8,455
1926	5,318
1927	over 9,000
Total	over 22,773

Sources: *Interior Department Appropriation Bill, 1927,* 398; *Problem of Indian Administration,* 208;
Interior Department Appropriation Bill, 1929, 575.

ment, Guthrie sent a draft of a proposed circular to each of the OIA's district medical directors. Because the Office had given its field physicians "teachings which apparently were more in favor of radical procedures than otherwise," he wrote, any order from him would have "to be expressed cautiously and diplomatically." Consequently, the proposed circular did not ban the tarsectomy operation, but merely instructed physicians to be more careful about employing it. Guthrie requested that the medical directors comment on the draft, and, after receiving favorable replies, issued it in final form on July 22. Like its predecessor, the Chief Medical Director's official directive urged caution, but did not forbid OIA doctors from performing the operation.[47] It was not until September that Guthrie decided to ban the procedure outright, although even then he allowed physicians to perform it when they obtained written authorization from Washington.[48] OIA physicians, as a result of this proviso, requested, and received, permission to perform an occasional tarsectomy until as late as 1931.[49]

Assessing the Damage

The trachoma campaign had ended in utter failure. But just how widespread was the damage? How common were tarsectomies? Official OIA statistics indicate that between fiscal years 1925 and 1927 a total of over 22,773 eye surgeries were performed (see table 4.1). But these included grattage operations, other milder forms of trachoma surgery, and surgical procedures for other eye conditions. To determine what proportion of this total was represented by tarsectomy, we must turn to the monthly statistical reports filed by the OIA's traveling trachoma specialists, which included specific breakdowns by type of procedure. These reports reveal that tarsectomies constituted 26.25 percent of all trachoma operations (see table 4.2).[50] Applying this percentage to the total of 22,626 operations produces a total of 5,978 tarsectomies performed.[51]

It is possible, of course, that other OIA doctors were less aggressive in their use of tarsectomy than were the traveling ophthalmologists. But even if one assumes, conservatively, that they performed tarsectomies only half as frequently as did the ophthalmological specialists (that is, in 13.13 percent of the cases) we are still left with a total of 2,989 tarsectomies performed. There is abundant evidence, furthermore, that suggests that tarsectomized patients frequently experienced severe complications, which could include an untreatable recurrence of trachoma, lagophthalmos, entropion, scarring, or blindness. The chair of the AMA's Advisory Committee on Trachoma reported observing "numerous" cases in which patients who had been tarsectomized suffered untreatable and disfiguring reoccurrences of trachoma. The operation had been performed, he added, "even in very recent cases of the disease and in young children before any other treatment had been used. Some overzealous enthusiasts even went so far as to advocate the operation as a preventive of the disease."[52]

As early as August 1926, H. V. Hailman, one of the OIA's traveling trachoma specialists, reported that he was having difficulty persuading Hopi patients to accept medical care. An OIA doctor had already performed tarsectomies on many Hopis, with devastating consequences, and tribal members showed no desire to repeat their mistake and entrust their eyes to the care of another government doctor. Hailman found it necessary to treat several patients for the side effects of tarsectomy, a task to which he attached great importance. "Every effort," he said, "should be made to save from blindness an eye that has been operated upon . . . every eye that goes blind following an operation, makes for more contention and op[p]osition among the Indians to whom the facts are known. For this reason I am giving more of my personal time to a number of Indians who have had their tarsal cartilege [sic] removed in order to save them, if possible, from blindness."[53]

Tarsectomized patients at Laguna and Acoma Pueblos also experienced severe complications. In April 1927 Dr. Ralph Ross, who had been one of the three ophthalmologists who began the trachoma campaign in the Southwest, visited both Pueblos and made a startling discovery. Among the 133 people who had received tarsectomies, Ross found 87 cases in which the physician performing the operation had left trachomatous granules remaining in the folds of the eyelid, a condition that made further treatment "very difficult." And in thirty-five more cases the tarsectomized patients showed "no indication" of ever having had trachoma at all. "It seems unfortunate," Ross said, "that tarsectomies should have been performed in such a promiscuous, wholesale and reckless manner. The result on the patient has been prejudicial to having anything more done to their eyes. Nearly all the cases . . . in which tra-

Table 4.2
TARSECTOMIES PERFORMED BY OIA SPECIAL PHYSICIANS, 1926 THROUGH SEPTEMBER 1927

Physician	1926			JANUARY–SEPTEMBER 1927			TOTAL		
	Operations Performed	Tarsectomies Performed	Percent Tarsectomies	Operations Performed	Tarsectomies Performed	Percent Tarsectomies	Operations Performed	Tarsectomies Performed	Percent Tarsectomies
J. L. Collard	220	12	5.5%	97	8	8.2%	317	20	6.3%
L. L. Culp	134	6	4.5%	206	166	80.6%	340	172	50.6%
J. L. Goodwin	3	0	0.0%	12	0	0.0%	15	0	0.0%
H. V. Hailman	121	12	9.9%	99	0	0.0%	220	12	5.5%
J. S. Perkins	292	182	62.3%	193	103	53.4%	485	285	58.8%
R. H. Ross	–	–	–	79	0	0.0%	79	0	0.0%
C. E. Yates	513	77	15.0%	343	41	12.0%	856	118	13.8%
TOTALS	1,283	289	22.5%	1,029	318	30.9%	2,312	607	26.3%

Source: Reports of Special Physicians, Records of the Health Division, RG 75, NA.

choma granulations still remain, have told me their eyes are in worse condition since the operation; although told beforehand that the tarsectomy would cure their condition." He concluded that the physicians who had performed the operations had not been competent enough either to diagnose the disease correctly or to perform the procedure properly.[54]

The implication was, of course, that more skillful doctors could have done a better job. The OIA responded to Ross's report by requesting the names of the supposedly incompetent physicians, which he quickly furnished. The Office then directed the medical director for the Southwestern District, H. J. Warner, to investigate Dr. Ross's charges. Warner examined the same patients as had Ross, although he noted that it was "hardly necessary" for him to do so, as he had "looked over many such cases during the last year in every section of the Southwest." He concluded that Ross's assessment of the tarsectomy campaign's horrible consequences was correct. In Warner's view, however, it was unfair for Ross to assign blame to the local physicians, who were simply following official policy by performing tarsectomies. "All the Indian Service physicians, including Dr. Ross, were taught to do tarsectomies," Warner noted. "They were instructed at the time that tarsectomy was a cure for trachoma. All of them did tarsectomies in wholesale numbers on all classes of trachoma." One should not, therefore, cast "any reflection" on the doctors who treated the Lagunas and the Acomas. "Their technique was good," Warner said, "and in accordance with the teachings of their preceptor. Both physicians have learned by experience and are now following conservative methods of treatment. You can go into any district of the Southwest where specialists have worked and see the same deplorable results from wholesale tarsectomies."[55]

Far from ending the trachoma epidemic, OIA doctors had caused even more suffering for American Indian patients. The reasons for their reliance on such an extreme, untested procedure are quite complex. Part of the motivation was a wrongheaded, albeit genuine, belief that tarsectomy was an effective, even humane, form of treatment. The year after the campaign began, members of the Board of Indian Commissioners declared emphatically that it warranted "the strong hope that in a comparatively few years our Indian people will be clear eyed and reservations will be rid of the disease which has made blind men and women common objects in Indian communities." Perkins believed that one hundred ophthalmologists using the Fox technique could eradicate trachoma among Southwestern Indians in only one month.[56] And one OIA physician held clinics at least twice where he operated on whites as well as Indians suffering from the disease.[57]

Still, the good intentions of some campaign officials do not by themselves explain why tarsectomy was selected as the preferred method of treatment. Fox and OIA medical administrators knew that medical therapies and public-health programs could also be used to treat the disease. Moreover, professional ophthalmological opinion on tarsectomy's merits was sharply divided, as evidenced by the harsh dissents that accompanied the publication of pro-tarsectomy articles written either by Fox or by one of the handful of other proponents of the procedure.[58] Nowhere can one find an example of another instance of widespread use of the procedure, even by the Public Health Service in its Appalachian trachoma control program.[59] Why, then, did the OIA come to rely so heavily on a radical, untested program of surgery?

The answer lay in the racial and cultural beliefs of the campaign's originators. Throughout the 1920s, federal policy-makers and their allies consistently defended attacks on Indian health programs by invoking the refrain of racial and cultural difference. According to the chief of the OIA's construction division, Indian hospitals did not need to be built to the same standard as comparable white facilities. There were, he said, "many differences contrasting the Indian from the white race" that made the provision of top-quality facilities less important for Indian patients. Medical Director Newberne expanded on this point in 1924. While the level of care provided in OIA hospitals was not, he noted, equal to that available "in the hospitals of large cities, in some respects it suit[ed] the Indians better." Superior medical facilities would be wasted on American Indian patients, who in Newberne's view were inclined to disobey their physicians' orders. "We are dealing," he said, "with a primitive people."[60]

The idea that radical surgery was the only suitable method for treating American Indian trachoma patients flowed naturally from such racially based justifications for differential treatment. In the minds of OIA officials, alleged racial deficiencies would render all alternative approaches to treating trachoma ineffective. Thus John McMullen, the PHS trachoma specialist who had designed the initial stages of the campaign, rejected public-health measures as unsuitable for Indian patients. To prepare his recommendations for the campaign, McMullen had taken temporary leave from his regular position as director of PHS trachoma programs in the Appalachian region. An important part of the PHS effort, which served mostly lower-income whites, was a public-health education campaign. Under McMullen's direction, teams of nurses traveled from place to place, lecturing on the etiology of the disease and holding clinics on techniques of trachoma prevention.[61] But McMullen specifically rejected the use of such measures among the Indians. The Navajos, he argued, lived in hogans where they practiced "appalling" sanitary habits, and such alleged problems would present what he claimed to be an insurmountable barrier to any program of health education.[62]

McMullen also rejected the use of medical treatments, arguing that what he labeled the Navajo peoples' "backward" taboo against revealing family names would complicate the practice of keeping medical records.[63] Fox, similarly, claimed that reliance on medicines would be ineffective, citing what he believed to be the particular virulence of trachoma among the Indian population. American Indians did not, he argued, possess "the natural immunity to [trachoma] of the North American negro." And while whites experienced trachoma in varying degrees of severity, each case in Indians seemed "to be worse than the preceding one," which made medical remedies "a waste of time." Even if medicines had been capable of producing results, there remained what Fox saw as the intractabilities of Indian behavior. American Indian patients could not be, he argued, "considered as in the class that will stand for protracted treatment of any kind." Tribal members would not return for applications of medicine "more than a very few times," and refused to apply the medicine themselves inside their own homes. "The Indian," he noted, "is a born skeptic anyhow, and must be handled by those familiar with his temperamental vagaries."[64]

Fox also noted that he had treated trachoma sufferers even among "the highest type" of Indians, students at the Carlisle Indian School, a place where "the very best hygienic conditions" prevailed. That the disease could flourish in such a scrupulously clean environment, and among such relatively assimilated tribal members, demonstrated, for Fox, the futility of using public-health measures to control the disease. "It is extremely difficult," he wrote, "to teach these ignorant Indian women that the bottom hem of their skirts is not the proper thing with which to wipe their noses and their babies' eyes. The urging of health journals, such as *Hygeia*, on them would be ridiculous, and even the talks to the youngsters accomplish very little."[65]

Fox's opinion about American Indian personality traits was shared by many medical observers. The average Indian person's history, according to one of the OIA's traveling ophthalmologists, was "that of taking things as they come, and leaving the morrow for its own problems. . . . To prevail upon him as we say, 'to take his medicine in broken doses,' or to be persistent in continuing any treatment or preventive measures over an approp[r]iate period of time has been a hard matter, because it did not coincide with his earlier conception of propriety."[66] Others went even further, comparing Indian men and women to children who responded at best only marginally to health-education efforts. "It is exceedingly difficult," said one of the OIA's traveling trachoma specialists three years before the campaign began, "to induce the Indians to adopt hygienic measures for their own protection. They are very much like children, and one is obliged to keep at them continually, teaching them the dangers of neglecting these matters." "The Navajo," added another, "is a wonderful child of intellect and his ignorance of diseases and his superstitions make him pathetic."[67]

That those responsible for federal Indian programs held racist attitudes will, of course, evoke no surprise from those familiar with the history of federal Indian policy. What may be more startling, though, is that in this case such attitudes shaped the creation of a health campaign organized by health professionals who were supposedly dedicated to principles of humanitarianism and scientific objectivity. Yet as Vine Deloria has noted, scientific interpretations of Indian cultures have had the impact of "precluding Indians from having an acceptable status as human beings, and reducing them in the eyes of educated people to a pre-human level of ignorance."[68] The trachoma campaign was clearly a case in point. The physicians responsible for the campaign had used their racial beliefs to justify the use of a dangerous, invasive surgical procedure.

For these doctors, Western medical science held the power to overcome alleged racial failings and to propel American Indians towards "civilization." So strong was their faith in the power of so-called scientific medicine that even witnessing firsthand the horrible consequences of the tarsectomy campaign did not alter their world view. Instead, they assigned the blame for tarsectomy's failure to their Indian patients. H. V. Hailman, for example, devised a simple explanation to explain why complications from tarsectomy were so common among Hopi trachoma sufferers. These patients, he argued, bore sole responsibility for what had happened to them because they had, "for many and varied reasons, real or imagined," discontinued their postoperative care. Another OIA ophthalmologist, John Hewitt, made the same argument about Ute patients on the Uintah and Ouray reservations. The reason these patients required up to five months of hospitalization to correct postoperative eye damage was, he said, because they had refused to accept "regular aftertreatments" following a tarsectomy.[69]

H. J. Warner, who had investigated the consequences of the tarsectomy operation at Laguna and Acoma, likewise continued to portray Indian behavior as the biggest obstacle to OIA trachoma-control efforts. Working with what he called "the primitive Indian population" presented OIA physicians, Warner said, with a range of problems. "Personal cleanliness and sanitary conditions" were, he said, "at their worst" in Indian communities. Further, "the Indians' adherence to the medicine man and his [sic] suspicion of the white man's innovations in matters of medical treatment" necessitated that the physician first "gain the confidence of the Indian" before attempting to provide medical assistance. Even then success was not assured. Warner argued that Indian patients generally would not continue to seek treatment for trachoma once their immediate symptoms had been relieved, and consequently "[f]ield work by ophthalmologists among adult Indians of the nomadic type," was "unsatisfactory and usually a waste of time."[70]

The racial beliefs that had been used originally to justify the tarsectomy campaign now provided Warner and other OIA physicians, when confronted with evidence of the campaign's failure, with an airtight alibi. Indian peoples' supposed backwardness, which had been the reason given for using tarsectomy in the first place, now could be used to absolve OIA physicians from any blame for what they had done. At least three thousand people had their eyesight destroyed or damaged. Yet it was not the physicians or the OIA that were at fault, but the behavior of the very patients who had been harmed. This was cultural arrogance of breathtaking proportions. From the very beginning, government physicians had demonstrated an absolute faith that medical science could compensate for alleged Indian racial inferiority and provide a cure for trachoma. Then, when the campaign failed, those same supposed racial defects served as a convenient scapegoat. It was an ingenious formulation.

Notes

1. H. J. Hagerman to Commissioner of Indian Affairs (hereafter CIA) Charles Burke, Dec. 15, 1924, 25663 (Pt. 1)-24-700-Navajo, Central Classified Files, Record Group 75, National Archives, Washington, DC (hereafter CCF, RG 75, NA); Polk Richards to H. J. Hagerman, Nov. 22, 1924, ibid. The nomenclature of Bureau of Indian Affairs did not come into official use until 1947. See Francis Paul Prucha, *The Great Father: The United States Government and the American Indians*, vol. 2 (Lincoln: University of Nebraska Press, 1984), II: 1227–29.

2. Ibid.

3. Burke to Hagerman, Dec. 22, 1924, ibid.

4. Hagerman to Burke, Jan. 21, 1925, 93221-24-734-General Service (hereafter GS), CCF, RG 75, NA.

5. Circular no. 2122, June 22, 1925, Roll 13, Series 6, Microfilm publication no. 1121 (hereafter Mfilm 1121), NA. No reply to Hagerman's letter could be located.

6. Ales Hrdlicka, *Tuberculosis among Certain Indian Tribes of the United States*, Bureau of American Ethnology Bulletin no. 42 (Washington, DC: Government Printing Office, 1909); *Contagious and Infectious Diseases among the Indians*, 62nd Cong., 3rd sess., 1913, S. Doc. 138, Serial 6365; *Trachoma in Certain Indian Schools*, 60th Cong., 2nd sess., S. Rep. 1025, Serial 5380. For general discussion of health conditions on reservations and in boarding schools in the late-nineteenth and early twentieth centuries, see Virginia E. Allen, "'When We Settle Down, We Grow Pale and Die': Health in Western Indian Territory," *Journal of the Oklahoma Medical Association* 70 (1977): 229–30; Virginia E. Allen, "The White Man's Road: The Physical and Psychological Impact of Relocation on the Southern Plains Indians," *Bulletin of the History of Medicine* 49 (1975): 156–60; Gregory R. Campbell, "Changing Patterns of Health and Effective Fertility among the Northern Cheyenne of Montana, 1886–1903," *American Indian Quarterly* 15 (1991): 339–58; idem, "The Epidemiological Consequences of Forced Removal: The Northern Cheyenne in Indian Territory," *Plains Anthropologist* 34 (1989): 85–97; Bernice N. Crockett, "Health Conditions in the Indian Territory from the Civil War to 1890," *Chronicles of Oklahoma* 36 (1958): 34–37; R. Palmer Howard and Virginia E. Allen, "Stress and Death in the Settlement of Indian Territory," *Chronicles of Oklahoma* 54 (1970), 357–58; Wallace B. Love and R. Palmer Howard, "Health and Medical Practice in the Choctaw Nation, 1880–1907," *Journal of the*

Oklahoma State Medical Association 63 (1970): 126; Diane T. Putney, "Fighting the Scourge: American Indian Morbidity and Federal Policy, 1897–1928" (Ph.D. diss., Marquette University, 1980), 201–9; Peter Thompson, "The Fight for Life: New Mexico Indians, Health Care, and the Reservation Period," *New Mexico Historical Review* 69 (1994): 145–61; Clifford E. Trafzer, *Death Stalks the Yakama: Epidemiological Transitions and Mortality on the Yakama Indian Reservation, 1888–1964* (East Lansing: Michigan State University Press, 1997); idem, "Invisible Enemies: Ranching, Farming and Quechan Indian Deaths at the Fort Yuma Agency, California, 1915–1925," *American Indian Culture and Research Journal* 21 (1997): 83–117; Robert A. Trennert, "The Federal Government and Indian Health in the Southwest: Tuberculosis and the Phoenix East Farm Sanatorium, 1909–1955," *Pacific Historical Review* 65 (1996): 61–63.

7. *Contagious and Infectious Diseases* 19, 29–31, 37; Fitzhugh Mullan, *Plagues and Politics: The Story of the United States Public Health Service* (New York: Basic Books, 1989), 65; M.C. Guthrie, "The Health of the American Indian," *Public Health Reports* 44 (April 19, 1929): 950, 952. By comparison, a 1912 survey by the Public Health Service (PHS) found 8 percent of whites in the Kentucky backcountry to be suffering from the disease, a figure that Congress deemed so alarming that it authorized the PHS the following year, for the first time ever, to treat trachoma patients. See Mullan, *Plagues and Politics*, 65.

8. Hrdlicka, *Tuberculosis among Certain Indian Tribes*, 3. See also Joseph A. Murphy, "Health Problems of the Indians," *Annals of the American Academy of Political and Social Science* 37 (1911): 104; idem, "The Work of the United States Indian Medical Service," *Survey* 33 (1915): 446; Jon F. Rice, Jr., "Health Conditions of Native Americans in the Twentieth Century," *Indian Historian* 10 (1977): 15; Burke to Kober, Oct. 13, 1921, 96343-21-732-GS, CCF, RG 75, NA; Guthrie, "Health of the American Indian," 949; Florence Patterson, "A Study of the Need for Public-Health Nursing on Indian Reservations," printed in Senate Committee on Indian Affairs, *Survey of Conditions of the Indians of the United States* (Washington, DC: GPO, 1928–1943); 3:959. National statistics are drawn from Bureau of the Census, *Historical Statistics of the United States, Colonial Times to 1970*, vol. 1 (Washington, D.C.: GPO, 1975), 58–59.

9. Putney, "Fighting the Scourge," 1–22; Prucha, *The Great Father*, II: 842–43.

10. Two excellent accounts of these developments are Frederick E. Hoxie, *A Final Promise: The Campaign to Assimilate the Indians, 1880–1920* (Lincoln: University of Nebraska Press, 1984), 147–87; and Janet A. McDonnell, *The Dispossession of the American Indian, 1887–1934* (Bloomington: University of Indiana Press, 1991).

11. *Annual Report of the Commissioner of Indian Affairs* [hereafter *ARCIA*], 1908, 24. The authors of a PHS survey of Indian health conditions went even further by arguing that Indians represented the single biggest threat to the nation's health. "[T]he danger now," they concluded, "is not so much the transmission of contagious and infectious diseases from immigrants to inhabitants of the United States, but from Indians to immigrants settling on lands in the West." *Contagious and Infectious Diseases among the Indians*, 70.

12. *ARCIA*, 1904, 36.

13. *Trachoma in Certain Indian Schools*, 2; *Contagious and Infectious Diseases*, 19.

14. House Committee on Appropriations, Subcommittee on the Interior

Department, *Interior Department Appropriation Bill, 1930*, 70th Cong., 2nd sess. (Washington, DC: GPO, 1928), 657; Putney, "Fighting the Scourge," 98–201; Prucha, *The Great Father*, vol. 2, pp. 852–55; Frederick L. Hoffman, "Conditions in the Indian Medical Service," *Journal of the American Medical Association* [hereafter *JAMA*] 75 (Aug. 14, 1920): 494.

15. Prucha, *The Great Father*, II: 855–56.

16. Mullan, *Plagues and Politics*, 40–65; James Tobey, *The National Government and Public Health* (1926; reprint, New York: Arno Press, 1978), 39.

17. Hubert Work, "Speech before the Advisory Council on Indian Affairs," Dec. 12, 1923, reprinted in House Committee on Appropriations, Subcommittee on Interior Department, *Interior Department Appropriation Bill, 1925*, 68th Cong., 1st sess. (Washington, DC: GPO, 1924), 9, 188; House Committee on Appropriations, Subcommittee on Interior Department, *Interior Department Appropriation Bill, 1926*, 68th Cong., 2nd sess. (Washington, DC: GPO, 1924), 667.

18. This description of trachoma draws heavily on Larry Schwab, *Primary Eye Care in Developing Nations* (Oxford: Oxford University Press, 1987), 51–54. For contemporary discussions of what was known about trachoma, see J. A. Stucky, "Trachoma: Suggestions as to Diagnosis, Etiology, and Treatment," *Southern Medical Journal* 19 (1926): 140–44; and Daniel W. White and Peter Cope White, "The Medical and Surgical Treatment of Trachoma," *Texas State Journal of Medicine* 20 (May 1924): 33–37.

19. Schwab, *Primary Eye Care*, 51–54. Entropion was also one of the disturbing aftereffects of tarsectomy that led Polk Richards initially to express his concern to Hagerman. See introduction of this chapter.

20. Stucky, "Trachoma," 140–44; White and White, "Medical and Surgical Treatment of Trachoma," 33–37; Mullan, *Plagues and Politics*, 65. A few years earlier, during the 1910s, the OIA had relied on public-health methods as its primary weapon against trachoma. See Putney, "Fighting the Scourge," 109, 165–66.

21. For a discussion of the methods used by the PHS, see Mullan, *Plagues and Politics*, 65; Paul B. Mossman, "The Clinic Control of Trachoma," *Eye, Ear, Nose and Throat Monthly* 6 (1927): 404–5; idem, "Trachoma," *Journal-Lancet* 47 (1927): 544–45; Joseph S. Waldman, "Trachoma: A Review of the Literature," *Illinois State Medical Journal* 54 (1928): 143.

22. Burke to J. S. Perkins, June 14, 1924, 25663 (Pt. 1)-24-700-Navajo, CCF, RG 75, NA; Perkins to CIA, Sept. 24, 1924, ibid.

23. "Program for Eradicating Trachoma among the Indians," John McMullen to CIA, May 15, 1924, ibid.; Malcolm McDowell to George Vaux, May 17, 1924, ibid.; Waldman, "Trachoma," 143.

24. Burke to Perkins, June 14, 1924, 25663 (Pt. 1)-24-700-Navajo, CCF, RG 75, NA; Perkins to CIA, Sept. 24, 1924, ibid; Walker to CIA, Aug. 12, 1924, ibid.

25. "Program for Eradicating Trachoma," McMullen to CIA, May 15, 1924, ibid.

26. Ralph Ross to CIA, Aug. 1, 1924, ibid.; Perkins to CIA, July 21, 1924, ibid.

27. G. Oram Ring, "Lawrence Webster Fox, M.D., 1853–1931," *Archives of Ophthalmology* 6 (1931): 598; Beatrice Fox Griffith, *Pennsylvania Doctor* (Harrisburg, PA: Stackpole Company, 1957).

28. L. Webster Fox, Letter to the Editor, *JAMA* 81 (1923): 1545; idem, "Trachoma

among the Blackfeet Indians," *Archives of Ophthalmology* 53 (1924): 166; idem, "The Trachoma Problem among the Indians," *Medical Searchlight* 1 (1925): 17; *Annual Report of the Board of Indian Commissioners, 1925,* 13; Walter Stevens to CIA, [Oct.] 10, 1924, "From Feb. 1, 1922" File, Box 1, Records of the District Medical Director, Muskogee Area Office, Record Group 75, National Archives, Southwest Region, Fort Worth, Texas [hereafter RDMD, MAO, RG 75, NAFW]. Stevens mistakenly dated his letter September 10.

29. Stevens to CIA, Oct. 10, 1924, "From Feb. 1, 1922" File, Box 1, RDMD, MAO, RG 75, NAFW; L. Webster Fox, "Trachoma at Its Worst among the Blackfeet Indians," *Journal of the Indiana State Medical Association* 17 (1924): 371.

30. Stevens to CIA, [Oct.] 10, 1924, "From Feb. 1, 1922" File, Box 1, RDMD, MAO, RG 75, NAFW; Fox, "Trachoma at Its Worst," 373.

31. Perkins to CIA, Oct. 2, 1924, 25663 (Pt. 1)-24-700-Navajo, CCF, RG 75, NA; Perkins to CIA, Sept. 24, 1924, ibid.; Stevens to CIA, Oct. 10, 1924, "From Feb. 1, 1922" File, Box 1, RDMD, MAO, RG 75, NAFW.

32. Stevens to CIA, [Oct.] 10, 1924, "From Feb. 1, 1922" File, Box 1, RDMD, MAO, RG 75, NAFW.

33. Ibid.

34. Ibid.

35. Burke to Stevens, Sept. 12, 1924, "From Feb. 1, 1922" File, Box 1, RDMD, MAO, RG 75, NAFW; Burke to Stevens, Oct. 19, 1924, "Oct. 10, 1924" File, Box 1, ibid.; Stevens to CIA, Oct. 15, 1924, ibid.; E. B. Meritt to Stevens, Oct. 24, 1924, ibid.; *Interior Department Appropriation Bill, 1926,* 672. The last of the two letters cited describes and gives official approval for the organization of the clinic, but predates it. There is no reason, however, to doubt that the actual method of pedagogy differed from what was planned, especially since Meritt gave Stevens's ideas the OIA's official sanction.

36. House, *Interior Department Appropriation Bill, 1926,* 671–73.

37. Burke to R. E. L. Newberne, Dec. 19, 1924, 93221-24-734-GS, CCF, RG 75, NA; Burke to J. R. Collard, Jan. 5, 1925, ibid.; Burke to L. L. Culp, Jan. 5, 1925, ibid.; Burke to L. Webster Fox, Feb. 5, 1925, ibid.

38. Perkins to OIA, Jan. 18, 1925, ibid.

39. Burke to Fox, Feb. 5, 1925, 93221-24-734-GS, CCF, RG 75, NA; Walter S. Stevens, "Indian Service Doctor Replaces the Medicine Man," *Nation's Health* 7 (1925): 385; *Annual Report of the Board of Indian Commissioners,* 1925, 13–14.

40. W. C. Barton to CIA, Sept. 11, 1924, "From Feb. 1, 1922" File, Box 1, RDMD, MAO, RG 75, NAFW.

41. Work to Guthrie, March 29, 1926, Marshall C. Guthrie personnel file, U.S. Office of Personnel Management, St. Louis, Missouri; House Committee on Appropriations, Subcommittee on the Interior Department, *Interior Department Appropriation Bill, 1928,* 69th Cong., 2nd sess. (Washington, DC, GPO, 1927), 327; House Committee on Appropriations, Subcommittee on the Interior Department, *Interior Department Appropriation Bill, 1927,* 69th Cong., 1st sess. (Washington, DC: GPO, 1925), 398; "The Southwestern Trachoma Campaign among Indians," *Santa Fe New Mexican,* Oct. 10, 1925, copy in 25663 (Pt. 2)-24-700-Navajo, CCF, RG 75, NA; Walker to CIA, Jan. 20, 1926, ibid.

42. William Wilder to CIA, "Outline of Suggestions for the Control and Treatment of Trachoma among the American Indians," April 24, 1925, 78136-24-732-GS, CCF, RG 75, NA.

43. Meritt to Wilder, May 18, 1925, ibid.

44. Richards to Knapp, Nov. 5, 1926, "Polk Richards—Special Physician" File, Box 452, Correspondence of Medical Officers, Phoenix Area Office, Record Group 75, National Archives, Pacific Southwest Region, Laguna Niguel, California [hereafter PAO, RG 75, NALN].

45. P. Richards, "Results in Treating Trachoma among Indians," *Archives of Ophthalmology* 56 (1927): 202–4.

46. "Report of the Advisory Committee on Trachoma among the Indians," *JAMA* 88 (April 9, 1927): 1175; "Report of the Advisory Committee on Trachoma among the Indians," April 13, 1927, 40506-25-732-GS, CCF, RG 75, NA; William Posey, "Trachoma among the Indians," *JAMA* 88 (May 21, 1927): 1618–19.

47. Mark Guthrie to District Medical Directors, July 2, 1927, 36655-27-734-GS, CCF, RG 75, NA; H. J. Warner to Guthrie, July 5, 1927, ibid.; Stevens to Guthrie, July 8, 1925, ibid.; Paul D. Mossman to Guthrie, July 11, 1927, ibid.; Emil Krulish to Guthrie, July 13, 1927, ibid.; Circular no. 2347, July 22, 1927, Roll 13, Series 6, Mfilm 1121, NA. A copy of this circular can also be found in 36655-27-734-GS, CCF, RG 75, NA. Positions for four district medical directors, each with responsibility for several states, were created when the OIA reorganized the medical division in 1926 and officially established it as a separate unit. Previously, medical activities had been conducted as part of the activities of the education division. See Department of Health, Education, and Welfare, Public Health Service, Division of Indian Health, *The Indian Health Program from 1800 to 1955* (Washington, DC: Public Health Service, 1959), 5.

48. Circular no. 2369, Sept. 20, 1927, Roll 13, Series 6, Mfilm 1121, NA.

49. See the correspondence between Paul G. Eilers and Burke in 24166-29-734-Southern Navajo, CCF, RG 75, NA, and between Culp and Commissioner Rhoads in 27501-31-734-GS, ibid. Special physician C. E. Yates was performing tarsectomies as late as 1932, although it is unclear whether or not he received official authorization to do so. See C. E. Yates, *Annual Report*, 1932, Box 8, Reports of Special Physicians, 1925–32, RG 75, NA.

50. The special physicians' reports reveal great variation in the frequency with which each doctor utilized the procedure. This should not invalidate the final result, however. These were, after all, specialists in treating the disease. One can assume even greater variation among inexperienced agency physicians: for every local M.D. reluctant to try surgery, there was probably another who used the tarsectomy operation at the first hint of trachoma infection.

51. Since Fox did not present his tarsectomy clinic at Blackfeet until late September 1924, and since the OIA's clinic at Fort Defiance was not held until just over a month later, it could be argued that roughly one-third of the trachoma operations performed in fiscal year 1925 could not have been tarsectomies, and that the total of 22,626 should be reduced correspondingly. Counterbalancing this, though, is the fact that this total figure does not include any trachoma operations performed after June 30, 1927, even though Guthrie did not ban tarsectomies until September 1927.

The historian Robert Trennert has attributed the failure of the OIA trachoma program to "[c]ultural problems," which, he says, "interfered with the campaign," creating a climate in which "radical surgery for large numbers of adults appeared to be impossible." But the large number of tarsectomies performed contradicts this assertion. It also appears as if Trennert bases this conclusion solely on contemporary descriptions of the campaign by OIA doctors, whose explanations for the campaign's failure were quite biased. See his "Indian Sore Eyes: The Federal Campaign to Control Trachoma in the Southwest, 1910–1940," *Journal of the Southwest* 32 (1990): 129–34 (quotations at 131 and 132).

52. William H. Wilder, "Trachoma among the Indians: Report of the Advisory Committee of the American Ophthalmological Society," *American Journal of Ophthalmology* 13 (1930): 387–89 (quotation, 387).

53. H. V. Hailman, Monthly Statistical Report, August, 1926, Box 7, Reports of Special Physicians, Records of the Health Division, RG 75, NA.

54. Ross to CIA, April 13, 1927, 19278-27-734-Southern Pueblos, CCF, RG 75, NA. Ross believed that in the remaining eleven cases of tarsectomy had been needed and had proven successful.

55. CIA to Ross, May 3, 1927, 19278-27-734-Southern Pueblos, CCF, RG 75, NA; Ross to CIA, May 14, 1927, ibid.; Warner to CIA, June 15, 1927, ibid. Warner noted that Dr. J. S. Perkins, who had directed the trachoma campaign in its initial stages, continued to perform tarsectomies. Perkins "still insists," Warner said, that the operation was "a cure for trachoma."

56. *Annual Report of the Board of Indian Commissioners, 1925*, 14; Burke to Perkins, July 3, 1925, 75270-24-735-GS, CCF, RG 75, NA.

57. Yates to CIA, Oct. 2, 1926, Box 7, Reports of Special Physicians, 1925–32, RG 75, NA; comments by G. F. Drew on Paul D. Mossman, "Trachoma," *Journal-Lancet* 47 (1927): 547.

58. For articles in favor of tarsectomy, see, in addition to the Fox articles cited above, H. H. Turner, "The Combined Excision of the Tarsus in Trachoma," *Atlantic Medical Journal* 28 (1925): 369–71; and S. Lewis Ziegler, "The Surgery of Trachoma: Practical Problems," *JAMA* 86 (Feb. 6, 1926): 404. For attacks on the procedure, see the comments by J. A. Stucky on Fox, "Trachoma Problem," 406, and by Edward A. Shumway on Turner, "Combined Excision," 373. See also Waldman, "Trachoma," 143.

59. For a discussion of the approach taken by the PHS, see the works cited in note 25, above.

60. Arthur E. Middleton, "Supplanting the Medicine Man," *Modern Hospital* 19 (1922): 42; Robert E. Lee Newberne, "A Review of Miss Patterson's Report Entitled 'A Study of the Need for Public Health Nursing on Indian Reservations,'" in Senate Committee on Indian Affairs, *Survey of Conditions of the Indians of the United States*, vol. 3 (Washington, DC: GPO, 1928–1943), 1013. Louis Cramton, who as chair of the House budget subcommittee on the Interior Department had more influence over OIA funding than any other member of Congress, made a similar argument in 1928 in justifying why OIA hospitals received only a $1.50 per diem per patient versus a figure of $4 for Public Health Service hospitals and $5 for Veteran's Bureau facilities. "Is

there not," he said, "a distinction in the facilities that should be provided, as between those who have been used to a life of comfort, and living on a pretty high plane, and those who have been living in wikiups [*sic*] and hogans, with their uncertain food supply, and perhaps accustomed to having their food cooked in a few tomato cans over a little fire. When they suddenly are taken into a hospital, not only do they not appreciate it, but the same food program for them that we gave our veterans, very possibly would not be the best thing for them." *Interior Department Appropriation Bill, 1930*, 655.

61. Mullan, *Plagues and Politics*, 65

62. "Program for Eradicating Trachoma among the Indians," McMullen to CIA, May 15, 1924, 25663 (Pt. 1)-24-700-Navajo, CCF, RG 75, NA.

63. McDowell to Vaux, May 17, 1924, 25663 (Pt. 1)-24-700-Navajo, CCF, RG 75, NA; "Program for Eradicating Trachoma among the Indians," McMullen to CIA, May 15, 1924, ibid.

64. Fox, "Trachoma among the Blackfeet Indians," 170; idem, "The Trachoma Problem," 405–6.

65. L. Webster Fox, "Trachoma: Its Surgical Treatment," *Northwest Medicine* 25 (1926), 493 (order of quotations reversed); idem, "Trachoma Problem," 406.

66. L. L. Culp, "Chippewas Affect Medical and Public Health Work," Paper read before the 23rd annual session of the Minnesota State Sanitary Conference, St. Paul, Minn., Nov. 6–7, 1924, in 33171-24-732-GS, ibid. Burke thought that Indians were naturally lazy. "It is astonishing," he said, "how difficult it is to get Indians to apply themselves diligently to an occupation that requires attendance." [*Interior Department Appropriation Bill, 1925*, 144.]

67. Quoted in "Medical Party Hopes to Save Sick Indians," San Francisco *Chronicle*, July 7, 1921, p. 6, copy in 48093-21-732-GS, CCF, RG 75, NA; Hailman to Burke, July 14, 1926, "H. V. Hailman" file, Box 449, General Correspondence, PAO, RG 75, NALN.

68. Vine Deloria, Jr., *Red Earth, White Lies: Native Americans and the Myth of Scientific Fact* (New York: Scribner, 1995), 19.

69. H. V. Hailman, Monthly Statistical Report, August, 1926, Box 7, Reports of Special Physicians, Records of the Health Division, RG 75, NA; John E. Hewitt, "Remarks," n.d. [ca. November, 1927], Box 2, ibid. For Hailman's description of conditions at Hopi, see above, pp. 16, 18.

70. H. J. Warner, "Notes on the Results of Trachoma Work by the Indian Service in Arizona and New Mexico," *Public Health Reports* 44 (1929): 2913, 2919.

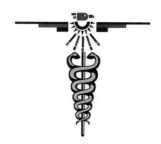

Infant Mortality on the Yakama Indian Reservation, 1914–1964[1]

The Yakama Indian Reservation is located on the Great Columbia Plateau of central Washington State.[2] It is the home of fourteen diverse tribes and bands of Native Americans who once spoke several dialects of three distinct languages, including Sahaptin, Salishan, and Chinookan. These Indians form the Yakama Nation, and their health has been closely related to the creation and execution of the reservation system of the United States since 1855 when a few chiefs signed the Yakima Treaty. Beginning in the 1870s, the Office of Indian Affairs placed a large number of Indians onto a limited land base and during the late nineteenth and early twentieth centuries restricted their access to traditional foods and medicines off the reservation.

Confinement on the reservation led to changes in subsistence, child care, and housing that contributed to infant deaths resulting primarily from pneumonia and gastrointestinal disorders. The modal age (the age that appeared most often) of death on the Yakama Reservation during the era from 1914 to 1964 was children under one year of age, with 631 (16 %) of the 3,899 deaths arising from this age group. This was the largest number of deaths suffered by any age group on the reservation.

The Yakama Treaty of 1855 and its ratification by the Senate in 1859 set into motion a series of events and circumstances that undermined the health of the Yakama people. As a result of the treaty, the various people placed on the Yakama Reservation secured a small portion of their traditional homelands in central Washington Territory. Other segments of their former land became part of the public domain, which the United States opened to white settlement after 1859. The government placed people from several tribes—Yakama, Palouse, Klickitat, Wishram, Wenatchee, Wasco, Wanapum, and others—on the Yakama Reservation, forcing approximately two thousand Native Americans onto the reservation where they competed for limited traditional-food resources.

During the early twentieth century, the federal government limited the movement of Plateau Indians onto lands they had long used for fishing, hunting, and gathering. Although Plateau Indians had acquired seeds from Hudson Bay Company and had planted gardens, they continued to maintain their traditional economic life. During the early reservation era, some of the people ranched and farmed, but most continued traditional seasonal rounds until white settlers destroyed root grounds, salmon, and game. Indians then turned more to ranching and farming in the 1920s and to wage earning by the 1940s.[3] The reservation system ended seasonal rounds and traditional housing of mat lodges and tipis, and both of these changes affected Indian health.[4] Whites farmed, ranched, and logged the inland Northwest, destroying animal habitats, berry patches, and root grounds. In time whites dammed the rivers, preventing salmon from running up the Columbia River and its tributaries.[5] Moreover, whites demanded that the United States restrict the movement of Native Americans across the public domain and private property, thereby restricting hunting, gathering, and fishing. The United States confined the fourteen tribes and bands of the Yakama Nation to a small geographical area, encouraging them to live in settled households and farms.[6]

By the 1920s and 1930s the seasonal rounds largely gave way to agriculture, farm labor, and government rations. Rather than living in mat lodges and tipis, most Yakamas lived in small, wood-framed dwellings that were overcrowded, unventilated, and unsanitary. The change in Yakama diet, housing, and settlement patterns contributed to the ill health of Yakama people. Poverty crippled the health of all Yakama, including pregnant women, infants, and small children. The breakdown in seasonal rounds also prohibited women from helping one another, from educating each other about prenatal care, birthing, and child care. Western medicine did not fill the void of sharing cultural knowledge, and the Office of Indian Affairs never had sufficient money to hire physicians and field nurses capable of compensating. Infant deaths and high infant mortality rates resulted.[7]

Under the terms of the Yakama Treaty, the United States agreed to provide the Indians with medical care. However, in spite of the fact that the Health Division of the Office of Indian Affairs provided some medicines and medical attention, it was not sufficient to protect the Yakama Indians from death and disease. Moreover, the Office of Indian Affairs did not initiate professional medical supervision of Indian health until 1908 with the position of chief medical supervisor, and it did not create the Health Division until 1921, two factors that contributed to infant deaths among the Yakama. As early as 1913, Yakama Indian Agent Donald M. Carr asked the Indian Office to fund a hospital at Fort Simcoe, a project that was not completed until 1928. Carr did not have a hospital, and the best education program he could provide addressed infant and child health.

For a short period of time, field matron Esther Sprague worked as an outreach nurse, instructing "younger women with children" about "cleanliness and proper feeding." Sprague worked among the Yakama, meeting with twenty-six women in May 1917, talking "to them on caring and proper feeding of children and cleanliness." Along with Carr, Field Nurse Sprague targeted mothers and babies, recognizing the devastation of infant mortality on the Yakama Reservation. In spite of sincere concerns about infant deaths, Carr and Sprague did not have sufficient funds to hire the needed medical personnel, educators, or doctors. They did not have enough money to build, maintain, and staff a clinic or offer mothers programs about the spread of bacteria and viruses. Without a sufficient medical staff and health clinic, the Yakama Agency could not adequately address infant deaths.[8]

Health conditions affecting infant mortality on the Yakama Reservation were indicative of Indian health throughout the United States. Before the 1930s, Lewis Meriam deemed government efforts relating to Indian health to be "curative and not . . . educational and preventive."[9] Sufficient funding for educational programs, doctors, nurses, medicines, hospitals, and clinics was never available, in spite of the fact that agents and health officials on reservations continually requested funding for health-related expenditures. The Health Division of the Office of Indian Affairs was a failure, in part because Congress refused to fund Indian health or consider the consequences of their budget-saving agendas. In short, Indian health was not a priority in the United States during the first half of the twentieth century.

Before the arrival of whites, medicine men and women healed the people and helped them prevent illnesses. Midwives counseled women about pregnancy, birth, delivery, and postpartum. Medicine people and midwives had less influence on what Yakama Indians termed "white man's diseases," and the Indians received little attention from white doctors and nurses. In fact, Indian agents on the Yakama Reservation reported that Indian doctors did "a great deal of harm" and the Indian Office urged agents to "do whatever you can to prevent the practice [of Indian doctoring]."[10] If the lack of adequate medical attention was detrimental for Indians as a general population, it was devastating for infants. Of the 631 infant deaths on the reservation between 1914 and 1964, 327 (52%) infants died of five major causes: pneumonia, gastrointestinal disorders, tuberculosis, heart disease, and syphilis.[11]

Death certificates of Yakama people, generated by employees of the Indian

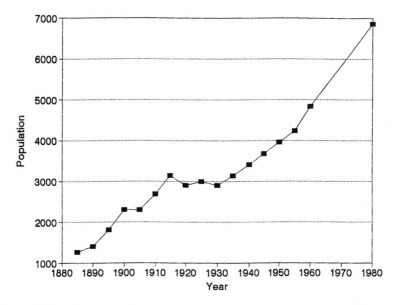

Figure 5.1 *Yakima population growth, 1885–1980. (Note: Population totals for 1935, 1940, 1945, 1950, and 1955 are estimates based on the assumption of linear population growth between 1932 and 1960.)*

Office and authorized by Yakima County, form the basis of this study. These records are sparse before the 1920s, when the agents began making a sincere effort to preserve death certificates. A few death records from the Yakama Reservation are available for the years from 1888 to 1924, although these data are poor, few in number, and do not represent the number or causes of deaths among Yakama people.[12] Unfortunately, there is no way of knowing how many mothers and fathers quietly buried their infants without notifying the agency or how many agency officials failed to record infant deaths. Like other Native Americans, many Yakama disliked and distrusted agency employees, and they simply did not notify the government of their losses. Many Yakama families buried infants in their traditional fashion, without contacting government employees.

The Yakama agency began recording births in 1914, and the infant mortality rate can be calculated for many years in the twentieth century.[13] The archives contain the Yakama Indian censuses, but these are only available for selected years from 1880 to 1931, and information regarding deaths within the various censuses is incomplete, inadequate, and unreliable in comparison to death certificates.[14] The censuses offer the best information on the Yakama Indian Reservation population, indicating that the population ranged from a low of 1,272 in 1885 to a high of 3,149 in 1914.[15] The population rise during the late nineteenth and early twentieth centuries was due to the migration of

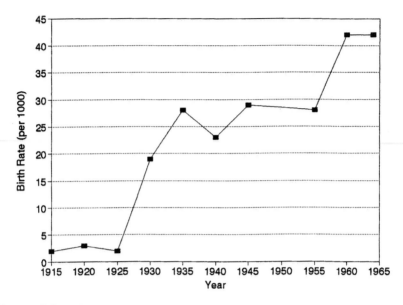

Figure 5.2 *Yakima birth rates, 1915–1964.*

non-reservation Indians from many diverse tribes onto the reservation where they could live with friends and relatives away from the white population that encroached on former Native lands (figure 5.1).

The rise in population on the Yakama Reservation was also due to the fact that the government refused to recognize Indian ownership of most lands off the reservation. If Native Americans had not filed homesteads, then most lands were open to white settlement. During the late nineteenth century, many Indians gave up hope of "owning" their aboriginal lands, so they moved to reservations where they could live in common with other Indians or take up an allotment. In the early twentieth century, the government allotted portions of the Yakama Reservation, and to do so they carefully counted and recorded the names of Indians. Some Indians farmed and ranched allotments, while others worked in the fields or on ranches run by non-Indians. The reservation system of the United States forced Indians to seek new livelihoods, for with each passing year, Indians became more confined by whites who destroyed plant, animal, and fish habitats. The growth of the Yakama population on the reservation was also influenced by an ever-increasing birth rate from 1925, when the Yakama birth rate was 2, to 1964, when the birth rate reached its zenith at 42 (figure 5.2).

The most complete data regarding Indian deaths on the Yakama Reservation were recorded between 1924 and 1946, a time period that corresponds with national reforms in Indian affairs. The demand to investigate American

Indian affairs culminated with an in-depth research project probing health, education, and administration. The result was the publication in 1928 of *The Problem of Indian Administration*, commonly called "the Meriam Report."[16] The publication was a far-reaching document that fueled the national reform of Indian affairs that had started earlier in the 1920s. In 1932, Americans elected Franklin Roosevelt as president, who selected John Collier as commissioner of Indian Affairs. Collier served in this capacity from 1933 to 1946, and as a reformer, he followed some of the recommendations made in the Meriam Report, including an improvement of Indian health.[17]

According to the report, "taken as a whole practically every activity undertaken by the national government for the promotion of the health of the Indians is below a reasonable standard of efficiency." Meriam added that "health work of the Indian Service falls markedly below the standards maintained by the Public Health Service, the Veterans' Bureau, and the Army and the Navy."[18] The Meriam Report had reported that "accurate figures based on reasonably complete records are not yet secured" because the Office of Indian Affairs, which "for many years had rules and regulations requiring the collection and tabulation of some vital statistics," had failed to collect the data.

Meriam was particularly concerned that the Office of Indian Affairs had not recorded Indian deaths. He specifically pointed out that "no report is made to the Indian Office" for "many of the Indian deaths which occur on reservations." When deaths were recorded, the information was often "defective in that some of the essential items are missing." Among the missing data were the cause of death and age of the person at death.[19] Before the 1920s, Yakama agency officials had little interest in keeping accurate and complete records, but after the 1920s they made a greater effort to do so. Since the "statistics and records of medical activities at present are incomplete and as a rule unreliable," Collier demanded that the agencies keep better records.[20] After the 1920s the death records on the Yakama Reservation were more numerous and complete than previous years, and this fact corresponds with the national reform of Indian affairs.

The best data on Yakama deaths are these death certificates, which provide such variables as the person's name, maiden name, gender, age, tribe, blood quantum, informant, marital status, date of death, place of death, and cause of death. Records during the 1950s and 1960s included additional information not found in the earlier documents such as the deceased's residence, date of birth, place of birth, mother's maiden name, father's name, patient's doctor's name, registrar doctor's name, name of funeral home director, and name of cemetery. The variables coded for this study included the deceased's age, gender, year, and cause of death with the purpose of examining in depth these variables relating to infant deaths.[21]

An analysis of this data from 1914 to 1964 reveals that the under-one-year age group showed the most marked number of deaths than any age group. In

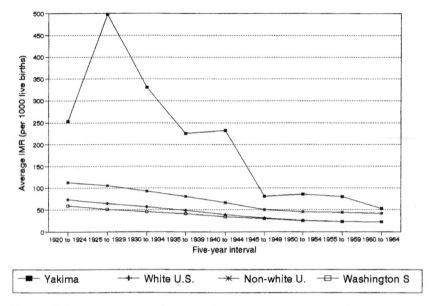

Figure 5.3 *Comparative infant-mortality rates (moving averages).*

spite of the fact that death certificates exist and inform us about infant deaths, many of the death certificates did not indicate the cause of death for a child, or the space provided for cause of death was left blank or offers the word "unknown."[22] The unknown or unrecorded deaths of Yakama children are not addressed in the narrative, but they are used to address the overall number of deaths and are briefly mentioned in the notes. This study examines the most important causes of death among infants, comparing their deaths to those suffered by the general population of Washington, whites in the United States, and the combined "non-white" population of the country that included African Americans, Asian Americans, Latinos, Native Americans, and others. The work also compares infant mortality rates among these various populations (figure 5.3).

One of the foremost factors leading to the death of infants on the Yakama Indian Reservation was poverty.[23] Poverty, disease, and death thrived on the reservation, and Native Americans died in large numbers, particularly infants. Indians lacked natural biological immunities to many diseases, and they died from smallpox, viruses, and measles. The Yakama had little "medicine" with which to combat diseases brought by whites, and they did not have sufficient space to use indigenous methods of quarantine. Reservation officials could not and did not provide enough medicines or cutting-edge health-care systems. Yakama people continued to be at risk in terms of death on the reservation during the first half of the twentieth century, and this was particularly true of infants.

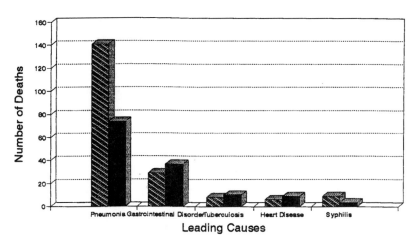

Figure 5.4 *Cause of death by gender for infants under one year, 1888–1964.*

Infant Deaths

The foremost killer of Yakama infants was pneumonia, which took the lives of 215 children (34%) under one year of age. Of these deaths by pneumonia, 141 males (66%) died, while 74 females (34%) succumbed to the disease (figure 5.4). Pneumonia sometimes was brought on by influenza or a viral infection of the lungs. Infants living in substandard and unsanitary housing with inadequate health care fell victim to pneumonia and died.

Between 1925 and 1964, pneumonia was the most dangerous disease among Yakama infants and children, who died of viral or bacterial pneumonia. The disease was generally an inflammation of the lungs, although other organs and parts of the body could become inflamed. In addition, infants with pneumonia ran high fevers, alternately experiencing chills and sweats. The disease was characterized by chest pains, coughing, and difficulty in breathing. Death resulted more often if infants had an underlying condition such as malnutrition, infection, tuberculosis, or heart disease—all of which thrived on the Yakama Reservation. In these cases, pneumonia was the primary cause of death, but other problems contributed to the body's weakened state, which made the child susceptible to pneumonia. For Yakama infants lacking a minimal standard of living, pneumonia was deadly.[24]

Gastrointestinal disorders caused the death of 66 infants (10%) during the era under examination. This was the second leading cause of death among children under one year of age. Gastrointestinal disorders took the lives of 37 females (56%) and 29 males (44%). Yakama infants died often of gastrointestinal disorders resulting from gastroenteritis, vomiting, diarrhea, and infections of the stomach, intestines, and other areas of the digestive tract. Yakama infants died of dehydration and diarrhea, two major elements of gastrointestinal disorders that took the lives of many infants and children—and continues to do so among poverty-stricken children from diverse populations around the world.

Disorders of the digestive tract proved fatal, particularly when infections developed. Antibiotics were scarce on the reservation or simply not available, and children without medicines to fight bacterial infections often died. Thus, bacilli and infections struck many organs of Yakama infants. The stomach, intestines, and other parts of the digestive tract contain essential bacilli for life, but sometimes dangerous bacilli invade the body, multiply rapidly, and infect the gut wall before entering the bloodstream and spreading to other parts of the body. Gastrointestinal infections were nearly always caused by bacterium, and children infected with the disorder suffered abdominal and intestinal pain, cramps, diarrhea, fever, and vomiting. Most often infants became dehydrated, and although they were thirsty, they were unable to keep fluids in their stomachs.[25] Among Yakama infants, gastrointestinal disorders were the second leading cause of death, followed by tuberculosis (figure 5.4).

Between 1914 and 1964, a total of 18 infants (3%) died of tuberculosis. Officials recording these deaths through the death certificates most often indicated that infants had died of "tuberculosis," rarely specifying the type. Occasionally the certificates indicated that the infant had died of "pulmonary tuberculosis," even though the disease could attack brains, lungs, kidneys, bones, or other parts of the body. Although Alexander Fleming discovered penicillin in 1928, the antibiotic was not readily available on the reservation until the late 1930s and early 1940s. Politics played an enormous role, as white politicians determined the fate of many Native people by refusing to fund health care for Native Americans as stipulated in treaties. After all, the people living and dying on the Yakama Reservation were only Indians who did not vote and who had little political influence. Of the 18 Yakama infants who died of tuberculosis, 10 (56%) were females and 8 (44%) were males. Throughout the Yakama population, deaths resulting from tuberculosis were the result of malnutrition, unsanitary living conditions, and inadequate medical care.

Although tuberculosis normally takes time to develop, it was one of the most important causes of death among Yakama infants. Tuberculosis is caused by airborne bacilli, which generally spread from one person to another, landing in the lungs where the bacilli multiply and destroy tissues. The bacilli are usually attacked by natural antibodies, but they can spread to other body parts. The bacilli may react to antibodies, but if children have a low resistance, the tubercle bacilli can travel to other parts of the body through the blood, attacking other organs. For months or years the tubercle bacilli can travel about the body or lay dormant. This process can occur for some time as bacilli remain inactive, but they can also become active at any point. In small children, the tubercle bacilli can take hold quickly, particularly if mothers and infants are ill, undernourished, or living in unsanitary or overcrowded housing.[26] According to Selman Waksman, an authority on tuberculosis, American Indians suffered severely because they were "confined to barracks or permanent reservation quarters" where they showed "a marked rise in tuberculosis rate[s] which far exceed that of either negro or white persons." He also argued that the semino-madic life of many Native Americans was conducive to good health, free from the ravages of tuberculosis.[27]

Infants affected by tuberculosis experienced fatigue, fever, and loss of appetite. They usually had a dry cough producing phlegm filled with blood and pus. Tuberculosis spread as a result of contact with phlegm, pus, and blood. Patients coughed and spit, spreading the bacilli onto others, bed clothing, blankets, and other material items. Dishes, eating utensils, and cups became contaminated, and the disease spread uncontrollably from patient to family to friends. Children carried tuberculosis to school, social events, and church, spreading it innocently among the larger reservation population. When tuberculosis struck, infants lost weight and could develop lumps in their bodies from swollen lymph nodes. Tuberculosis ravaged Native American populations during the first half of the twentieth century because of poor living conditions, malnutrition, and a host of other diseases that preyed on Native peoples (figure 5.4).[28]

Heart disease was the fourth major cause of death among Yakama infants, taking the lives of 16 children (3%) under one year of age. Of these infants, 9 (56%) were females and 6 (44%) were males, with 1 infant's gender unknown. Most of the heart-related deaths that occurred within the Yakama population occurred among the very young and the old. Within that group of Yakama under four years of age, 20 (6%) deaths occurred, and of this number, 16 were suffered by infants under one year of age. Heart diseases of all types were responsible for many deaths among infants under one year of age and children under four.

Heart disease includes many disorders such as diseases of the valves, congenital heart disease, heart attacks, heart failure, and others. Most infant deaths involving the heart were from congenital heart disease or abnormalities of the heart at the time of birth. Congenital heart disease was caused in the fetus, particularly when the mother had an infection or contracted German measles (rubella) while she was pregnant. Some disorders of the heart were genetic, including Down's Syndrome and Marfan's Syndrome, the latter of which is a disorder of the collagen or protein fibrous tissue that strengthens the vessels, valves, and heart. Because of the lack of prenatal care, poverty, and the lack of traditional foods, mothers were not nutritionally fit and their fetuses could develop in an unhealthy manner. The syndromes mentioned above likely developed among Yakama infants, but death certificates were not specific about these syndromes, providing only general, descriptive, nonmedical causes of death.[29]

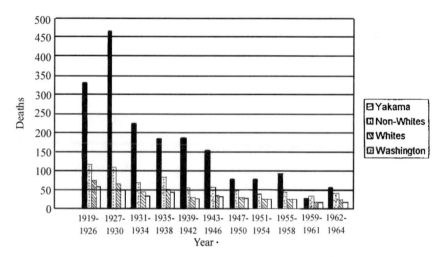

Figure 5.5 *Yakama infant-mortality rate comparisons per 1,000 live births, 1919–1964.*

Finally, syphilis was the fifth leading cause of death among Yakama infants. All of them contracted the deadly disease while in utero. A total of 12 children (2%) under one year of age died of syphilis, and of this number, 9 (75%) were males and 3 (25%) were females. During the years between 1888 and 1964, a total of 19 Yakama people died of syphilis. Thus, 79 percent of all Yakama that died of syphilis were children who had contracted the disease from their mothers. Of this number, 12 were infants and 15 were children in that group under four years of age. During the same period, only two adults died of the disease. Syphilis is a sexually transmitted disease caused by a bacterium known as "treponema pallidum." On the Yakama Reservation, syphilis was transmitted from mothers to their fetuses, and when the disease went untreated among mothers and their infants, it killed the infants (figure 5.4).

A total of 70 percent of all infant deaths among Yakama people occurred between 1924 and 1945, and the largest number of infant deaths in a single year occurred in 1931 during the darkest times of the Great Depression, when 36 children under one year of age died on the Yakama Reservation. Only 28 percent of the infant deaths on the reservation occurred between 1946 and 1964, and the number of infant deaths dropped dramatically after World War II as a result of antibiotics, improved sanitation and health care, and an improved economy in part due to wage labor (figure 5.5).

Infant Mortality Rate

Birth records for Native peoples living on the Yakama Indian agency were available for all the years between 1914 and 1964, except for the years 1915, 1916, 1917, 1920, 1922, 1924, and 1925.[30] For years in which sufficient data was available, an infant mortality rate was calculated and compared to whites and non-whites in the United States as well as the general population of Washington—the state surrounding the Yakama Nation (figures 5.3 and 5.5). The most complete data on births and deaths on the Yakama Indian Reservation were found between 1926 and 1964, during which time the Yakama experienced their highest infant mortality rate (in 1927): 684 per 1,000 live births. That same year, whites in the United States had an infant mortality rate of 61, nonwhites had a rate of 100, and the people of Washington had a rate of 50. The Yakama had an infant mortality rate markedly higher than that of other populations within the United States. Although this comparison is between a small population and three larger populations, the comparison is useful as a way of illustrating the high rate of infant mortality on a reservation (figures 5.3 and 5.5).

An examination of the infant mortality rates experienced by Yakama people and whites within the United States demonstrates that, over a period of forty years (with the exception of 1948), the Yakama always had a higher infant mortality rate than whites. This trend is also relevant when comparing the infant mortality rate of the Yakama with the people of Washington. Again, except for the year 1948, the Yakama had an infant mortality rate higher than the people of Washington; most years the infant mortality rate of the Yakama was many times higher, and this may well have been the result of poor record-keeping. Although the difference is not as great, over a period of four decades the Yakama experienced an infant mortality rate per 1,000 live births higher than that of nonwhites in the United States. However, the Yakama infant mortality rate declined generally between 1926 and 1964, dropping continually below the 100 deaths per 1,000 live births after 1955. This was likely due to a general improvement in health in the 1940s and early 1950s, better health care administered by the Public Health Service after 1954, and a decline in deaths caused by infectious diseases (figures 5.3 and 5.5). This trend was marked with a dramatic decline in the number of deaths caused by gastrointestinal disorders and tuberculosis, both of which were nearly eradicated in the 1940s. In addition, although infant deaths caused by pneumonia continued, the number of these deaths declined.

Infant mortality rates for the Yakama are erratic, because the Yakama constitute a small population in which the ebb and flow of deaths fluctuated greatly. Therefore, moving averages (an average of death rates during a four-year period) of infant mortalities were calculated for the years in which data was available from 1920 to 1964 (figure 5.5).[31] The data show a general and steady decline in the infant mortality rate of Yakama from 1925 to 1964, except for a slight rise between 1940 and 1944. This rise in the infant mortality rate may have been related to World War II, a time when Yakama men and women went off to war or worked in defense-related activities that may have placed fetuses and newborn babies at risk. This was also a time of drought in the American West, which may have affected food supplies, a complication that influenced food rationing. Overall, the moving averages depicting infant mortality rates on the Yakama Reservation declined from a high of 497 per 1,000 live births during the years from 1925 to 1929, to 52 per 1,000 live births during the years from 1960 to 1964. This important decline in the infant mortality rate was due to an improved standard of living on the reservation and better health care. The moving average of infant mortality rate demonstrated that the infant mortality rate within the Yakama Indian population was consistently higher than that of whites and nonwhites within the United States as well as the people of Washington State (figure 5.5).

The moving averages of infant mortality rates show that the highest rates of death occurred from roughly the 1920s to 1945. In part, this was the result of the Great Depression, which struck rural areas in the 1920s before the stock-market crash. The general health of the Yakama people was poor during this era, and this was, in part, connected to the economic problems of the state and nation. The Yakama Nation was situated in an area heavily tied to ranching and agriculture, and since both of these economic pursuits suffered in the 1920s and 1930s, so did Yakama people. The lives of Yakama people were also tied to the national reforms in Indian affairs during this same time period. The reformers did not push their agenda until the 1920s, and their efforts did not bear fruit until the late 1930s and early 1940s. However, their efforts had many tangible results, including an improvement in economic, political, and educational matters pertaining to Native Americans.

Another factor that had a bearing on infant mortality rates on the Yakama Reservation was the passage in 1954 of Public Law 83-568, a bill known as the "Transfer Act," which transferred the health care of American Indians and Alaska Natives from the Bureau of Indian Affairs in the Interior Department to the Department of Health, Education, and Welfare—known today as the Department of Health and Human Services. Throughout most of the twentieth century, the Public Health Service had aided the Interior Department in its efforts to deliver health care to Native Americans, but after 1954 it took full command of health delivery among Indian people. The Public Health Service had a great deal of experience and expertise in dealing with public-health issues, and the public entity had more resources to devote to prenatal and postnatal care for both mother and baby. These factors soon contributed to the decline of infant mortality. Health care improved during the 1950s on the Yakama Reservation, and this is evident in lower infant mortality rates in comparison to most years of the previous decades. Still, over the course of much of the twentieth century, the Yakama witnessed numerous infant deaths. During the course of forty-two years, from 1922 to 1964, the Yakama experienced an average infant mortality rate per 1,000 live births of 198, while during the same years whites in the United States had an infant mortality rate of 41. Thus, the Yakama infant mortality rate was roughly double that of nonwhites in the United States and nearly five times greater than that of whites in the country (figures 5.3–5.5).

Conclusion

Yakama infants constituted the largest number of deaths recorded in the death certificates for any age group among Native people living on the Yakama Indian Reservation between 1914 and 1964. Infants died primarily of pneumonia, gastrointestinal disorders, tuberculosis, heart disease, and syphilis. All of these causes were significantly influenced by removal to and life on the reservation, where poverty flourished. Poor diets, unsanitary housing, and social anomie contributed to infant deaths. In addition, the health division of the Office of Indian Affairs did not adequately educate or care for Native people, particularly pregnant mothers.

Infants on the reservation were at risk because of the lack of medicine, doctors, nurses, and hospitals. They were at risk because mothers received little or no prenatal care or basic education about sanitation, disease prevention, disease control, and techniques of quarantining infants and other patients. Before the United States created the reservation in the Pacific Northwest, midwives and elders among the Native population advised and assisted women and babies on a number of health-related issues, but with the destruction of the seasonal round, women of child-bearing age were often without the old health support group. Furthermore, wage earning off the reservation, boarding school experiences, the decline of Yakama language use, and isolation from elders contributed to the loss and transference of traditional knowledge among Yakama women.

Mothers and babies were also at risk because parents no longer ate as many traditional foods or served them to their children. The Yakama Reservation became a host for bacilli and viruses that preyed on infants who were undernourished and who lived in cramped, unsanitary homes. Bacilli spread rapidly through the air and on such material items as blankets, bedding, cups, flatware, dishes, and clothing. They thrived in homes where people were unaccustomed to cleaning themselves or material items with soap and disinfectants, since they had never needed to do so before the introduction of so many new and deadly bacterium. They did not understand germ theory, and, as a result, bacilli spread quickly from person to person, spreading pneumonia, tuberculosis, and a variety of gastrointestinal disorders.

When the government of the United States forced fourteen diverse tribes and bands onto the reservation, the government broke a pattern of life that had been established at the time of Yakama creation, when humans formed a spiritual, physical, and cultural relationship with salmon, deer, roots, berries, and other foods. In the early twentieth century the government ended seasonal rounds of Indians, forcing them to remain on the reservation rather than move from root to fishing to hunting grounds. The government broke the natural cycle of the people, which had profound health implications. In addition to a detrimental change in diet, the government altered familial and band relationships. As Indians became more sedentary, grandmothers, mothers, aunts, and other relatives who once shared in the caring of children no longer banded together as regularly to travel from the rivers to the plateaus and from the plateaus to the mountains.

The relationship between women in the care of each other's children through extended families and extended relationships was changed by the reservation system, which encouraged or required Indians to remain in certain areas where extended family and friends may or may not have been located. Furthermore, the reservation altered the role of women who had once gathered a predominant amount of natural fruits and vegetables. Although women gathered some roots and berries, they generally ran their family's affairs on the reservation through ranching, farming, and wage earning. Women gradually did not share as many child-care duties, even though they had to work outside of the home for the family's survival. Many men also worked outside the home, often traveling great distances to work on ranches or pick hops and fruit. Some men hunted and fished, but racism and state game and fish officers ignored sovereign treaty rights of Native men by jailing them for continuing a traditional way of life.

The reservation system of the United States destroyed the standard of living of Native peoples and introduced a host of bacilli and viruses among the Yakama population. Poverty resulted and with it came ill health and death. Once the United States destroyed much of Indian culture, the government failed to enrich the body and bodies of Yakama people with nutritious foods, medicine, doctors, nurses, and health systems in accordance with trust and treaty responsibilities. Without housing, sanitation, education, hospitals, and medical staffs—and living in a state of social disarray—Yakama infants were at risk for many diseases, the most aggressive and deadly being pneumonia. These circumstances contributed to the ill health and deaths of Yakama people of all ages. Death was particularly pronounced among Yakama infants who fell victim to pneumonia, gastrointestinal disorders, tuberculosis, heart disease, and syphilis. Death stalked all Yakama people during the 1914 to 1964 era, but babies under the age of one suffered the most.[32]

Notes

1. This study was made possible in part by a research grant provided by the National Council of Learned Societies, National Endowment for the Humanities, and the Ford Foundation. The author thanks the following scholars, physicians, and public-health officials for reading portions of the manuscript and verifying the accuracy of medical information about diseases. These include Edgar W. Butler, John Weeks, Neal Hickman, Terry Smith, Lisa Firth, and Brad Richie. For information on the Yakima Treaty, see *Documents Relating to Negotiations Ratified and Unratified Treaties of the United States*, National Archives, Record Group 75, Microfilm T494, Reel 5. Also see Charles S. Kappler, *Indian Affairs, Laws and Treaties* 2 (Washington, DC: Government Printing Office [GPO], 1940), 698–702. Article five of the Yakima Treaty specifically mentions hospitals and medicine to be provided for twenty years. The government did not provide the Yakama with minimum health care until the 1950s.

2. In 1994 the Confederated Tribes of the Yakama Nation changed the spelling of their name from Yakima to Yakama. Thus, throughout this work, "Yakama" is the form used in describing the tribe, reservation, agency, and people. However, the treaty, city, valley, and river is presented here as "Yakima." The term "Yakama" is used to denote all of the Native people living on the Yakama Reservation, since the death certificates almost never delineate the diverse tribes and bands of individuals who died on the reservation. Fourteen distinct tribes and bands, three distinct languages, and several dialects of these languages are represented on the Yakama Reservation.

3. For the most detailed treatment of traditional foods among Indians of the Columbia Plateau, see Eugene S. Hunn, *Nch'i-Wana, The Big River: Mid-Columbia Indians and Their Land* (Seattle: University of Washington Press, 1990), 138–200. Also see Helen Hersh Schuster, *Yakima Indian Traditionalism: A Study in Continuity and Change* (Ann Arbor: University Microfilms International, 1975), 68–87, 204, 238, 262.

4. Schuster, *Yakima Indian Traditionalism*, 46–50. According to Lucullus McWhorter, a white neighbor and rancher in the Yakima Valley, in 1913 most Yakama lived in one- or two-room shacks with a "lean-to kitchen" outside. See Lucullus Virgil McWhorter, *The Crime against the Yakimas* (North Yakima, WA: Republic Press, 1913).

5. For destruction of salmon through irrigation projects, see *Yakima Tribal Council, The Yakimas: Treaty Centennial, 1855–1955* (Yakima, WA: Republic Press, 1955), 36, 48.

6. Hunn, *Nch'i-Wana*, 270–72, 292–93. For general studies on dams located on the Columbia River and its tributaries, see U.S. Department of the Army, *Review Report on Columbia River and Tributaries*, Corps of Engineers, North Pacific Division, October 1, 1948; U.S. Department of Interior, "The Columbia River," House Executive Document 473, 81st Congress, 2nd Session, 1950; Bureau of Indian Affairs, *Report on the Source, Nature and Extent of the Fishing, Hunting and Miscellaneous Related Rights of Certain Tribes in Washington and Oregon* . . . (Los Angeles: Office of Indian Affairs, Division of Forestry and Grazing, 1942); and T. W. Mermel, ed. and comp., *Register of Dams in the United States: Completed, Under Construction and Proposed* (New York: McGraw-Hill, 1958).

7. Schuster, *Yakima Indian Traditionalism*, 270–75.

8. A brief history of health agencies dealing with Native Americans is found in

"Comprehensive Health Care Program for American Indians and Alaska Natives," U.S. Department of Health and Human Services, Washington, DC, n.d., p. 6. For information about duration programs on the Yakama Reservation, see Carr to Commissioner of Indian Affairs, June 7, 1917, and Sprague to Carr, May 5, 1917, "Health and Hospitalization Records and Reports, 1912–1940," Box 264, National Archives, Pacific Northwest Region, Seattle, Record Group 75 (hereafter cited as NA, PNWR, RG 75).

9. Lewis Meriam, *The Problem of Indian Administration* (New York: Johnson Reprint Corporation, 1971), 259. Meriam asserted in the narrative that the health delivery of the Bureau of Indian Affairs "has to a great extent been merely palliative in practice," which was certainly the case on the Yakama Reservation.

10. Schuster, *Yakima Indian Traditionalism,* 165–76. Schuster states that the Yakama recognize that some illnesses are caused by traditional factors, such as spirit sickness, contact with powerful totems or places, and witchcraft. Other sicknesses are classified as "white diseases." One of Schuster's informants stated: "We get sickness from white man: measles, chickenpox, smallpox, whooping cough, flu, and all from white man." Ibid., 176. Information on Indian doctors is taken from Meritt to Carr, January 24, 1916, "Medicine Men," NA, PNWR, RG 75.

11. In 1884 the U.S. House and Senate passed an appropriations bill that required the Office of Indian Affairs to keep vital statistics on Indian reservations. Nevertheless, most agencies failed to comply with the law, including agents on the Yakama Reservation until 1888. However, the statistics kept did not reflect the births and deaths on the reservation. No birth records were kept until 1914, and the death records were almost nonexistent until 1924. Information regarding the appropriations bill of 1884 was provided by Lee Francis (Laguna Pueblo), who worked for the Bureau of Indian Affairs in Washington, D.C. The death certificates used in this study originated after 1907 when Washington became a death-registry state, and the Yakima County Health Office began recording the certificates of death. County officials recorded some Indian deaths on the reservation, but not many. County health officials relied on agency employees to notify them of deaths, and apparently this did not happen to any extent until 1924, when the Yakama agency made a major effort in reporting deaths.

12. Death Certificates, Yakima Indian Agency, 1888–1964, NA, PNWR, RG 75. Death Certificates for the Yakima Reservation number a total of 3,899 cases and are found in the National Archives, Pacific Northwest Region, Seattle, under the Records of Yakima Indian Agency.

13. The infant mortality rate is the number of deaths of infants under one year of age per 1,000 births. The National Archives, Pacific Northwest Region, contains birth records for most years after 1914. These vital statistics were kept by the Yakama Indian agency.

14. Death data found in the censuses do not provide information on primary or secondary causes, date of death, place of death, blood quantum, or other variables commonly found on death certificates. The census data run from July 1 to June 30, and it is often difficult to ascertain in which year a person died. Also, the censuses do not provide information on deaths after 1900, and it is intellectually hazardous to assume that because a person appeared on one census and not on the next that the person died. Some Yakama moved off the reservation to live on another reservation, a common

practice among the Plateau Indians. Thus the best data dealing with deaths on the Yakama Indian Reservation in the twentieth century are found in the death certificates.

15. Yakama Indian Censuses, 1885–1931, NA, PNWR, RG 75.

16. Meriam, *The Problem of Indian Administration*, 170–82. An analysis of the statistical information is found in this segment of the report. The reform of Indian affairs received a boost when John D. Rockefeller, Jr., provided a grant to the Institute for Government Research—later renamed the Brookings Institute. The Institute appointed Lewis Meriam to conduct the research, who in turn appointed a team to help him deconstruct the workings of the Office of Indian Affairs. Their report is an indictment of policies and led to many reforms.

17. Kenneth R. Philp, *John Collier's Crusade for Indian Reform, 1920–1954* (Tucson: University of Arizona Press, 1977), 114, 126–27, 130, 134.

18. Meriam, *The Problem of Indian Administration*, 189.

19. Ibid., 189, 266. This is in reference to eleven reservations surveyed for their death records, none of which was the Yakama Reservation. However, the principle is accurate for the Yakama Reservation.

20. Ibid.

21. Yakama Death Certificates, NA, PNWR, RG 75. This work is part of a larger social and cultural study that will deal with Yakama deaths between 1888 and 1964, including all age groups.

22. Cases 4537, 4540, 4541, 4542, 4543, 4552, 4558, Yakama Death Certificates, NA, PNWR, RG 75. Others could be cited but this run provides an example of a series of unknown or unrecorded deaths on the Yakama Reservation. The author chose not to include the names of the deceased in order to protect the privacy of the Yakama families.

23. Clifford E. Trafzer and Richard D. Scheuerman, *Renegade Tribe: The Palouse Indians and the Invasion of the Inland Pacific Northwest* (Pullman: Washington State University Press, 1986): 93–102; Hunn, *Nch'i-Wana*, 138–200; Schuster, *Yakima Indian Traditionalism*, 243–46, 249–51. For a historical perspective of the importance of disease, see Alfred W. Crosby, *The Columbian Exchange: The Biological and Cultural Consequences of 1492* (Westport, CT: Greenwood Publishing, 1972); Frederick Fox Cartwright, *Disease and History* (London: Hart-Davis, 1972); Howard Simpson, *Invisible Armies* (Indianapolis: Bobbs-Merrill, 1980); and Ann F. Ramenofsky, *Vectors of Death* (Albuquerque: University of New Mexico Press, 1987). Some Yakama children died of suffocation, which, in some cases, was the recording official's assessment of sudden infant death syndrome or "crib death."

24. Wesley W. Spink, *Infectious Diseases: Prevention and Treatment in the Nineteenth Century* (Minneapolis: University of Minnesota Press, 1978), 209–12; Frank MacFarlan Burnet and David O. White, *Natural History of Infectious Diseases* (Cambridge: Cambridge University Press, 1972), 32–43, 52–69; Andrew B. Christie, *Infectious Diseases: Epidemeology and Clinical Practice* (Edinburgh and London: E. and S. Livingstone, 1969), 269–99; and Jeffrey R. M. Kunz and Asher J. Finkle, *The American Medical Association Family Medical Guide* (New York: Random House, 1987), 365, 695.

25. Kunz and Finkle, *AMA Family Medical Guide*, 467, 664, 702; Christie, *Infectious Diseases*, 122–167; Spink, *Infectious Diseases*, 246–47; Burnet and White, *Natural History of Infectious Diseases*, 70–87.

26. Tuberculosis was the leading killer of all Yakama ages 0 to 99, during the 1888–1964 era. See Ales Hrdlicka's, "Tuberculosis among Certain Indian Tribes in the United States," *Annual Report of the Bureau of American Ethnography* 42 (Washington, DC: Smithsonian Institution Press, 1909), 31–32; Spink, *Infectious Diseases*, 220–21, 224; Burnet and White, *Natural History of Infectious Diseases*, 213–24; Jay Arthur Meyers, *Captain of All These Men of Death* (St. Louis: Warren H. Green, 1977), 73–83, 142–58; Selman A. Waksman, *The Conquest of Tuberculosis* (Berkeley: University of California Press, 1964), 24; Kunz and Finkle, *AMA Family Medical Guide*, 574, 719, 748; Spink, *Infectious Diseases*, 220–22. The most significant work on the subject in recent years is Barbara Bates, *Bargaining for Life: A Social History of Tuberculosis, 1876–1938* (Philadelphia: University of Pennsylvania Press, 1992).

27. Waksman, *The Conquest of Tuberculosis*, 24.

28. Waksman, *The Conquest of Tuberculosis*, 24; Meriam, *The Problem of Indian Administration*, 204–8; *San Bernardino Sun*, March 15, 1994, 15. According to this article, a recent study of lung and lymph tissue taken from the body of a Peruvian Indian woman believed to have lived 1,000 years ago indicates "that tuberculosis was not introduced to the Americas by Europeans" but that it was native to this land. This is a theory long held by some scholars, but the physical evidence of the tissue is revealing. Although tuberculosis existed in the Americas prior to 1492, there is no evidence that it existed among the Yakama. Wilmar L. Salo, a scholar working for the University of Minnesota, pointed out that "the harsh treatment of the Indians undoubtedly contributed to the American epidemic of the disease." *San Bernardino Sun*, March 15, 1994.

29. Waksman, *The Conquest of Tuberculosis*, 24.

30. An infant mortality rate is the number of deaths of children under one year of age per 1,000 live births in the population, excluding premature births and stillbirths.

31. Moving averages are used when the data are erratic, which is often the case when dealing with a small population like that of the Yakama. In such cases, infant mortality rates or crude death rates for a number of years are added together and divided by the number of years. This tends to smooth out the data so that it may be read more easily.

32. Clifford E. Trafzer, *Death Stalks the Yakama: Epidemiological Transitions and Mortality on the Yakama Indian Reservation, 1888–1964* (East Lansing: Michigan State University Press, 1997), 158–65.

SIX

NANCY REIFEL

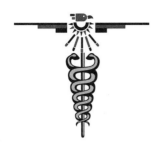

American Indian Views of Public-Health Nursing, 1930–1950[1]

American Indians, like many people of minority cultures in the United States, have access to the health-care system of the traditional culture as well as hospitals and clinics operated in the biomedical model. Administrators and providers of health care in the federally funded Indian clinics are continually faced with the question of how to manage the persistence of traditional healing practices. Beginning in the second half of the nineteenth century, government officials viewed Western medical services as an instrument of assimilation. The self-defined role of the federal Indian service was to assist the Indians to live in the white society.[2] Medical personnel argued for the construction of Indian hospitals because the use of Indian hospitals would diminish the influence of medicine men.[3] Not until the mid-twentieth century was the value of traditional healing practices recognized by physicians.[4] Since then, Indian health programs have experimented with consultation with traditional healers,[5] facilitation of the use of traditional healing, provision of funds to hire and train traditional healers,[6] and incorporation of traditional health beliefs in health education.[7] These efforts demonstrate that traditional health does have a legitimate role in the delivery of health care by government institutions. Unfortunately, little is known about what Native people consider when choosing between traditional medicine and biomedicine. Nor is there an understanding of how people perceive the role of the two systems of medical practice. An examination of responses from Indian people from one Sioux reservation area regarding integration of biomedical practices into their traditional system of health care will serve as an example of how people make choices about health care. From 1930 to 1950, the Bureau of Indian Affairs (BIA) stationed public-health nurses at Indian reservations throughout the country. The Sioux people offer their views of these nurses. The field nurses brought health care in the biomedical tradition (white medicine) to small, rural, isolated reservation communities.[8] At this time, many Indian people relied on traditional medicine for health care and demonstrated poor cooperation with recommendations from the non-Native, government physicians.

Traditional Indian Health Care

Prior to contact with Western society, American Indian tribes had developed a medical system based on Indian concepts of health, illness, and death causations. Although there were more than five hundred Indian tribes in North America, most tribes seem to have had similar theories about the causes of disease. Two general disease classifications[9] include those from an environmental cause, like injuries, intestinal disorders, and rheumatism. Indians had treatments for these ailments based on medicine plants, animals, and minerals found in the natural environment. The successful treatment of scurvy used by Cartier's expedition in 1534 is an example of this level of medicine.[10] Usually the more common natural remedies were kept in supply in the home and dispensed by a knowledgeable family member.[11] In the case of illness or injury, home remedies and natural remedies were used first. The second type of disease for which Indian tribes developed treatment included those whose origins were attributed to supernatural forces. Because these diseases had spiritual origins, they required cures affecting spiritual forces. Most American Indian tribes had health practitioners trained in treating the natural diseases and another class of health practitioners trained to treat diseases of spiritual origin. One of the major qualifications for becoming a healer was that the person lead a "blameless life of honesty, bravery, and humility."[12] When home and natural remedies did not cure the patient, a spiritual healer was called.

During the nineteenth century, infectious diseases of European origin devastated Indian populations. To account for this type of disease some Indian tribes added a third classification of disease commonly called "white disease." Tribal healers sent people with white diseases to white doctors for treatment.[13] This is consistent with the American Indian practice of matching the treatment of a disease to the origin of the disease.

From 1900 to 1950 medical staff and facilities of the Indian Bureau expanded tremendously. Appropriations for health services grew from $40,000 in

1911 to $18 million in 1955.[14] It was during this period, in 1924, that public-health nurses were added to the staff of the Bureau of Indian Affairs. These "field nurses" were stationed at agency substations throughout a reservation until the mid-1950s. Field nurses maintained some of the traditions of public-health nursing such as autonomy, personal contact, and an emphasis on teaching "right living."[15] To better understand how American Indian people viewed medical services offered by the field nurses and how they made choices about health care, Indian-reservation residents who had contact with the field nurses in the 1930s and 1940s were interviewed.[16]

Data-Collection Methods

Two adjacent South Dakota reservations were selected as the primary data-collection site. This site was selected for several reasons: (1) Indian people currently residing on reservations represent the largest population likely to have had contact with field nurses in the 1930s and 1940s; (2) the author had recently conducted a community-based survey of elders at this site (familiarity with the population and the geographic area is critical to the success of the data collection); and (3) familiarity with the site improved our ability to select a reliable interpreter/translator.

The research team conducted in-depth interviews with twenty-three individuals (seventeen women and six men) currently residing on the Pine Ridge and Rosebud reservations. The team recorded interviews that lasted one to two hours. The semistructured interviews consisted of questions designed to elicit information in the following categories: (1) the community of residence of the interviewee from 1930 to 1950; (2) the degree of contact with the field nurse. Whenever possible the field nurse was identified by name; and further information was solicited regarding (3) attitudes about the field nurse and the services she provided; (4) the use of Indian medicine; and (5) how or if Indian medicine and white medicine were integrated.

Most of the respondents were seventy years or older and were asked to recall events that took place between 1930 and 1940.[17] The interviews often followed a rambling indirect route to the discussion of the field nurses. Researchers investigating attitudes and beliefs among American Indian populations find that conversational situations elicited better responses from this population.

The research is limited since researchers asked elders to recall events that occurred fifty years ago. Memories could be colored by intervening events and maturity of the individual. Some of the respondents were children when they met the field nurses and may have been unaware of the reasons their parents had for the actions they took on behalf of the child. The data are limited geographically to South Dakota and to the Sioux people; thus, it may not be representative of American Indians throughout the country. Nevertheless, the interview data will identify salient impressions and attitudes, critical events in a person's life, and fundamental family beliefs regarding the field nurses.

All but one of the interviews were conducted in English, but elders occasionally used Lakota words. The researchers transcribed the interviews and reviewed them all with an interpreter. This proved valuable because the interpreter often clarified sections in which the respondent used words and syntax unique to the reservation, in addition to translating the smattering of Lakota words in most interviews. Researchers then edited the interviews following recommendations from the interpreter. These data were used to identify major themes to describe how American Indians used the services of the nurses.

Use of Remedies

Native health care in Indian communities was usually provided in the patient's home. When the family determined that assistance was needed, they sent for the appropriate healer. The field nurses provided home-based health-care services, and in some ways Indians responded to the nurses as they did to Native healers. This was because Indians viewed the field nurses as providing some of the same services as traditional healers. The nurses did not have the powers of spiritual healers, but they used medicines and had medical knowledge. The Sioux elders spoke of similar medicines offered by the field nurse and natural healers. Dispensing cough syrup was the most commonly mentioned service the field nurses provided. Indians may have asked for cough syrup because they were accustomed to using a syrup remedy for relief of cough. White medicines were fit into existing classifications and used in a similar manner as the Indian medicine. The following statements illustrate how white medicines were commonly viewed as equivalent to frequently used Indian remedies.

> White remedy: I always got eye drops, you know. From the nurse.
>
> Indian remedy: My grandma was good at that too. She gives some kind of, she boils some stuff and gives for eye drops for the eye.
>
> Indian remedy: If we had a cold, we were doctored right away. It was given cough syrup or skunk oil. And, you know, they kept that on hand. They even kept their [wild choke] cherries. That's why they cherish their cherries because it's like a cough syrup. They give you a teaspoon of cherry jelly or feed you cherry jelly and bread. They made it like a syrup and they used them for pancakes in the morning.
>
> White remedy: They give that [cough syrup] to everybody who's got a cough and is coughing. There's an old guy that went after cough syrup almost every day. Finally the nurse asked him how he used that cough syrup. Too much

cough syrup. He said that the reason why I come after my cough syrup is I like it with my pannycake.

Ten of the twenty-four Indian people interviewed remembered using both Indian medicine and white medicine from nurses. For the people who had access to both kinds of medicine and used both, the two main reasons given for choosing or rejecting one or the other were convenience and efficacy. When both Indian and white medicines were equally available, people tended to use the remedies that worked. Some elders spoke of their families using only Indian medicine, even though they had daily contact with the field nurses. As long as remedies worked, they saw no need to abandon the Indian medicine. "If it looked to them like it was doing the trick, if it was getting better, they would just go ahead and do it." Other people had equal confidence in both types of medicine and used whichever they had easier access to. "Took it for granted that they knew what they were doing. . . . I went both ways. . . . It just happens that I was there when I had an ailment of some sort." The medicine offered by the nurses was held to the same standards and used in the same way as the traditional medicines. White medical treatment, rather than replacing Indian traditional medicine as some medical personnel had hoped, was selectively incorporated into the existing Indian system of natural remedies.

Character of the Healer

The personal character of the nurse was critical in determining how well the Indians accepted her services. Eighteen of the twenty-three persons interviewed talked about the character of the nurses they knew. Often that was their first response when asked if they remembered the field nurses. Those who had used the nurses' services generally described them as being of good character, dedicated to helping people, responsive to the people, and respectful. Some of the most frequent types of comments included nurses being dedicated to the needs of the Indian people:

> She's working for the people.
> She's pretty busy. Good worker. She helped people.
> I think she really worked. Worked hard. For the people.
> She was a lot of help to us. Like I said she was always there when we need.

Comments about the good character of the nurses is an important theme repeated by everyone who used their services. In most tribes the primary requirement of the healer, both supernatural and natural, was that the person be of good character. Since healing powers could be used to inflict illness and death as easily as to cure, it was essential that the healer be a good person dedicated to the well-being of the people. These same criteria were applied to the field nurses. They had to be of good character and dedicated to helping the people before they were respected as healers. As one person stated, "People just upheld them in the communities and they really were sensitive to the needs of the people. They took pride in their station in life. In return, they got a lot of respect in every community."

The nurses came to an Indian community to practice medicine. In order to be successful they had to meet the standards applied to all Indian healers. One of the respondents described a nurse who did not meet these standards:

> And when we're ready to leave the boarding school she'll say . . . You're better off in school. Stay for the summer. She was that mean. She didn't want [the school children] to come home because their family are poor and they have outdoor toilet and no bathtub and like that. She talks like that. She's very rude mean woman.

This nurse was not seen as dedicated to helping the people. She fell short of meeting the standards of an Indian healer and her services were not used by the family.

In 1900 the Indian Bureau issued a directive requiring physicians to make home visits and "to do his utmost to educate and instruct them in proper methods of living."[18] Home visits and instruction in home health care would promote assimilation to white culture and adoption of white standards. Ironically, when the field nurses fulfilled the 1900 directive thirty years later, their work was accepted only if they were deemed worthy by Indian standards of "proper methods of living."

Filling the Gap

The types of white medicine that did not fit into the Indian organization of health care included immunizations and surgery. By 1924, when the field nurses began practicing on reservations, Indians were familiar with the dangers of smallpox and other communicable diseases and with the benefits of surgery. By 1924 the Sioux accepted immunizations and surgery even though they had no equivalent in the Indian medical system.

Indian people who had some contact with field nurses were cooperative in receiving immunizations. Most of the people interviewed had a sense that the immunizations were given as part of an organized program. Five people talked about school-based immunization programs. One of the local day school's immunization programs was described with typical Indian humor:

They broke a glasses and put alcohol on here and they scratch it down like that. Ow, ow, ow, I said. That time they used the glasses. Those school kids when the doctors come everybody run away. Run to the field. When the doctors come the teachers locked the door and snap all the windows and everybody stay in the school. They cry and try to break the window.

Many people found smallpox immunizations unpleasant, so much so that fifty years later they still remembered the circumstances surrounding the inoculation. But most people said, "I take it." As the illustration above shows, those who were children at the time saw the school-based immunizations as mandatory and accepted the treatment.

Field nurses also gave immunizations in other settings. Eight people talked about methods the nurses used to deliver immunizations outside of the school-based programs. Parents brought their children to the nurse's station or to the school when the nurse made her regular visit. Nurses vaccinated families at their homes. From 1937 to 1939 the federal government conducted a mass chest–X-ray survey for tuberculosis.[19] Families received vaccinations when they were brought to town for screening exams as part of a health-status survey.

The field nurses brought families to a central station for the health survey. One woman, who was ten years old at the time, related this story of the screening:

There was a big tent put up, like a circus tent. And that's where we were all given shots. Everybody stand there and hovered like stand in line. And boy, when they stuck me why I'd really scream. I really embarrassed myself. And then my mother handed my baby brother into my arms. And here I was holding him and he didn't even cry.

The field nurse arranged for people in her district to come to town for the screening. "For a couple weeks there she kept hauling people, well, every day until everybody is checked." During this survey nurses performed mass inoculations, treating families together. There was a general feeling among the Sioux that every family in the community participated in this health-related event. One of the women interviewed had been hired by the field nurse to drive people to this screening. She also reported that most people went to town for the screening exams. "As far as I know [most people came in]. She [the field nurse] made the arrangements. She would tell me where to go and who to pick up and when." Most Indian families accepted the immunization services offered at this program.

It is illuminating to examine the comments of people whose families primarily used Indian medicine. Three of the people interviewed had close relatives who were traditional healers. None of these three regularly used the field nurses' medical services, although they did accept rides from them, assistance with boarding-school arrangements, and were generally welcoming when the nurses visited their homes. These people received primary medical care from relatives who were Indian healers. However, all three people vividly described getting smallpox inoculations:

> We had our Indian doctors and our, my grandad was an Indian doctor. And he believed in herbs and everything for us so why when we got sick why mamma just took us to him. I don't remember us ever giving any medication. She [the field nurse] never gave medication. We depended on our grandad. The only thing they allowed us I remember they vaccinated us. They took a needle and they scraped our [arm]. He did allow that.

Vaccinations were accepted as an addition to traditional Indian health-care services. Smallpox was a disease of white origin. The prevention and treatment legitimately fell within the scope of white medicine, and there was no equivalent in the Indian health-care system. Vaccinations were readily incorporated into the Indian health-care system because they filled a need that Indian healers were unable to meet within their scope of practice.

Surgery was another service white medicine offered that was not well developed within the Indian health-care system. Corlett described some early surgical techniques of North American Indians, but they are primarily related to wound suturing. The Indian medical system lacked surgical skills and Indian people recognized this deficit.[20] One man, who was an adult at the time, recounted this story of seeking surgical assistance:

> I remember early '30s, there was a nurse, Field Nurse. She's stationed at Norris [approximately thirty miles away and on a different reservation]. She can surgery, she can do it. Big woman, tall one. She had skillful hands. I had a nail sticking through here [thigh]. Got it patchin'. I ride horseback over there. She look at it and said tie your horse up. Over here and I'll stitch it. She boil water and hot. She have a can and stick a kind of a knife. And I remember this. Why they tied me to this chair and some womans get ahold of my leg. Put oxide in there get that cleaned out and get that hot. She took it out and said "boil everything now." Boy, it was hot. But she put salve there. Cold pack. Rub it. Then she put me to bed. Sleep for I don't know how long. I woked up and it's alright. I got on horseback and I come [home].

Both immunizations and surgery filled a gap in the Indian health-care system. People who primarily used Indian medicine incorporated these two services into their own health-care system.

Tuberculosis

Between 1920 and 1940 the number of beds in tuberculosis hospitals operated by the Bureau of Indian Affairs increased from 573 to 1,200. Institutional treatment was a primary component of the Bureau's tuberculosis-control program among Indians during the 1930s.[21] The field nurses were instrumental in referring afflicted American Indian children and adults to nearby sanatoria. Three of the women interviewed had tuberculosis as children. Their relationships with the nurse and subsequent admission to the sanatorium differed.

The first woman recounted a history characterized by compliance with the recommendation for institutional treatment:

> My mother contracted pneumonia. I didn't think she was really that sick, but she died. And then, after that, I was lonely and really feeling bad. And then it just seemed like I didn't feel good at all. And that was when the Field Nurse took me in to the clinic and they run a series for tests on me and they said I had TB. So what did they do, they sent me to [an adjacent state]. It's on a [different tribe's] reservation. And the reason I was sent there was when my dad was in [boarding school], he befriended a man from there and became blood brothers, more binding than birth brothers. So anyway there he knew that he and his wife would give me good attention because he wrote him a letter explaining that my mother had died. So then I was in the hospital in there.

The family did eventually send their daughter to the sanatorium, but they had a high degree of choice in the matter. The father had a regular job at the sub-agency and his wife had died just one month prior to his daughter's diagnosis. The father did not have the resources to care for his daughter at home. He did, however, take an active role in selecting a sanatorium where he felt his daughter would be looked after by a trusted friend. The father was able to maintain some control over care for his daughter while following the recommendations of the field nurse.

The family of the second woman who had tuberculosis as a child was not as compliant with the nurse's recommendations. However, she eventually went to the sanatorium:

> The Field Nurse saw that I got to the hospital. I had to go periodically. Because I had. At that time, you know, TB was going through the reservation. My mom was a good nurse. She kept me clean. There was a whole bundle of bandages there. Denver mud. That's what they treated me with. Part of the time I stayed at home. But there was a time that my dad took me to [the sanatorium in a nearby city] on the train and left me over there. I really cried so bad they put me to, you know, I went to bed. There was another girl that was with me at that time. And she didn't go and she's dead. So my dad thought you better go for that, so I went. And I survived.

This family initially decided to treat their daughter at home and the field nurse supported them. She made periodic home visits bringing supplies and she transported the child to the hospital whenever necessary. It was only when the family saw the disease as life-threatening that they agreed to send their daughter to the sanatorium. They were able to send her to a sanatorium about 150 miles away. In this case the family maintained control of the medical care their daughter received. The field nurse supported them when they decided to care for her at home. They decided when the daughter would be hospitalized.

The third woman contracted tuberculosis and was cared for at home:

> One time I was about 17 years old I was really sick. At that time the people really have it TB. And I had it too, at that time. So those [field nurses] tell me I should go to the government sanatorium. I didn't go, I stayed home. And I'd get up early in the morning to go outside and go for a walk and come back. And I was all right. [Field nurse], she was there. She give me clothes or stuff that I drink in the morning. [She wanted me to go to the sanatorium] but grandma didn't want me to go so I didn't. Stayed home.

In this case the family did not accept the recommendations of the field nurse. However, the field nurse continued to follow the girl's condition and support her. There were only three members of the household: the grandmother, the uncle, and the woman. Unlike the previous two cases, the family was able to care for this girl at home. She and the caregiver were relatively isolated from other family members, and there did not appear to be any immediate threat to her life. The family decided it was unnecessary to institutionalize her for treatment.

These three cases illustrate how families used white medical services as an adjunct to home care for family members with tuberculosis. In all three cases the family maintained control of the treatment choice and the field nurses supported the families in their choice.

Conclusion

By the mid-1920s American Indian people had survived two centuries of dramatic changes. The population had been reduced by 80 percent. Many tribes had been forcibly moved so that white people could occupy their lands. The natural resources of the land had been destroyed. Federal law, missionaries, and the Bureau of Indian Affairs suppressed their cultural and religious practices. The people residing on reservations when the field nurses arrived in the 1930s came from a long tradition of maintaining a viable culture in spite of these assaults. The people were survivors.

Indians treated the imposition of white medicine in much the same way as they did other aspects of their interactions with white people. They incorporated what was necessary for survival into their cultural practices. They evaluated the services according to their own standards and accepted white medicines that were useful to them. They only used advanced medical services if they judged that such use would be more beneficial than traditional home care. They accepted and appreciated the nurses as healers, holding them to the rigorous standards applied to the American Indian healers. They also held white treatments and remedies to Indian standards: the remedy was used as the equivalent to Indian medicine, and it had to work. If white medicine offered an effective treatment for diseases that Indian medicine was unable to cure, the white treatment was incorporated into the Indian medical-care system. They made reasoned decisions about the use of institutionalization for tuberculosis. Indian people used the services of the nurses on their own terms. They took an active role in evaluating and selecting from alternate treatment regimens.

The Sioux people who interacted with the field nurses in the early twentieth century evaluated the nurses' work, their medicines, and their character against standards of traditional Sioux medicine. They recognized the contributions the nurses could make to Indian people and made a place for field nurses within their own medical-care system. Field nurses became an integral part of the federal Indian health system after the 1930s. In 1996 public-health nurses made more than 380,000 health-care visits to American Indians on reservations. More than 50 percent of these were for health services provided to people in their homes.[22]

Notes

1. This project was funded by the Institute of American Cultures, University of California, Los Angeles, and conducted under the guidance of Dr. Emily Abel, UCLA School of Public Health, and with the assistance of Phoebe Little Thunder.

2. Lewis Meriam, *The Problem of Indian Administration* (Baltimore: Johns Hopkins University Press, 1928), 112.

3. Ruth Raup, *The Indian Health Program from 1800–1955* (Washington, DC: Department of Health, Education and Welfare, 1959), 4.

4. Everett Rhoades, Lillie McGarvey, and Luana Reyes, *Report on Indian Health, Task Force Six: Indian Health* (Washington, DC: Government Printing Office, 1976), 74–83.

5. John Adair and Kurt Deuschle, *The People's Health: Medicine and Anthropology in a Navajo Community* (New York: Appleton-Century-Crofts, 1970), 33. The Indian Health Service from time to time engages in special initiatives to investigate methods of incorporating traditional healing practices into its health-care-delivery system. In 1998 a description of the Traditional Medicine Initiative could be found at the Internet address http://www.his.gov/2Co/Tradup.html.

6. Robert L. Bergman, "A School for Medicine Men," *American Journal of Psychiatry* 130 (June 1973): 663–66.

7. M. Dignan, P. Sharp, K. Blinson, R. Michielutte, J. Konen, R. Bell, and C. Lane, "Development of a Cervical Cancer Education Program for Native American Women in North Carolina," *Journal of Cancer Education* 9 (winter 1995): 235–42.

8. Elinor D. Gregg, *The Indians and the Nurse* (Norman: University of Oklahoma Press, 1965), 105.

9. William Thomas Corlett, *The Medicine Man of the American Indian and His Cultural Background* (Springfield, IL: Charles C. Thomas, 1935), 68; Stephen J. Kunitz, *Disease Change and the Role of Medicine: The Navajo Experience* (Berkeley and Los Angeles: University of California Press, 1983), 119; Ake Hultkrantz, *Shamanic Healing and Ritual Drama: Health and Medicine in Native American Religious Tradition* (New York: Crossroad Publishing, 1992), 133–37.

10. Virgil J. Vogel, *American Indian Medicine* (Norman: University of Oklahoma Press, 1970), 249.

11. Jennie R. Joe, "Traditional Indian Health Practices and Cultural Views," in *Native North American Almanac*, ed. Duane Champagne (Detroit: Gale Research Inc., 1994), 803.

12. Barbara Melosh, *"The Physician's Hand": Work Culture and Conflict in American Nursing* (Philadelphia: Temple University Press, 1982), 134.

13. John Adair and Kurt Deuschle, *The People's Health: Medicine and Anthropology in a Navajo Community* (New York: Appleton-Century-Crofts, 1970), 33.

14. Raup, *The Indian Health Program*, 29.

15. Melosh, *"The Physician's Hand."*

16. This research was conducted by Drs. Emily Abel and Nancy Reifel, with funding provided by the Institute of American Cultures at the University of California, Los Angeles. Dr. Abel obtained copies of monthly reports submitted by the field nurses working on Indian reservations from 1930 to 1950. Dr. Reifel interviewed reservation residents in South Dakota who had interacted with the field nurses. See Emily Abel and Nancy Reifel, "Interactions between Public Health Nurses and Clients on American Indian Reservations during the 1930s," *Social History of Medicine* 9 (January 1996): 89–108. For a discussion of the field nurses, see Emily Abel, "'We are left so much alone to work out our own problems.' Nurses on American Indian reservations during the 1930s," *Nursing History Review* 4 (1996): 43–64.

17. At times, extensive probing was necessary to spark a memory of these events. Whenever possible, names of field nurses were suggested. One useful probe was to describe the usual uniform of the field nurses, which was distinct from that of the hospital nurses.

18. Raup, *Indian Health Program*, 4.

19. Ibid., 14.

20. In 1925, on a field visit to the Navajo Reservation, Elinor Gregg, the first public-health nurse hired to work for the Bureau of Indian Affairs, reported this incident: "I was interviewed by two old Navahos who had heard by the grapevine that I was coming, and they had ridden one hundred miles from Bluff, Utah, on horseback, to ask 'Washington' to send them a new doctor who 'could cut.' They had only an internist. Their own Navaho medicine men could take care of other illnesses, but they had only a piece of glass to cut with. They wanted a surgeon, not an internist. The

Indians knew the difference." Elinor D. Gregg, *The Indians and the Nurse* (Norman: University of Oklahoma Press, 1965).

21. The Bureau of Indian Affairs operated tuberculosis hospitals (sanatoria) and special school sanatoria for Indian children with tuberculosis. From 1911 to 1941, the number of tuberculosis hospital beds increased from 227 to 1,400. See Raup, *The Indian Health Program*, 13.

22. *1966 Trends in Indian Health* (Rockville, MD: U.S. Department of Health and Human Services, Indian Health Service), 134.

SEVEN

DIANE WEINER

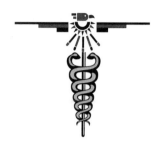

Interpreting Ideas about Diabetes, Genetics, and Inheritance[1]

Genetic inheritance is a multilayered concept enveloped by cultural assumptions. The idea of genetic inheritance is given diverse meanings by physicians who serve American Indians and by their patients. Unfortunately, providers and clients are often unaware of the different perceptions each have. Ethnographic data about perceptions of inheritance enhances an understanding of notions of diabetes and its causes. A broader view of this topic reveals that subtle and explicit cross-cultural misunderstandings are common to individuals and to topics of all sorts, consequently effecting associated prevention and treatment courses.

The words "genetics" and "inherited" are used frequently during discussions of diabetes. Due to the prevalence of Type 2 diabetes[2] among American Indians, Alaskan Natives, and Native Hawaiians, it is a common subject of communications between providers and their American Indian clients. The age-adjusted Indian Health Service diagnosed-diabetes prevalence rate for American Indians is 69 per 1,000,[3] whereas the overall U.S. rate is 24.7 per 1,000.[4] Results from the Strong Heart Study reveal that among Arizona American Indian participants, for example, the age-adjusted rates of Type 2 diabetes are 65 percent in men and 72 percent in women.[5] Thus diabetes is the second leading cause of outpatient visits to Indian Health Service facilities, after the common cold.

Of as much importance, diabetes is diagnosed by physicians (as opposed to laypersons or native diagnosticians and healers) with the aid of medical knowledge and technology. When confronted by this medical information and technology, laypeople rarely remain passive. They actively interpret and evaluate illnesses and treatments. Interpretations are greatly impacted by historical, social, linguistic, cultural, and educational factors as well as by the genders of providers and clients. Members of California and Arizona tribes whom I interviewed often explain inheritance as a part of biological, social, and cultural ethnic identity. Their providers define inheritance in a biological context. Multiple interpretations of a single concept by professional and laypeople alike may represent underlying disagreements about etiologies that in turn influence healthcare behaviors.

In my research, doctors, nurses, and physician assistants seemed stunned by clients' notions of diabetes causation. They were particularly surprised that native people interpreted "genetic inheritance" to have social and or learned aspects.

Clients are often unaware that medical professionals do not interpret inheritance in manners similar to their own. Importantly, geneticists themselves have multiple views of the relationships between genetics and particular medical conditions. Scientists create and negotiate competing perceptions due to institutional, political, and economic conditions. Nevertheless, notions of genes are perceived and presented by scientists and health professionals as "culture-free facts" rather than social constructs. Even though there exists "no fixed agreement" among biological scientists "about what a gene is and how genetic control works,"[6] information about genetics is passed to biomedical practitioners as if non-negotiable truth exists. Challenges to a particular scenario or theory concerning genetics will only occur if and when a competing alternative gains attraction.

Using the study of the terms "genetics" and "inherited" as an example, one can assess conditions of power and authority as part of cross-cultural communication processes. An analysis of the various interpretations of inheritance enables us to understand intricate constructions of diabetes etiologies. Examining doctor–patient communication about diabetes helps to account for offered, requested, and enacted treatment behaviors. At a macroanalytical level, this study investigates two scientific systems: professional and lay theories of etiological knowledge. These "two ways of knowing" are based on observations, empirical tests, and validated responses. Furthermore they are dynamic —based on paradigms that are influenced by ideas internal and external to the distinct knowledge systems.

To identify the ways doctors and American Indian patients define "genetics" and "inheritance," I will examine who creates particular definitions, what makes definitions persuasive or unconvincing, and the processes and factors that motivate people to develop, ignore, or act in particular understandings.

This analysis will aid in the establishment of a framework for assessing competing realities of biomedicine.

This chapter is based on six years of research on chronic-illness beliefs and behaviors among two Indian communities—one in southern California and one in southern Arizona (all names included are pseudonyms).

In the California study, 121 individuals between the ages of 18 and 91 years participated in face-to-face, open-ended interviews; 91 people were female. Thirty people (9 males and 21 females) claimed to have diabetes. These individuals were members of the same American Indian tribe, who resided on, or were enrollees of, three neighboring reservations. Data-collection techniques included a questionnaire, informal interviews, combined genealogical and medical-history maps, and participant observations.

In the Arizona study, 33 people between the ages of 45 and 71 years were informally interviewed. Seven were male. Three of these men and 17 of the women had diabetes. These individuals, who are members of the same tribe, were contacted through a tribal diabetes clinic for senior citizens that met weekly. In addition to conducting interviews, I participated in and observed clinic and senior-center activities two to three days per week for 13 months. Participants who did not have diabetes were contacted through senior-center events such as daily meals, arts and crafts, and exercise programs. Interviews were conducted in both English and Spanish. Frequently, one of two trilingual women would assist as interpreters for interviews that included the native language.

My observations of and informal interviews with medical providers from American Indian health programs in California (10 individuals) and Arizona (14 individuals) enabled me to garner data about practitioner and client communication practices. All of the providers from California are, or were, affiliated with one Indian Health Service contract-branch facility. Three of these practitioners were doctors, although none of these physicians were American Indian.

In contrast, all but 2 of 14 providers with whom I had contact in Arizona were American Indian. The two physicians were career Public Health Service doctors who have each had contact with the research population for several decades. These doctors are stationed at two separate Indian Health Service facilities in Arizona. Both doctors reportedly maintain social and medical service contacts with their former clients. Two other providers were associated with nonprofit health organizations that serve indigenous populations throughout the nation.

California

Members of the three California reservations live in a rural area that is approximately 60 miles from a metropolitan area. Most members 65 years of age and younger speak English in public. Although the majority of tribal members embrace the tenets of two religions, their Native religion and Catholicism, Christian Evangelical churches also attract congregants. Due to geographic remoteness, employment opportunities are often limited to seasonal and/or part-time tribal programs and businesses and local non-Indian operated services.

The diet of these people has changed drastically during a period of 200 years. The consumption of wild foods, including game, fish, nuts, fruits, and vegetables, was supplemented by horticultural and ranch practices through the early part of this century. Access to water and land for agricultural is currently quite limited. Since World War II, few people hunt, fish, or collect wild foods on a regular basis for personal consumption. However, household gardens of varying sizes are maintained by some individuals, especially retirees.

Historically, members of this ethnic group tended to attribute illness to accidents, sorcery, and the transgression of social rules, believing that reactions to events may occur instantaneously, or take place weeks, months, years, or generations later. The intentional or inadvertent social transgressions of kin of one generation could influence the health of an individual of a distinct or similar generation. Like many aspects of life, certain illnesses were considered to have mysterious etiologies and courses. The American Indian physician, John Molina, explains:

> Native American people are a spiritual people. Their lives have meaning and a purpose. Events are hardly ever random or accidental and many times warrant an interpretation. . . . Knowing the meaning of an illness may then guide the performance of a ritual or ceremony.[7]

The goal of most preventive and curative therapies performed by "Indian doctors," diagnosticians, and herbalists was to address the social, physiological, and emotional imbalance of a person and members of his/her social network.

In this view, contemporary analyses of health are often causal. These cause–effect linkages are frequently said to effect many acute and chronic health conditions. Some health problems have observable causes, while others do not. Similarly, some health situations may be traced to accidents or mysterious circumstances. Mystery may be perceived as a sacred, willful, and humanly uncontrollable power or object that may aid in the creation of social system violations. It is not uncommon to hear parents state that when a child cut her foot while bicycling without shoes, the child or her caretakers are deemed to be responsible for this injury. This episode is analyzed as a circumstance of visible causal relations. These same parents may also attribute this accident to the improper social behavior of the victim or her kin, or to mysterious causes.

People who are perceived to be mature are believed to consistently create and negotiate causal relationships. Each action may create a distinct reaction. An astute member of this tribe learns to make such connections throughout his/her life. Not everyone chooses to react in similar manners to a situation and distinct approaches mirror the actions of the primordial beings, or First People. Of great importance is the ability of an individual to make linkages of some sort.

Arizona

Unlike California, tribal members in Arizona reside on and near a "suburban" reservation—in close proximity to a city. Everyone interviewed spoke English and Spanish, and at least 11 of these individuals were trilingual, also speaking their Native language. Like their neighbors to the west, almost all the individuals from Arizona say that they practice both their Native and Catholic religions. Two exceptions are members of Protestant denominations. Senior-center clients tend to be retirees; they are almost all former agricultural, manufacturing, or domestic laborers.

These seniors often proclaim that their diets have changed little since their youth, although they report that more hunted meat was eaten in the past. Diets tended to consist of store-purchased foods and items grown in household gardens. The population density and size of this reservation seems to constrict individual or collective agricultural practices. Wild foods, such as cactus fruits, are still collected for personal use, and sometimes traded, given, or sold to other seniors.

Traditionally, members of this group shared many illness etiologies with tribal people interviewed in California. All illnesses had causes, and multiple etiologies were commonplace. Treatment was provided by lay individuals through prayer, ritual song, dance, vows, and/or herbs. Professional herbalists, divinely inspired healers, masseurs, saints, and guardian spirits also assisted the ill and members of their social networks. Health in all its facets was and continues to depend on familial support and care. According to senior-center clients, social, emotional, physical, or spiritual isolation greatly contributed and continues to contribute to unwellness.

Health-Care Resources

Both in California and in Arizona, tribal members have many treatment options. Most utilize medical providers associated with local community-operated programs and Indian Health Service facilities. People also seek the care of practitioners associated with Veterans' Affairs hospitals, urgent-care units, and private-practice physicians. In California, health maintenance organizations were also used. Often people also obtain assistance from laypersons, clergy, herbalists, masseurs, and/or "Indian doctors" or healers. People often utilize several health-care systems at once.

The Indian Health Service has operated a variety of diabetes-prevention projects throughout the United States since 1979. People with whom I had contact in California were able to receive care from an Indian Health Service contract-branch clinic operated by a consortium of reservations. This clinic offers dental, medical, social service, nutrition, psychological counseling, and pharmaceutical care.

In contrast, Arizona tribal members with whom I had contact had access to services operated by the tribal health department. The tribal health department employed nurses, social workers, psychologists, and community health workers. All other needs were referred to specified contract care facilities. These programs offer those with diabetes their only direct contact with doctors associated with the tribal health-care-delivery system.

Medical Perceptions of Inheritance, Genetics, and Diabetes

Basic scientific assumptions about "genetic inheritance" equate this idea with biological heredity. Yoxen asserts that constructions of biological heredity depend on the ability to

> perceive organisms both as individuals with distinct characteristics and as members of sets of like individuals. If all organisms were regarded as utterly distinct, or as similar in all essential respects, it would make little sense to try and explain patterns of resemblance between them.[8]

Other analysts view the body as divided into minuscule discrete parts rather than as a whole entity or a human being.[9] Genetic mechanisms serve as bodily codes or texts[10] that may be interpreted in distinct manners by different individuals. Various constructions of genetic diseases are continuously negotiated and described by groups of research specialists who offer their knowledge to clinicians. Information about genetics and associated conditions may be distributed in a variety of forms such as journal articles, videos, or educational forums. These interpretations are purportedly reassessed by clinicians and then dispersed to clients and sometimes members of their health- and social-support networks as scientific, value-free, and authoritative information.

From 1993 through 1995 the Indian Health Service distributed the *IHS Physician's Introduction to Type 2 Diabetes*[11] and its *Standards of Care* to diabetes-control officers and coordinators[12] in each of the 12 Indian Health Service Area offices.[13] In California, all Indian Health contract facilities are annually sent these items as well as patient-education curriculums.[14] According to one of the authors, this "concise booklet" was developed in order to: (1) familiarize providers with American Indian experiences of Type 2 diabetes; and (2) standardize diabetes treatment practices.[15] In California and throughout the nation, Indian Health Service staff attrition rates are relatively high with the average stay of doctors of approximately two years. The authors considered this book to be an orientation aid. Tribal health employees in Arizona, who are community members, claim to be unfamiliar with *IHS Physician's Introduction to Type 2 Diabetes*. Instead, they read *The Diabetes Forecaster*.

Based on 20 years of medical and epidemiological research with members of the Pima tribe of Arizona, the 1993 guide defines Type 2 or noninsulin-dependent diabetes mellitus (NIDDM) as a "genetic disorder characterized by insulin resistance and subsequent relative deterioration of insulin secretion. . . . Recent studies suggest that insulin resistance is inherited in a codominant fashion."[16] This information is linked to the "thrifty gene theory," embraced by the majority of Indian Health Service doctors and nurses.[17] Data also suggests that Arizona Pima may increase their risk of diabetes if the mother or both parents have diabetes, in addition to a personal high waist–hip circumference.[18]

The 1993 and 1995 *Indian Health Service Introduction to Type II Diabetes* both note that factors including obesity, age, family history, blood quantum, impaired glucose tolerance, and a parental or personal history of gestational diabetes purportedly increase an American Indian's risk of developing diabetes. In the 1993 *Physician's Guide*, genetic processes are represented as the central feature of this mixture. However, in the 1995 general providers' guide, "genetic tendency," "inactivity," "obesity," and "levels of insulin in blood" are listed as discrete factors that all aid in the development of insulin resistance.[19] Ideas about genetics and diabetes are partially updated through a packet distributed to physicians in California as part of their on-going "orientation." Some articles on the pathogenesis of diabetes decree the significance of genetic events.[20]

Providers' Explanations of Diabetes and Genetic Processes

Providers communicate American Indian genetic predilection to diabetes in two ways: through verbal interactions with clients and through the distribution of written materials. Although each facility has its own education programs and protocols, the *Physician's Guide* states that "it is very important that all health care providers have the same message for the patients."[21]

During a visit to the California clinic in 1996, I asked a physician to explain the relation between diabetes and genetic inheritance. This doctor said:

I usually say [to patients], if there's a lot of diabetes in the family, there is a predisposition to get it—that's genetic. [Through] dietary habits and care for one's self, they may never get it, but if they do, they can control it. The genetic part of it is—if a lot of family members have it the [clients] are more predisposed.

And obesity [has a role]. A couple of hundred years ago it was good to be able to put weight on in a hurry. It was good to have low metabolism. If a person had that ability, she could survive. The skinny ones died. It was good one hundred years ago, but not now, with unlimited fast food.[22]

This explanation demonstrates a linkage between genetics and what is often referred to in the Indian Health Service–sponsored literature as "environmental factors." Dietary habits are often felt to be especially critical by providers in California and Arizona who note the connection between obesity and the consumption of "carbohydrates," "sweets," and "fast foods" among their clients. According to practitioners in California and Arizona, this situation is exacerbated by limited exercise and physical activities performed by adults, especially women.

Physicians are requested by Indian Health Service diabetes-control officers and coordinators to inform their patients that "diabetes is a disorder in which the body is unable to use food properly." Requests are also made for providers to teach clients, among other things, the ways family members can prevent diabetes.[23] Apparently, no mention is made to providers to inform their clients that "diabetes is genetic" or that "diabetes is inherited genetically."

In addition to informing their patients verbally about diabetes, providers tend to distribute a variety of written materials that are generally in English and designed for national or regional distribution. These items are rarely developed for a particular ethnic, age, or language group. Pamphlets, flyers, and books are usually geared toward the fourth- or fifth-grade reading levels. The authors of these materials often link the onset of diabetes to food consumption and physical activity and topics focus on symptoms and/or treatment methods, such as food preparation and choice. Passages about diabetes etiologies are also included. *Diabetes and American Indians*,[24] found in clinics in Arizona and California, explains that diabetes "is mainly due to changes in eating and exercise" and is attributed to high blood sugar, which according to this text, "you are more likely to get . . . if you are heavy, . . . inactive, over age 30, have family members with high blood sugar, had high blood sugar during pregnancy." The booklet emphasizes that siblings and "children of people with diabetes tend to get high blood sugar."

Doctors, nurses, dieticians, and community health workers distribute other education tools with similar information. California providers whom I interviewed claim that they discuss the ideas expressed in these materials with their patients. During the few clinical encounters between health professionals and patients witnessed by the author, providers did not distribute written materials.

Nurses and community health workers in Arizona tended to distribute items during diabetes clinics. Sometimes information was discussed at the individual level, while at other times groups of 10 to 30 people were asked if they had any questions. In such situations, questions rarely arose from the participants. Similar scenarios occurred when guest speakers made health-care presentations one to two times per month. These talks rarely generated public inquiries. Instead, Native people saved their questions for post-presentation, either one-on-one or in small-group interactions.[25] For instance, a diabetes educator who is a member of this tribe made a presentation about the interaction between dietary practices and blood sugar levels. During and after the slide presentation lay audience members made comments such as "I love to eat squash." However, no questions were asked by the audience. Later, almost all the people in attendance approached this presenter and made inquiries about ways to obtain and prepare a variety of foods. This education communication method greatly varies from that used by Natives of California. The latter frequently make comments and inquiries during presentations.

Written health-education materials that I have seen circulated among American Indian laypeople do not use the term "genetic." Instead diabetes is reported to "run in families." The term "genetic" is used by some providers and is found in public health and medical literature. In these forms, "genetic" is a synonym for biological inheritance. Users of this social construct seem unaware that lay explanations of "genetic," like the term "inherited," encompass varied meanings.

Lay Explications of Genetics

Among Native people interviewed in California, diabetes is often reported to be genetic and/or inherited. In this vein, "genetic" or "inherited" refers to an object, idea, or condition that is passed between or within generations. Since interviews were open-ended and unstructured, not everyone discussed diabetes etiologies. Due to the nature of these interviews, people had the opportunity to discuss more than one cause of diabetes.

As in Arizona, members of this California tribe also may associate the onset of diabetes with weight gain,[26] collective dietary changes of the past century,[27] and/or alcohol consumption. Aging is thought to be a possible cause of diabetes by certain people interviewed in California.

Although several people in California claimed that pancreatic disruption is a function of diabetes, only one woman, a diabetic from Arizona, reported that her pancreatic malfunction caused her diabetes. Another person in Arizona

TABLE 7.1
LAY ETIOLOGIES OF DIABETES[28]

Causes of Diabetes	California Natives		Arizona Natives		Totals
	diabetics	*not diabetics*	*diabetics*	*not diabetics*	
weight gain	12	13	2	1	28
inheritance	11	33	5	2	51
emotions	1	1	1	1	4
aging	2	2	0	0	4
alcohol	4	8	0	1	13
diet	17	21	5	4	47
don't know	0	0	2	2	4
no response	0	0	2	0	2
pancreas	0	0	1	0	1
pollutants/pesticides	0	0	0	1	1
tumors	0	0	1	0	1

stated that pollutants contributed to diabetes. A daughter of a former cancer patient said that tumors caused diabetes. Only in Arizona did individuals assert that they did not know what caused diabetes. Two seniors from Arizona with diabetes did not respond to this question.

Diabetes was also attributed to emotional conditions. In California two people said that stress and depression, provoked by pressures to perform numerous activities, caused diabetes. In Arizona, two people claimed that stress, depression, frustration, and fears related to social isolation caused diabetes.

People from both states felt diabetes has multiple causes, including genetics and weight gain. Individuals from California mentioned five causes of diabetes, and people from Arizona noted eleven different causes, having relatively more idiosyncratic perspectives of diabetes causation. Table 7.1 shows the diversity of etiologies described by interviewed individuals from California and Arizona.

In California, the *biological* consequences of diabetes are frequently mentioned by laypeople with reference to genetics. Yet this term is confusing. A person may state during an interview, "diabetes is genetic," but within minutes the person may inquire, "what does 'genetic' mean?" The speaker will inevitably follow this question with the message that diabetes is, according to doctors, inherited. Indeed, four people who have diabetes and five people who do not have diabetes mentioned the biological transmission of this condition. Twenty-nine individuals, seven of whom are diabetic, as well as seven others from Arizona, feel that diabetes "runs more or less through families." On the surface, this view mimics that of the health-education materials, and in-depth interviews reveal a wealth of information on this notion. Some people propose that even if one ancestor has or had diabetes, this illness may be passed to members of the next generation, like a viral contagion spreading through the populace. Indeed, diabetes is sometimes called "contagious" because it may be "caught" from a family member. In this context, "contagious" refers to something that is easily passed from a person in one generation to an individual in the next generation.

Diabetes is also perceived to have a *social* basis for inheritance. Social lines are said to bind people between and across generations through blood, marriage, and adoption. In addition to those people who believe "diabetes runs in families," four people without diabetes note the relationship between familial ties and the advent of diabetes. The idea that "all [members of our tribe are] related somehow," suggests that "if one person has [diabetes], you're gonna get it." Diabetes is considered to be quite commonplace. Sometimes this condition is clustered among members of a social geography—other times diabetes appears to be scattered throughout the group. The transmission of this condition is linked to collective social ties.

These social aspects are represented by individual and communal perceptions of identity. Those individuals who believe that "to be Indian is to be diabetic" (to quote one man in California), assert a symbolic identification with American Indians throughout the nation, but more specifically with the collectivity of other tribal members. Ethnic relations become entwined not merely with physiological markers but also with invocations of distinct history, lineage,[29] and immersion into the nation-state.[30] One elder, Margaret, is the only one of nine siblings who does not have diabetes. She and many of her peers feel that diabetes is partially a result of being economically, politically, and socially dependent upon outsiders. Margaret claims the major problem, health or otherwise, among members of her reservation is

a lack of proper nutrition due to economics. If you only have three dollars in your pocketbook, you'll probably go buy potatoes and flour and maybe that will feed your family for five days.

I think [diabetes is] just a weakness of the system to me of digesting processed food. I think there's definitely ties to the modern times of packaged food. In my grandmother's time they were eating wild, they were eating rats, birds, they were eating possums, wild things. I think this was in the 1860s when they started bringing food and Indians were sent to the reservations.

In this perspective, the advent of diabetes is linked to communal dietary changes. Stories about the relationship between food, politics, and history are repeated during conversations among band members of different generations.

Social bonds concerning diabetes are partly framed by health circumstances that are delineated by medical providers who initially make diabetes diagnoses. If (as another person claims), "very few people here [on my reservation] can say they aren't diabetic," then issues of medicine, illness, and well-being perceptually link one person to another. These bonds are both infiltrated by and embrace changes in the health status of group members. For instance, those with diabetes may discontinue certain jobs such as farming and domestic service due to neuropathic damage. These same individuals may instead babysit grandchildren, nieces, and/or nephews. Households may expand or contract as chores shift. Modifications in employment, household responsibilities, and residence reflect the fluidity of these social networks.

The intergenerational transfer of diabetes purportedly also has *cultural* components. Interest in and taste for foods are said to be acquired by seven persons, three of whom have diabetes. Arizona seniors frequently agreed with this notion. Knowledge of diet and food preparation is also thought to be learned. In the California population, beef, potatoes, rice, tortillas, tacos, enchiladas, and "sweets" are all publicly acknowledged by those with diabetes as desired foods. Favored luxury food items reportedly include deer, rabbit, wood rat, acorn, and particular wild mushrooms. In Arizona some of the favorite foods of the interviewed seniors include wild spinach, flour tortillas, enchiladas, potatoes, beans, sodas, candies, and cakes. Foods such as jackrabbit and cactus fruits are also extremely well-liked, but sometimes difficult to obtain due to physical infirmities and collection restrictions. A frequent topic of conversation among women, especially, was their inability to obtain permits from federal, county, and intertribal agencies to collect wild foods. Political restrictions purportedly decrease access to desert fruits and nuts that often grow on lands other than those of the reservation.

The views of many men and women, nondiabetics and diabetics alike, are reiterated by one woman's description of diabetes:

> Bad food habits, I think that's what it is. They say it's inherited, right? You inherited it from your mother. Well, of course, you watched your mother cook and all the things she gave you to eat, and now you serve yourself that and the kids that. And they say it's inherited. Yes, it's inherited that way.

In this context, susceptibility to diabetes is learned from members of prior generations. One does not inherit diabetes per se, but rather one inherits the dietary habits that increase the possibility of developing diabetes. Teaching cultural knowledge is part of the pathway of diabetes. Elders pass down recipes, and youth use these recipes.

Four elders from one reservation discussed another "cultural factor" that purportedly contributes to the onset of diabetes. These two men and two women described the importance of serving food to guests and the demonstration of respect offered by guests who accept such food. Those with diabetes often find themselves in difficult situations. They do not want to feel physically sick by consuming certain foods, yet they do not wish to place themselves nor their hosts in cultural or spiritual jeopardy by refusing food. Earl, who has had diabetes for more than 25 years, remarked that even when "you stick to your diet, someone hands you a candy bar and you feel you can eat it, cause he *gave* it to me. You can eat a candy bar, but just a bite of it."

Gifts of food are offerings. To refuse food is insulting. Many other people taught me this lesson, but only these elders verbally linked this cultural more to the advent of diabetes.

The intergenerational distribution of knowledge is apparently one of the pathways of diabetes. Inheritance also involves biological and social modes. Importantly, these lay models of inheritance stress transmission from one person, or whole being, to the next. This view differs from that of the Mendelian slant, which describes the passage of coded messages created by and delivered to body parts. None of the providers with whom I spoke were aware of these multifold interpretations of inheritance by their clients. Clients' assumptions about inheritance apparently are not shared with providers.

Some Roots of Competing Realities

What might account for these seemingly subtle differences in understanding and expressing the transmission of diabetes? Numerous factors may contribute to belief systems; however, two interconnected possibilities are considered: health-care communication practices and education approaches.

Communication Practices

Many sociolinguists have noted the differences between physician and client communication practices. Providers and their clients tend to form two speech communities. Agreement on the interpretations of words and on associated social values may be limited. This disagreement may be due in part to the marginalization of social contexts during patient–provider interactions. Discussions between providers and patients about food preferences and preparations may occur, although talk about associated cultural meanings and behaviors may be absent.

In some cases, efforts may be made to incorporate cultural information into a medical encounter. One non-Indian physician from California suggested to a diabetic patient, Joy, that she attempt to lose weight by forgoing some of the food on her plate. "In your tradition," he remarked, "you leave some [food], a little offering, you don't have to lick your plate clean." Interestingly, Joy, who was in her mid-seventies, countered this statement, responding that this task was "kind of hard after all these meals and years." Joy was not asked why she considered this approach to be difficult. The provider assumed that his understandings of local cultural practices might be a means to solve a problem; however, the cause of the problem, as defined by the patient, remains unclear. In this way, the patient's thoughts are disregarded by the earnest attempts of this physician to include his perceptions of local cultural practices into the medical encounter.

Bewilderment on the part of both parties may exist as a result of conversational flow. Medical practitioners generally control information exchange through their manipulation of topic shifts.[31] Prior studies reveal that during medical-speech events women and ethnic minorities rarely direct the flow of communication.[32] When a patient's speech is interrupted by a provider's topic shift, there may be two consequences. First, like Joy, the view of the patient may be neglected, thus eliminating what the patient may perceive as useful information. Second, topic shifts, especially relatively rapid ones, may disrupt the ability of a patient to explicate an idea or term, such as "genetics," posed by a physician. Confusion may be increased if the provider and patient do not speak the same native language.

According to lay individuals, miscommunications occur when unfamiliar terms are not clarified, diagnoses are not precise, and details are not offered. "Sometimes," one woman explained, "you have to go look up terms in the dictionary or ask [another] person." Physicians, even when attempting to translate medical jargon into lay terms, have a tendency to frame their ideas in complex professional language. In some cases, terms are understood by participants in a dialogue, but topics are incongruent. At other times, similar vocabulary may be used, such as the word "inherited," but meanings are not shared.[33] If participants in a speech event are unaware of linguistic and cultural differences or methods to mend splits, disjunctures will continue.

Physicians in California reported to me that they often ask clients if they understand what is being taught. One doctor relates that after his explanations, he often requests clients to state in their words what he has said. Frequently blank stares are the response. Unfortunately, even if patients understand directives, providers may not be able to interpret silence or gazes made by clients. Silence may mean many different things. As used by local elders, silence may represent agreement with a statement, or it may reflect utter confusion. Health-care practitioners may also not recognize that comprehension of treatment directives by clients does not infer mutual understanding of underlying meanings of cause or therapy.

If a client is stumped by the ideas of a provider, the hierarchical nature of their relationship may sway clients from making inquiries. To do so might displease the practitioner.[34] Among many California and Arizona Indians, it is considered improper behavior to question people directly who offer knowledge and assistance.[35] However, according to many interviewed Californians about 50 years of age and older,[36] it is deemed appropriate to ask questions to garner precise explanations about information offered by practitioners. This situation reflects the status attained by these older persons.

Historically, California and Arizona Indians rarely expected an egalitarian relationship with their providers. Healers and Indian doctors of tribes in California and Arizona were considered and continue to be thought to have distinct expert knowledge[37] through which they direct the health-care encounter. Verbal input, especially in the form of patient inquiries or challenges, may be frowned upon or considered culturally irrational by clients. Even though power may not be evenly distributed in this relationship, providers and patients shared and continue to shape broad cultural knowledge, language, and associated goals. Medical personnel who have "earned power" through evidence of training, diagnosis, and healing will also frequently be accorded politeness behaviors that often include client silence and reticence. Individuals in Arizona often reiterate the ideas of one woman who, describing herself and her friends, says, that they have "trust in the doctors and the pills and shots for diabetes."[38] Trust and confidence are established and maintained through provider demonstrations of efficacious care, not necessarily through verbal skills. This stance may reflect shared health-care objectives but divergent linguistic and cultural orientations, whereby clients entrust their bodies to others in order to alleviate suffering.

Professional Health Education

The construction of competing realities may be due to the separate reasoning and language methods that professional and lay individuals employ. These approaches are effected by informal and formal education. Indian Health Service providers have undergone years of medical training in which the culture of biomedicine is espoused and ingrained. Through observation, interaction, memorization, and discussion, medical students learn medical categorizations. Bodily parts, functions, and conditions are classified through sequenced lists and contrastive modes.[39] This education enables students and providers to develop images and associated contexts to which lay individuals are rarely privy.

In clinical practice, doctors and other health professionals have access to jargon and data that is perpetually updated in relation to new medical procedures, technologies, and research. Physicians report that they draw upon medical literature and their experiences as both providers and as possible patients throughout the course of their training and practices in order to enhance their practices.[40] Unique experiences lead to varied interpretations, insights, and guidance. Four doctors who participated in interviews, two of whom are of American Indian descent, are career Public Health Service physicians. They use the knowledge gained from their work with members of other tribal and rural communities to care for their patients. In fact, these doctors may be unique in that three of them have traveled and worked throughout the United States and other nations. Experiences and interpretations of cultural, social, and medical variation expand the knowledge bases of these doctors who use this information to resolve clinical problems.[41]

All of the providers interviewed perceived socioeconomic conditions as partial influences upon diabetes-treatment approaches. They frequently cited poverty, limited infrastructural resources, household size and density, and substance abuse among community members as factors that may effect the health of an individual. I did not observe health literature or talk directed toward clients that focused on socioeconomic, cultural, or historical conditions.

Practitioners may be able to grasp and empathize with some client language and cultural beliefs, including agreement on diagnoses and the utility of a therapy. However, the ability to switch between professional and lay languages does not infer that all underlying meanings will be expressed or shared.[42] This situation may reflect the ability of medical workers to learn parts of lay health languages, without having full immersion in such. Some of these providers have, as Lave and Wegner note, learned to talk about a subject but not within a subject. This mode may unwittingly increase the transmission of skewed information by speakers.[43]

Lay Health Education

Lay health-care training about diabetes may take many forms. In addition to interactions with medical practitioners, some lay people claim to read popular and Public Health literature. Others obtain information from radio and/or television programs, forums, and conferences on diabetes. The most common educational method is discussion with and observations of extended family members, neighbors, and members of their tribe. In particular, conversations with and observations of diabetics who have visible symptoms are reported to be a major source of pertinent information. These individuals become teachers.[44]

Pieces of information garnered over a number of years mixed with common-sense cultural knowledge generally forms the experiential model of lay individuals.[45] This model includes empirical evidence noted by laypersons. Among individuals in California, diabetes information is generally requested to solve particular problems like "dizziness" or "the shakes."[46] Personal therapeutic approaches are then created or this knowledge is integrated with previously obtained information. People who do not have diabetes tend to acquire knowledge about diabetes during conversations with and through observations of diabetics.

Apparently data about the acquisition of diabetes is offered by providers without requests by clients. In California, only one person with diabetes interviewed stated that she initiated a conversation with a biomedical provider concerning the causes of diabetes. Nevertheless, physicians offer etiological information in the context of treatment descriptions. The apparent objective is to link the cause of diabetes to its control, much in the same vein as in the literature, so that patients may be more easily persuaded to pursue a particular treatment approach.

In the case of diabetes etiologies, doctors often employ physiological explanations while laypeople describe life events that might have made him/her the target of an illness.[47] As Jennie Joe has stated, providers frequently offer mechanistic data about *how* diabetes may develop, while patients and family often describe causal information regarding *why* diabetes develops.[48] Both types of explanations are rooted in the distinct cultures of the speakers. Providers initiate discussions of genetics and inheritance as vehicles for care options. Patients and their family members address genetics and inheritance as part of personal, collective, and cultural stories and histories.

Lay understandings of technological and medical terms may be incongruent with scientific meanings if the ideas have no strong foundation in daily experiences.[49] As was aptly noted by a participant in Emily Martin's study of the immune system, laypeople are not included in the conversations of scientists.[50] Thus, many people reinterpret ideas based on historical and cultural experiences.[51]

Inheritance may have biological, social, and cultural components because interpretations of these terms are based on lived experiences. Coupled with statistical and observational evidence that as one person claims, "diabetes is an Indian disease," diabetes and its causes are, not surprisingly, linked to local histories and cultures. In this perspective, diabetes is an illness that members of a group may have, share, discuss, teach, and live; it is not merely a biological condition influenced by social features.

Conclusion

These differences in perceptions espoused by providers and their American Indian clients are due *in part* to attempts by health professionals to assert authoritative control. According to B. Jordan, authoritative knowledge, frequently disseminated by those who control a dominant power base, is considered to be information that is objective, convincing, natural, official, notable, and consensually constructed.[52] Providers argue that biological explications of genetics and inheritance are the foundations of diabetes causation theories and treatment approaches. Genes and the environment create problems for bodies of individuals. Providers appear to propose such arguments for altruistic purposes, and the health professionals, believing in their version of truth, feel that patients will be healthier if they understand the causes of their illnesses.

Laypeople develop alternative models of diabetes causation, thereby partially revamping medical control of health-care knowledge. In some cases, people appear to accept the views of their providers. In other cases, clients seem actively to resist and reinterpret ideas espoused by medical practitioners. In still other situations, lay and professional people have translation problems. Breakdowns in the communication process encourage both providers and patients to create and adhere to separate truths. Laypeople think and act in a variety of manners. When lay individuals try to understand "genetics" and "inheritance," they give expert knowledge legitimacy but not complete authority.

Providers may attempt, though not always successfully, to render their knowledge authoritatively to clients. Indian Health Service diabetes researchers, control officers, and coordinators distribute data about Type 2 diabetes, presenting it as value free, official, facts. As the Indian Health Service declares, all providers are to deliver similar messages concerning the etiology of diabetes. Practitioners tend to disseminate etiological descriptions as produced and disseminated by the Indian Health Service. Providers who discuss the terms "genes" and "genetics" with patients may be, in a way, quite individualistic in a bureaucratic system. Whether or not these communication approaches are truly isolated remains to be clarified by additional research.

Diabetes is a medicalized condition. It is an illness that is labeled, defined, diagnosed, and treated by medical professionals. In their efforts to explain diagnoses, prognoses, and treatments to clients, Indian Health Service providers must intellectually and physically mediate the relationships between technology and bodies.[53] A hierarchical arrangement certainly exists whereby patients are offered parcels of information to aid them to control blood sugar levels and associated metabolic conditions. However, the providers in this project seemed willing to share additional knowledge with their clients. The former are willing to answer questions, and the author has witnessed that they will occasionally negotiate therapies. Providers rely on patients' views and behaviors as guides in the management of therapies. Perhaps due to their training,[54] these providers seem not to realize that some clients wish to participate in therapeutic decisions.

The hierarchical nature of diabetes care becomes compounded by verbal impasses. Health-care professionals are prone to using technical language, which obscures causes and associated solutions, thereby consciously or unconsciously exerting the need for additional technical and expert assistance.[55] Control is thus exerted, even though it may be expressed in an empathetic or friendly manner.

Lay responses to diabetes etiologies are diverse. Etiological sources are based upon technological screenings, the results of which are used by providers for diagnoses. Clients and the general health-service population tend to consider technological data to be reliable and authoritative.[56] For instance, urine and blood tests that reveal diagnoses are rarely doubted. Only one person interviewed refuted a medical diagnosis of diabetes. Months later this test, done in a local hospital, was also rebuked by Indian Health Service contract personnel. Nevertheless, clients, especially in California, counter the absolute influence of authoritative knowledge concerning diabetes causation through the creation of parallel or opposing knowledge. They cast doubt upon and, at times, redefine medical expertise. People interviewed in California in particular, actively and consciously produce, validate, and distribute ethnically and culturally based etiologies. Ideas about inheritance are reshaped in an effort to demystify the talk of medical professionals.

Perceptions of inheritance are embedded in individual and collective genealogies and culture.[57] Indeed, both California and Arizona Indians tend to incorporate and reshape ideas and behaviors to fit into their lives and social identity. Personal and group dynamics of cultural historical, political, and ethnic relations are reflected and, at times, forged.[58] This turn of events may illustrate community efforts to demystify and gain ownership of information and care.[59] Unlike the mainly middle-class participants in cancer and AIDS advocacy movements, Indian Health Service clients (even those whose facilities are managed by tribal representatives) have little political, social, or economic clout on health-care treatment protocols. However, assertions of locally and ethnically based social knowledge, intellect, and history provide a basis for ownership of the illness, the etiology, and the treatment.

Lave and Wegner explain that individuals create identities that are influenced by participation in a community of practice. People obtain the abilities to exchange information: (1) about a topic or practice; and (2) within the topic or practice. With the latter, a person acquires, through stories and community lore, ways to engage, focus, and coordinate approaches of communal memory, reflection, signals, and membership.[60] Similarly to medical students involved in schooling,[61] those laypeople that I interviewed are all participants in a communal understanding of diabetes. People gain a form of ownership, not merely as "people who have diabetes" or relatives thereof, but as those who create, shape, and comprehend local and shared views of etiologies. For certain individuals, from these ideas of causation, theories of treatment are established and/or understood. For some, the situation may resolve a frustration with the inability to control or cure their diabetes.[62] And, if biomedical experts can not cure diabetes, why should they have intellectual ownership over this condition? As one elder, Margaret, suggested, ideas about diabetes may be based on social interactions between members of her ethnic group partly because medical resources can only alleviate problems—they can not resolve them. Margaret maintained:

> I think that there's so much of [diabetes] it's not unusual for someone to
> come across another and say, "How are you?"

"You know I've got diabetes."

And they're young, maybe in the twenties. . . .

Myself, I don't go to the doctor and how would I typically say that? 'Cause I'm not interest in suppressing symptoms. Now if I crushed the tip of my finger here and it wasn't gonna work anymore I'd go to the doctor and have him cut it off or do whatever had to be done. I'd always do that, but I wouldn't be interested in having it hang there and take pain killers and aspirins and stuff that's going to—it's still there, but it's not cured.

I think maybe that's the part that hasn't convinced my people: they're not cured. But you could go to some wise person, and there's a lot of people that just talk to one another and minister to their mind and let them know they're all right and yet they could feel well. . . . I think the experience [with doctors' treatments of diabetes] is pretty well repetitious and . . . I don't think [my relatives] really see any hope of change.[63]

Lay explanations expand upon the medical sphere, but people can only negotiate data to which they are exposed. L. Garro and G. C. Lang contend that most of the individuals in their diabetes studies were "well informed about standard medical explanations."[64] Perhaps due in part to the prevalence of diabetes among American Indians, individuals seem willing to participate in medical discourse. Indeed, American Indian people in California pride themselves on their abilities to negotiate cross-cultural information and their associated meanings and behaviors. Remarks about etiologies are often made in assured and declarative tones. In contrast, in Arizona, a sense of bewilderment was common when discussing diabetes etiologies. Several seniors commented that they rarely ask their providers to explain confusing terms or ideas. I have observed that in group settings, health-care inquiries tend to be made only in the hearing of adopted or biological relatives. As Clifford Trafzer notes, these individuals may not wish to expose their ignorance to a doctor or to anyone else.[65] Perhaps for this reason, one woman claimed that "we all have diabetes and we don't even know where it comes from."

Some people may actively resist or reinterpret the beliefs of medical providers. As often, lay individuals do not understand the language, ideology, and culture of providers.[66] The former thus explicate and expand upon terms and ideas. However, technical knowledge that is not directly and observably tied to efficacious diabetes screening and care is not necessarily equated with fact or with authoritative information. Limited access to scientific and medical discourse through literature, lecture, and conversation obstructs public understandings of medical constructs of genetics and inheritance.[67] Communication becomes disrupted when sociocultural knowledge and linguistic tactics are not shared.[68] Clearly, those interviewed in Arizona are restricted participants in medical discourse. The case of genetics and inheritance partially represents an error in translation. Within this context, ideas about genetics may be a consequence of diverse realities but not of realities in competition for authority.

Significantly, although this chapter has been focused on "genetics" and "inheritance," other concepts and terms that providers and clients use are often confusing to participants in health-care encounters. Discourse about diabetes and its etiologies embraces more than one language and system of knowledge. Both the professional and lay perspectives have truths based on "scientific" observations and trial-and-error experiments. Neither perspective is culture-free and a key to understanding treatment objectives and courses relies on this "fact."

Notes

1. I am deeply indebted to all those individuals who participated in my research projects in southern California and southern Arizona. Special thanks to Susan Coutin, Annette Busby, and Mark Luborsky for their editorial comments. This chapter is based on anthropology field studies and writing financially supported by the following agencies: the American Association of University Women; the University of California Psychocultural Studies Program; the Institute of American Cultures; and the University of Arizona Health Sciences Center, Arizona Prevention Center.

2. Prior to July 1997 this condition was classified as Type II or non-insulin dependent diabetes mellitus. For additional information see, Anonymous, "New Recommendations for the Diagnosis and Classification of Diabetes Mellitus," *IHS Primary Care Provider* 22(8) (August 1997): 121–22.

3. This rate does not include individuals who chose not to use Indian Health Service facilities, people who have not received a medical diagnosis, nor members of tribes that are not federally recognized.

4. Dorothy Gohdes. "Diabetes in North American Indians and Alaska Natives," in National Diabetes Data Group, eds., *Diabetes in America* (Rockville, MD: National Institutes of Health, 1995).

5. Elisa Lee et al., "Diabetes and Impaired Glucose Tolerance in Three American Indian Populations Aged 45–74 Years: The Strong Heart Study." *IHS Primary Care Provider* 20(8) (1995): 97–109.

6. Max Charlesworth et al., *Life among the Scientists: An Anthropological Study of an Australian Scientific Community*, 49–51; see also Rayna Rapp, "Accounting for Amniocentesis," in Shirley Lindenbaum and Margaret Lock, eds., *Knowledge, Power, and Practice: The Anthropology of Medicine and Everyday Life* (Berkeley: University of California Press, 1993), 55–79.

7. John Molina, "Cultural Medicine," *Journal of Minority Medical Students* (spring 1997): 32.

8. Edward Yoxen, "Constructing Genetic Diseases," in Peter Wright and Andrew Treacher, eds., *The Problem of Medical Knowledge: Examining the Social Construction of Medicine* (Edinburgh: Edinburgh University Press, 1982), 145.

9. Ruth Hubbard and Elijah Wald, *Exploding the Gene Myth* (Boston: Beacon Press, 1993).

10. Max Charlesworth et al., *Life among the Scientists: An Anthropological Study of an Australian Scientific Community*, 41.

11. Indian Health Service Headquarters Diabetes Program, *IHS Physician's Introduction to Type 2 Diabetes* (Albuquerque: Indian Health Service, 1993).

12. A control officer is someone who operates an Indian Health Service Area program, whereas a coordinator manages a designated diabetes model program.

13. The *IHS Physician's Introduction to Type 2 Diabetes* was updated in 1995 as a guide for health-care providers; much like the earlier guide, the recent version emphasizes the differences between Type I and Type 2 diabetes as well as criteria for diagnosing and managing the latter among American Indians.

14. Kathy Kobus, personal communication (October 1996).

15. Beth Dabrant, personal communication (November 1996).

16. Indian Health Service Headquarters Diabetes Program, *IHS Physician's Introduction to Type 2 Diabetes* (Albuquerque: Indian Health Service Headquarters Diabetes Program, 1993), 2.

17. J. V. Neel, "Diabetes Mellitus: A 'Thrifty' GenoType Rendered Detrimental by 'Progress'?" *American Journal of Human Genetics* 14(1962): 3091; J. V. Neel, *The Thrifty GenoType Revisited: The Genetics of Diabetes Mellitus*, J. Koebelerling and R. Tattersall, eds. (New York: Academic Press, 1982); E. Benjamin et al., "Exercise and Incidence of NIDDM among Zuni Indians," *Diabetes* 42(suppl. 1) (1993): 203A; W. C. Knowler, et al., "Determinants of Diabetes Mellitus in the Pima Indians," *Diabetes Care* 16(1) (1993): 216–27; K. Weiss et al., "Diabetes Mellitus in American Indians: Characteristics, Origins and Preventive Health Care Implications," *Medical Anthropology* 11 (1989): 283–99.

18. M. Prochazka et al., "Linkage of Chromosomal Markers on 4q with a Putative Gene Determining Maximal Insulin Action in Pima Indians," *Diabetes* 42 (1993): 514–19; Peter Bennett, "Non-Insulin Dependent Diabetes Mellitus and Its Complications," Third International Conference on Diabetes and Indigenous Peoples: Theory, Reality, Hope. Winnipeg, Canada, 1995.

19. Beth Dabrant, Kelly Acton, and Bernadine Tolbert, *IHS Introduction to Type 2 Diabetes* (Albuquerque: IHS Diabetes Program, 1995), 3.

20. Hannele Yki-Järvinen, "Pathogenesis of Noninsulin-Dependent Diabetes Mellitus." *Lancet* 343 (1994): 91.

21. Indian Health Service Headquarters Diabetes Program, *IHS Physician's Introduction to Type 2 Diabetes* (Albuquerque: Indian Health Service Headquarters Diabetes Program, 1993), 5. The revised edition expands upon this theme. The authors state that "every facility should work towards providing systematic mechanisms to make culturally-relevant self-care information available for patients." Dabrant et al. (1995), 21.

22. Diane Weiner, field notes, 1996.

23. Indian Health Service, *Indian Health Service Basic Series Diabetes Curriculum* (Rockville, MD: Public Health Service, 1996).

24. Portland Area Indian Health Service Diabetes Program, *Diabetes and American Indians* (Bellingham, WA: Indian Health Service, 1987).

25. These "small groups" tended to consist of luncheon-table groupings that were basically rigid. Groupings of biological and social kin sat at the same tables during

almost every visit to the senior center. About a half-dozen individuals seemed to move from table to table without social compunction. Presenters who visited table groupings were asked questions by the seniors.

26. See also L. Garro and G. C. Lang, "Explanations of Diabetes: Anishinaabeg and Dakota Deliberate Upon a New Illness," in Jennie Joe and Robert Young, eds., *Diabetes as a Disease of Civilization: The Impact of Lifestyle and Cultural Changes on the Health of Indigenous Peoples* (Berlin: Mouton de Gruyter, 1994), 293–328; and Maryjane Ambler, "Dine College Students Research Diabetes for Their People," *Tribal College* 11 (fall 1999): 18–20.

27. See also Joan Marie Roche, *Sociocultural Aspects of Diabetes in an Apache-Choctaw Community* (Ann Arbor, MI: University Microfilms International, 1982); Garro and Lang, "Explanations of Diabetes," in Joe and Young, eds., *Diabetes as a Disease of Civilization*; Benjamin Kracht, "Diabetes among the Kiowa: An Ethnohistorical Perspective," in Joe and Young, eds., *Diabetes as a Disease of Civilization*, 147–68.

28. This table does not include data on gestational or Type I diabetes.

29. Fredrik Barth, "Introduction" in Fredrik Barth, ed., *Ethnic Groups and Boundaries* (Boston: Little, Brown, and Company, 1969).

30. See also Mathew C. Snipp, "The Changing Political and Economic Status of the American Indians: From Captive Nations to Internal Colonies," *American Journal of Economic and Sociology* 45(2) (1986): 143–55; Eric Wolf, *Europe and the People without History* (Berkeley: University of California Press, 1982).

31. Robert Hahn, *Sickness and Healing: An Anthropological Perspective* (New Haven, CT: Yale University Press, 1995); H. B. Beckman and R. Frankel, "The Effect of Physician Behavior on the Collection of Data," *Annals of Internal Medicine* 101 (1984): 692–96; Candace West, ed., *Routine Complications: Troubles with Talk between Doctors and Patients* (Bloomington: Indiana University Press, 1984).

32. Alexandra Dundas Todd, "Exploring Women's Experiences: Power and Resistance in Medical Discourse," in Dundas Todd and Fisher, eds., *The Social Organization of Doctor–Patient Communication*, 2d ed. (Norwood, NJ: Ablex Publishing, 1993), 267–85.

33. See also Veronica Evaneshko, "Presenting Complaints in a Navajo Indian Diabetic Population," in Joe and Young, eds., *Diabetes as a Disease of Civilization*, 357–78.

34. See also Dianna Garcia-Smith, "The Gila River Diabetes Prevention Model," in Joe and Young, eds., *Diabetes as a Disease of Civilization*, 471–94.

35. See also Tamar Kaplan, "An Intercultural Communication Gap: North American Indians versus the Mainstream Medical Professions," in Walburga von Raffler-Engel, ed., *Doctor–Patient Interaction* (Belgium: John Benjamins, 1989): 45–59. In a study of Midwestern urban and rural patients, 60 percent were found to want an active role in medical decision-making, yet only 47 percent of patients claimed to have challenged the ideas or recommendations of their doctors. M. R. Haug B. Lavin, "Practitioner or Patient—Who Is in Charge?" *Journal of Health and Social Behavior* 22 (1981): 212–29.

36. Individuals interviewed both in California and Arizona who are or have been cancer patients or who are in the field of education also tend to feel at ease making inquiries.

37. Lowell John Bean, "Power and Its Applications in Native California," in Lowell John Bean and Thomas Blackburn, eds., *Native Californians: A Theoretical Perspective* (Socorro, NM: Ballena Press, 1976), 407–20; Lowell John Bean and Sylvia Brakke Vane, "California Religious Systems and Their Transformations," in Lowell John Bean, ed., *California Indian Shamanism* (Menlo Park, CA: Ballena Press, 1992), 33–51.

38. This view is shared by others in Arizona and California who frequently contend that diabetes is a relatively new ailment mainly diagnosed and treated by physicians. Other studies reveal similar views. See Martin Hickey and Jannette Carter, "Cultural Barriers to Delivering Health Care: The Non-Indian Provider Perspective" and Garro and Lang, "Explanations of Diabetes," in Joe and Young, eds., *Diabetes as a Disease of Civilization*; and Scott Camazine, "Traditional and Western Health Care among the Zuni Indians of New Mexico," *Social Science and Medicine* 14B (1980): 73–80.

39. Byron Good and Mary-Jo Del Vechio Good, "'Learning Medicine': The Constructing of Medical Knowledge at Harvard Medical School," in Shirley Lindenbaum and Margaret Lock, eds., *Knowledge, Power, and Practice: The Anthropology of Medicine and Everyday Life* (Berkeley: University of California Press, 1993).

40. See also Hahn, *Sickness and Healing*.

41. Ibid., 151; see also E. Friedson, *The Profession of Medicine* (New York: Dodd, Mead, 1970), 170.

42. Anne Burson-Toplin, "Fracturing the Language of Biomedicine: The Speech Play of U.S. Physicians," *Medical Anthropology Quarterly* 3(3) (1989): 283–93; Cecil Helman, "Communication in Primary Care: The Role of Patient and Practitioner Explanatory Models," *Social Science and Medicine* 20 (1985): 923–31; Kathleen Huttlinger et al., "'Doing Battle': A Metaphorical Analysis of Diabetes Mellitus among Navajo People," *American Journal of Occupational Therapy* 46(8) (1992): 706–11.

43. Jean Lave and Etienne Wegner, *Situated Learning: Legitimate Peripheral Participation* (New York: Cambridge University Press, 1991), 109.

44. Ibid., 95.

45. See also Cecil Helman, *Culture, Health and Illness: An Introduction for Health Professionals*, 2d ed. (Boston: Wright Publishers, 1990); Arthur Kleinman, *Patients and Healers in the Context of Culture* (Berkeley: University of California Press, 1980); Hahn, *Sickness and Healing*.

46. See also L. J. Benett, "What Do People with Diabetes Want to Talk about with Their Doctors?" *Clinical Practice* (1993), 968–71.

47. Linda Hunt, Miguel A. Valenzuela, and Jacqueline A. Pugh, "¿Porque Me Tocó a Mí? Mexican-American Diabetes Patients' Causal Stories and Their Relationship to Treatment Behaviors," unpublished manuscript (1997), 6.

48. Jennie Joe, "Sociocultural Factors in Diagnosis and Treatment," in Jennie Joe and Robert Young, eds., *NIDDM and Indigenous Peoples: Proceedings of the Second International Conference on Diabetes and Native Peoples* (Tucson: Native American Research and Training Center, 1993), 47–49.

49. See Hickey and Carter, "Cultural Barriers to Delivering Health Care," 613.

50. Emily Martin, *Flexible Bodies: The Role of Immunity in American Culture From the Days of Polio to the Age of AIDS* (Boston: Beacon Press, 1994), 180. See also Rapp,

"Accounting for Amniocentesis," in Lindenbaum and Lock, eds., *Knowledge, Power, and Practice*.

51. See also, Joseph Kaufert and John O'Neil, "Biomedical Rituals and Informed Consent: Native Canadians and the Negotiation of Clinical Trust," in G. Weisz, ed., *Social Science Perspectives on Medical Ethics* (The Netherlands: Kluner Academic Press, 1990); Libett Crandon, "Medical Dialogue and the Political Economy of Medical Pluralism: A Case from Rural Highland Bolivia," *American Ethnologist* 13(3) (1986): 463–76.

52. See Brigitte Jordan, "Cosmopolitical Obstetrics: Some Insights from the Training of Traditional Midwives," *Social Science and Medicine* 28(9) (1989): 925–44; Brigitte Jordan, *Birth in Four Cultures: A Cross-Cultural Investigation of Childbirth in Yucatan, Holland, Sweden and the United States*, 4th ed. (Prospect Heights, IL: Waveland Press, 1993[1978]), 154.

53. See Monica S. Casper and Marc Berg, "Introduction to Special Issue: Constructivist Perspectives on Medical Work: Medical Practices and Science and Technology Studies," *Science, Technology, and Human Values* 20(4) (1995): 395–407.

54. Arthur Kleinman asserts that physicians are taught to consider the illness narratives and causal beliefs of clients with skepticism. Arthur Kleinman, *The Illness Narratives: Suffering, Healing, and the Human Condition* (New York: Basic Books, 1988), 17.

55. See Yoxen, "Constructing Genetic Diseases," in Wright and Treacher, eds., *The Problem of Medical Knowledge*.

56. See also Carole H. Browner and Nancy Press, "The Production of Authoritative Knowledge in American Prenatal Care," *Medical Anthropology Quarterly* 10 (1996): 141–56.

57. Garro and Lang, "Explanations of Diabetes," in Joe and Young, eds., *Diabetes as a Disease of Civilization*, 294.

58. See also Crandon, "Medical Dialogue and the Political Economy of Medical Pluralism"; and Kaufert and O'Neil, "Biomedical Rituals and Informed Consent."

59. See also Susan Di Giacomo, "Biomedicine as a Cultural System: An Anthropologist in the Kingdom of the Sick," in Hans A. Baer, ed., *Encounters with Biomedicine: Case Studies in Medical Anthropology* (Philadelphia: Gordon & Breach, 1987), 316; Steven Epstein, "The Construction of Lay Expertise: AIDS Activism and the Forging of Credibility in the Reform of Clinical Trials," *Science, Technology, and Human Values* 20(4) (1995): 408–37.

60. Lave and Wegner, *Situated Learning*, 109. See also, Aaron Cicourel, "Hearing Is Not Believing: Language and the Structure of Belief in Medical Communication," in Dundas Todd and Fisher, eds., *The Social Organization of Doctor–Patient Communication*, 64.

61. Hahn, *Sickness and Healing*, 157–58.

62. Kleinman, *The Illness Narratives*, 44, 48.

63. Diane Weiner, field notes, 1990–1993.

64. Garro and Lang, "Explanations of Diabetes," in Joe and Young, eds., *Diabetes as a Disease of Civilization*, 321.

65. Clifford Trafzer, personal communication, January 1998.

66. See also Epstein, "The Construction of Lay Expertise"; and L.M.L. Ong et al.,

"Doctor–Patient Communication: A Review of the Literature," *Social Science and Medicine* 40(7) (1995): 903–18.

67. Rapp, "Accounting for Amniocentesis," in Lindenbaum and Lock, eds., *Knowledge, Power, and Practice*, 73.

68. John Gumperz, "The Retrieval of Sociocultural Knowledge in Conversation," in John Baugh and Joel Sherzer, eds., *Language and Use* (Englewood Cliffs, NJ: Prentice-Hall, 1984), 129.

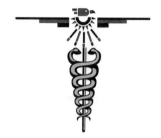

The Embodiment of a Working Identity

POWER AND PROCESS IN RARÁMURI RITUAL HEALING[1]

In a recent essay, Csordas and Kleinman call for studies that develop an analytic of *power* in conjunction with the examination of healing as *process*.[2] I take their directives seriously in this case study of ritual healing among the Tarahumara—or Rarámuri as they call themselves—an indigenous people in northern Mexico. I am concerned with examining the process whereby power is restored to a patient through the gradual embodiment of a working identity, that is, an identity that manifests a normative and corporeal self, capable of participating with others in the everyday give-and-take of society.

On the one hand, Csordas and Kleinman urge describing the "connection among therapeutic, political, and spiritual power in both the practice of healers and the experience of the afflicted." They recommend a method that strives to recognize "distinctions among healing as a form or reinforcement of oppression, healing as a[n] . . . attempt to address the misery of poverty and powerlessness, and healing as a mode of empowerment wherein small changes can mean the difference between effective coping and defeat." While an examination of the structures of power are significant, they go on to say: "Perhaps more important than any other principle for guiding research is the observation that the therapeutic process does not begin and end with the discrete therapeutic event." Like the analysis of power, they suggest that this also needs to be comprehended in several ways. "First, therapeutic systems and the events they generate exist in historical and social context, as both products of that context and performances that construct it. . . . Second, the therapeutic process cannot be understood as bounded by the therapeutic event precisely because it is ultimately directed at life beyond the event."[3]

Similarly, the interrogation of "power" has been linked with analysis of "the body." Both have drawn increasing attention, especially in the wake of Foucauldian perspectives, as loci for the development of critical social theory. In a seminal article, Scheper-Hughes and Lock brought together these two analytic frontiers for medical anthropologists in an approach that not only married micro- and macrolevels of analysis, but conjoined symbolic and interpretive perspectives with a gaze from political economy.[4] They wrote of the need to scrutinize the individual body, the social body, and the body politic as multiple and overlapping sites for the construction, arbitration, and subversion of meaning and experience. The phenomenology of health and illness was now understood not only via an idiom of intersecting bodies of power, but as a story whose significance was processual.[5] By situating a performative micro-analysis of a specific instance of religious healing within the broader frame of sociopolitical processes as they impinge upon the patient, I will show how the discussion of recovery is informed when an event-centered discussion is linked to the particularities of local history and world view.[6] Specifically, I shall demonstrate how a patient who presents symptoms of weakness, low energy, and a body in pain is gradually empowered by being brought into physical contact with agents, sites, and practices thought to embody power.[7]

If the "ascription of illness is one of society's ways of recognizing that individuals are not always able to fulfill all the socially prescribed behaviors," as suggested by Adams and Rubel in their classic discussion of sickness and social relations among indigenous peoples of Mesoamerica,[8] then well-being or health conversely implies a resumption and continuance of normative roles. The expression of normative behavior depends upon an ability to evidence an identity that "works," both socially and physically. In addition to the cognitive and emotional components of an individual's identity, a working identity also requires a body, as the corporeal manifestation of a temporal self. Conceptions of work and the body are of central importance to the definition of ethnic identity in Mexico, where indigenous peoples stereotypically are contrasted from the non-Indian population in terms of these dimensions of the self.

The Rarámuri

The Rarámuri are one of the largest indigenous ethnic groups in northern Mexico, about sixty thousand of whom live in the Sierra Madre Occidental of southwestern Chihuahua, a place often referred to as "the Sierra Tarahumara."[9] Despite being one of the most populous and "traditional" Native peoples in North America, the Rarámuri have been the subject of relatively few studies devoted to analyzing their systems of religious healing. Building on the works mentioned below, this chapter attempts to address this gap in the literature.

The fieldwork upon which this chapter is based was initiated in 1985.[10] Most research has been conducted in the gorges down river from a colonial mining town in the Cuervo area—a series of dispersed hamlets (rancherías) around El Cuervo Mountain and the adjacent Barranca de San Rafael to the south—among Rarámuri locally known as *gentiles* (unbaptized ones) or *cimarrones* (fugitives). For comparative purposes, some fieldwork also was conducted among the baptized Rarámuri, known as *pagótame* (washed ones) or *rewéame* (named ones), most of whom lived upriver from Batopilas.

Discussion of the differences between the *pagótame* and the *gentiles* is beyond the scope of this chapter, though research on the Rarámuri is empirically skewed in favor of the former subgroup. Suffice it to say that while the two groups in large measure share the same cultural pattern, *gentiles* reject baptism, inter their dead in ancestral burial caves, and are found only in rugged corners of the southwestern gorges; whereas *pagótame* exist in the central highlands as well as in the canyon country, bury their dead in cemeteries, and accept the Christian sacrament of baptism. Also, *gentiles* are a minority subculture comprising only about 5 percent of the total Rarámuri population.

Most importantly, *pagótame* orient their civil and religious life around colonial churches centered in a pueblo, even though they may live in outlying rancherías; while the *gentiles*, on the contrary, constitute communities that have severed most ties to nearby pueblos and churches. Instead, they have organized both their civil and religious life almost exclusively at the ranchería level. These features are related to historical forces shaping the present identity of the *gentiles*. As *cimarrones*, many *gentiles* are the descendants of apostates and fugitives who associated conversion to Christianity with colonial practices of forced labor. In conceptually linking the Jesuits' missions with the Spaniards' mines and haciendas, many sought refuge from European intrusion by retreating into more isolated regions.[11] To a great extent, therefore, the differentiation between *gentiles* and *pagótame* actually reflects a situation in which political and historical differences are articulated using religious nomenclature. In fact, both groups show influences from Christianity, though obviously these are much more apparent among *pagótame* than they are among *gentiles*. For our purposes, the salient point is that *gentiles* are the most marginalized minority of an indigenous ethnic group that is already dominated politically, economically, and numerically by the non-Indians, or Mestizos, in the region. Recalling that the language of illness often reveals how individual bodies bear witness to the impressions made upon them by the body politic, it is therefore significant that in the case of the "powerless body" I examine below, the patient himself is a *gentile*.

Emphasizing that *tesguinadas*, or drinking parties, are not only the most important form of social organization and labor recruitment existing above the level of the household, Kennedy also shows that they are basic to virtually all Rarámuri ceremonies.[12] Furthermore, curing and other kinds of rituals, insofar as they convey a sense of order and control, are a social and psychological response to the fear that arises from living under unpredictable environmental conditions.[13] Slaney's rich analyses of the most crucial rites of passage, specifically death rituals and "double baptism" in the *pagótame* community of Panalachi, highlight the significance of Rarámuri bodies in relation to intersecting symbolisms of ethnicity and gender.[14] Merrill, focusing on the relation between healing rituals and world view, demonstrates the centrality of concepts of the soul to curing, dreaming, inebriation, and the general maintenance of well-being in the *pagótame* community of Rejogochi.[15] Moreover, in following a single Rarámuri man through multiple diagnoses, etiologies, curing rituals, and eventual death, his monograph represents another case-study approach to discussions of the therapeutic process.[16]

This chapter builds on the above studies in several ways. First, I suggest that in addition to being "the house of the souls,"[17] the body is more than a passive receptacle for the active agents of Rarámuri personhood. The body itself merits serious attention in the analysis of Rarámuri healing rituals, as the locus of both symbolic and practical expressions of a working identity. To be sure, Rarámuri notions of life, vitality, and energy are linguistically and conceptually closely related to ideas about the soul, breath, and the imparting of strength, stamina, encouragement, and contentment.[18] But it is only through the possession of a physical body (*sapá*) that Rarámuri can manifest an empowered self, corporealizing the spirit of strength and ruddy health that each person seeks to radiate, communicating it through physical work and embodying it through social interactions. Second, this chapter presents comparative data on Rarámuri ritual healing, especially valuable since there is only one other source describing how these practices are performed among *gentiles*. Finally, this chapter includes the only full text in the literature, in both Rarámuri and English, of a complete healing chant that is contextualized in the analysis of ritual events.[19]

Processual Healing of the Powerless Body

Case History, Political Symptoms, and Social Antecedents

The healing ritual I shall describe took place on June 25, 1989, in the ranchería of Wa'eáchi, a highland community located at the rim of a steep side canyon off the Batopilas Gorge, but below the approximately 5,625-foot summit of Crow Mountain (Spanish, *El Cuervo*; Rarámuri, *Korachi*). I was living in the community and invited to attend the healing ritual by the ritual host and his son, the patient. The healing ritual was performed during the second phase of a *tesguinada*, or ceremonial drinking party, for a middle-aged man who was the eldest son of one of the region's respected leaders and elders. The patient, Felipe, reported suffering from great pain (*we okó*) all over his body, a condition that was especially acute in his neck and chest. He told me he had no strength (*tasi hiwera*), and generally described feeling weak, powerless, and lacking in energy. He first went to the government clinic in Yoquivo, but the personnel, according to Felipe, could find nothing wrong with him and were therefore unable to treat his symptoms. Subsequently, he sought the help of a family friend, who was also the senior shaman in the Cuervo area. The shaman said that he would perform a curing ceremony in the context of a *tesguinada*, and a date was set for the event.

Before describing the ritual, I believe some background information on the social and political events that were occurring in the community is relevant here. In many of the rancherías of the Cuervo district, unresolved issues of land ownership, community membership, and hazy geographical as well as administrative boundaries were perennial, albeit submerged, sources of social tension. Briefly, in the weeks preceding Felipe's illness and subsequent ceremony, the normally dormant issue as to who really controlled the craggy land where the *gentiles* lived was becoming a more pressing matter, especially in view of recent gold exploration by an international mining firm at Satevó in the gorge below them, the escalating pace of the timber industry operating on the mesas of Yoquivo above them, and a rash of unpunished thievery that was robbing the *gentiles* of their cattle, sheep, and goats. People from the old colonial pueblos of Satevó and Yoquivo were now coming into the district "reminding" the *gentiles* that they really were still part of their pueblos. Another set of competing claims came from Mestizos at the mining town of Tres Hermanos. But the most ominous assertion of rights to the rancherías below the summit of Cuervo was made by some members of a Mestizo family at a nearby ranch, whose patriarch was notorious throughout the region for allegedly having killed members of his own family in order to lay claim to a vast, if somewhat indistinct, tract of land.

These issues impinged on Felipe in meaningful ways that made the onset of his illness at this time especially poignant. Not only was he from the most prominent Rarámuri family in the area, with a ramified network of relationships with Indians and non-Indians throughout the region, but Felipe, and his father before him, recently had served as the *siríame*, or indigenous governor, of the Cuervo rancherías. As the chief community leader, this individual is regarded as morally upright and is charged with the responsibility for acting in the best interests of his community, which often requires intercession with outsiders on their behalf. And yet, during the simmering tensions in the summer of 1989, rather than struggling for the rights of his people, Felipe instead found himself embroiled in business dealings with a family at the ranch, sharecropping beans on some of their land and working as a day laborer in their cornfields. Felipe further distinguished himself from others in the community via an ethnically coded sartorial idiom. Rather than wearing the loincloth and handmade shirt that was the conventional attire of most Rarámuri men, Felipe almost always dressed in Western clothing.

Noteworthy also is that just days before his curing ceremony, Felipe misplaced his *bakánawi*, a personal power object carried by many Rarámuri in the region. *Bakánawi* are tuberous roots believed to have souls, which sometime appear in dreams in human form, such as Mestizos riding around on horseback, powerful Rarámuri men, or beautiful women. *Bakánawi* is identified as various plants in different parts of the Sierra Tarahumara, though often it is euphemistically glossed in conversation as "peyote" or *híkuri*.[20] The roots periodically must be fed cornmeal and tobacco, have traditional Rarámuri music played for them, and generally require being treated with utmost care and respect lest they endanger their owner. In return, the *bakánawi* impart health, power, and vitality, as well as bring luck in hunting and love. Yet *bakánawi* are especially prized for their ability to appear during nighttime dreams, singing beautiful chants and doing vigorous dances for the benefit of their owners.

The salience that these historical antecedents have for a social etiology of Felipe's illness is that they suggest the patient was manifesting in his own body the political symptoms of his community. Torn between the plight of his people, on the one hand, and his own predicament with the landowners at Los Novillos, on the other, while simultaneously feeling pressure from other competing factions as a prominent member of the community, Felipe increasingly led a pained existence. Irony was now heaped upon tragedy. Felipe was a community leader, a powerful man from a powerful family, albeit among the most marginalized minority of the already subordinated Rarámuri. And yet, he was powerless. Physically, he lacked energy, nor could he advocate politically. A servant of his people who was beholden to their opponents, Felipe's powerlessness seemed to be psychological retribution for his own ill-gotten attempts at acquiring the signs of power, wealth, and status. In dressing like a Mestizo, he sought to embody the garb of the local power elite, distancing himself from headbands, loincloths, and homespun blankets, icons of Rarámuri identity but also ethnically coded symbols of poverty. Yet in doing so, and in associating with the forces that would threaten Cuervo's well-being, he lost his moral authority and with it his community's backing, which were the unexamined sources of his strength and empowerment. Finally, as if to underscore the message that Felipe possessed a body that lacked energy and an identity that was incapable of working in normal social contexts, he misplaced his *bakánawi* just days before the ceremony. That is, he lost his power object. In no uncertain terms, Felipe was showing people through this final, and potentially dangerous, act of carelessness that he had literally "lost his power." By asking for a curing ceremony, however, Felipe was also showing that he wanted to get back on the right path, correct his improper behavior, and redress these insults to cultural, natural, and supernatural orders through normative ritual intervention.

The Work Party

Because Rarámuri *tesguinadas* require substantial expenditures of labor and resources from the households that host them, they usually cover several ritual functions.[21] Felipe and his father, Benito, who were the ritual hosts (*chokéame*) for this gathering, stipulated that this *tesguinada* was held for three reasons. It was convened as a work party to build a new corral for Benito (*nochama napawuka newama koralchi*, "to work together to make a corral"); as a curing ceremony for Felipe (*owema uchémera rehói*, "to cure by anointing a man"); and as the annual petition for rains needed for their summer crops (*bayésa ukwíki*, "call the rains"). For the occasion, three large earthenware pots (Spanish, *ollas*; Rarámuri, *sekorí*) brimming with sacred fermented maize beer (Spanish, *tesguino*; Rarámuri, *suwí* or *batári*) had been prepared, as well as a smaller *olla* that was hidden away, to be consumed by family and close friends at a more intimate party after the other guests had departed.

By 8:30 A.M. many men were on the hill above Benito's house, bringing poles and starting to build the corral for Benito's large herd of sheep and goats. Others joined gradually, and some men did not come until the drinking was about to begin. Because of his status in the region, Benito had an impressive network of people upon whom he could call for labor inputs or ceremonial duties. As the more than 70-year-old patriarch of his own family, this network included not only the families of his married children, but also those of his older and younger brothers, the extended kin group of a wide range of agnates, numerous friends and their families, as well as other community leaders and their close kin. For this event two notable men and their families arrived: Pedro, who was a shaman and *capitán*, and Rufino, who was both the eldest man and senior shaman in the vicinity. In all, about fifty people came for the occasion.

Work continued on the corral until around 11 A.M. Some men brought poles cut from the forest, some tied the poles together, some hauled poles from another corral—but many men just sat around. Even Felipe helped, as best he could. Benito was constantly working, so as to inspire the others to participate, he later explained. As is customary, however, he gave no work orders, even though he was the *chokéame*. Nor was anyone else directing the labor. People saw what needed to be done, knew what the task required, and either pitched in or did nothing as the spirit moved them. In this leisurely manner, the corral was finished.

140

It was now almost noon and people began to file down to the house, signaling the next phase of this social event, which consisted of the ceremonial drinking of *tesguino*. As the senior ritual host, Benito opened the ceremony by taking a small pot of the *tesguino* to the domestic dance patio (*awírachi*) outside the house and, before a four-foot cross erected for the occasion, performed the *wiróma*, offering *tesguino* to God (*Onorúame*, "The One Who Is Father") by tossing libations of the sacramental drink skywards and to the four directions.

Significantly, the domestic dance patio, the actions performed on it, and the associated ritual objects all index aspects of Rarámuri cosmology. As a physical representation of cosmography, it was explained to me that the circular dance ground replicates in miniature the *namókame*, the cosmic disks "stacked like tortillas" comprising the earth, the heavens, and the lower worlds. Most people reported that there exist three planes below the earth and three planes above, with God dwelling on the third and highest plane.[22] Benito explained that the wooden patio cross stood for God, which, in the Cuervo district, is unequivocally associated with the sun. Similarly, the pot of *tesguino* is always placed to the east just before the cross, or as Benito said, "*bachá, bachá!*" (meaning "first" or "in front"), pointing to the vessel containing the sacred drink with his index finger and then to the rising sun. *Bachá* connotes priority in any ordered sequence, and can refer to older brothers, earlier actions, original conditions, or seniority of people, things, times, and places. In this context, Benito indicated that *bachá* conveyed a fundamental principle of ritual primacy in Rarámuri world view by mapping spatial and temporal equivalents onto a single dimension of cosmological precedence, referenced by the sun, symbol of God, the primary giver of order.[23]

In like manner, Benito and others explained that when the host or shaman opens a ceremony by casting upwards with a drinking gourd droplets of sacramental maize beer in all directions around the dance patio, it is both an offering to God as well as a mimetic reenactment of the creation of the Rarámuri people. When the world was new, God himself stood in the center of the earth—on the middle cosmic plane in the middle of the disk, as people symbolically do to this day while standing in the center of the dance patio—tossing libations of *tesguino* in all directions, thereby sprinkling across the land scattered drops of maize beer. I was told this is why Rarámuri live in dispersed ranchos to this day. Thus, even a seemingly mundane work party is first sanctified by using *tesguino* to make connections between God, people, land, and maize; primordial space and sacred time; sun and the orders of existence.

Now, one by one, people were served the fermented maize beer. They sat tranquilly on the ground around Benito's house, talking peacefully and laughing in hushed tones, sun glinting through the trees. Soon everyone had drunk one gourd (*labáka*) full of *tesguino*. The pungent smell of *wipáka* (native tobacco; Spanish, *Nicotina*) began to waft through the air, as the men quietly puffed their corn-husk cigarettes (*péwari*). Just as the drinking gourd went round the crowd, touching each person's lips, so too smoking was a communal, ceremonial act. Like *tesguino* drinking, it is not a symbolic representation of something, but actually constitutes an essential commensal relationship.[24] Communal acts of smoking, eating, and drinking, especially of substances with psychotropic properties, are powerful modalities of body knowledge, corporeal gestures of sociality, sharing, and expressions of cultural identity. In contrast to Mestizos, it is significant that Rarámuri rarely smoke except in ceremonial drinking contexts, just as they never drink *tesguino* alone. In fact, smoking is so connected with the ceremonial consumption of maize beer that a conventional way to invite someone to a *tesguinada* is simply to ask them to bring some tobacco on a certain day, and even though no mention is made of *tesguino*, it is understood they are being asked to attend a drinking party.

Because *tesguino* drinking is an even more central embodiment of Rarámuri sociality than smoking, it conforms to a more formalized set of behaviors, particularly during the first half of a drinking party before people become intoxicated. This etiquette holds: (1) that one may serve others *tesguino* or be served by them, but should never serve oneself from the *olla*; (2) that a *labaka ro'ása*, a dipper or scattering gourd used for dedicating the maize beer, also be used to ladle *tesguino* from the *olla* into the *labáka bahísa*, or drinking gourd, but that the drinking gourd itself should not be dipped into the *olla* of *tesguino*; (3) that one should not dally when offered the drinking gourd, which usually holds almost a quart, but get on with gulping down as quickly as possible the tingling sweet-bitter liquid; so as to (4) say "thank you" (*natéteraba*) and pass the empty container back to the server, thereby allowing him to fill the gourd for the next person. The giving and accepting of *tesguino*, like all ritual gestures, is done with the right hand; only in the land of the dead, where everything is backwards, is the left hand used for these purposes.

Moreover, although one is always obliged to acknowledge being offered a gourd of *tesguino*, this by no means implies that one always must drink it. Nevertheless, given a norm stipulating that gifts are accepted unless one wishes to sever relations of reciprocity, people must be adept at skillfully manipulating certain verbal and bodily arts of social interaction if one should not want to drink, yet still remain on good terms. Such elaborate verbal and behavioral codes governing drinking etiquette may seem odd were it not for the fact that in addition to being the paradigmatic form of ritual *commensality* and public embodiment of reciprocity, *tesguino* also is regarded as the preeminent medicine (*owáame*) among Rarámuri. Rather than viewing *tesguino* as simply an alcoholic beverage, albeit a sacred one, I wish to highlight its Rarámuri conceptualization as their most basic *medicine*. From this perspective, it is therefore logical that Rarámuri would be as concerned with following precise prescriptions about how it should be properly administered as having recourse to a stock of socially acceptable excuses in the event they are not taking their medicine.

After the first round had been distributed, Benito's eldest brother, a man about 80 years of age, took me by the hand and led me inside the house where Benito's brothers and sons were now starting to serve a second helping of *tesguino* to the guests. The three large *ollas* full of *tesguino* were placed on the dirt floor in the middle of the inner room. Here, men were gathered outside around the front of the house, while the women sat on the ground beneath the trees on the other side of the wall towards the back end of the house. While Benito's sons served *tesguino* to the men who were waiting out front, Benito's elder brother meanwhile was passing gourds of maize beer through a large hole in the wall to the women on the other side. The first two *ollas* of *tesguino* were finished in several hours. People had three to four gourdfuls each, which allowed them to achieve the desired state of *bayóame rikú*, "beauteous inebriation." This rosy glow is one whereby celebrants are getting drunk but not getting out of hand.

It is the attainment of this physiological state, a biological condition having to do with the body but a mode of being inextricably linked to Rarámuri concepts of the soul, which permits the escalation of the event to the next phase of the ritual—the curing ceremony. For it is held that once participants become "beautifully drunk," some of a person's souls begin to leave the body, easing communication not only among the celebrants, but also between humans and supernaturals.[25] Consequently, people are more open to experience communion with the holy through the words and actions of the shaman. As such, they are also more receptive to the moods and images of beauty, sanctity, well-being, and order that are the goal of every curing ceremony through a felicitous performance.

The Curing Ceremony

Rufino opened the ritual with the ceremonial use of tobacco. Rolling a cornhusk cigarette, he silently took several puffs, held the *péwari* in his hand, and motioned around the top of the *olla* in circular movements, letting the smoke waft over the curing paraphernalia, thereby purifying the ritual space and blessing the objects. He then called upon God's help by offering the smoke skyward, holding the *péwari* with an outstretched arm above his head and then drawing it back to his chest, or *surachí*, literally, "place of the heart," an area of the body that is important in Rarámuri ritual and world view, often described, along with the head, as the seat of a person's largest souls.[26] The whole procedure was repeated several times before the *péwari*, beginning with the patient, was passed clockwise around the third *olla*, each member of the curing party smoking for a few moments while they prayed in silence or low tones.

Rufino and his wife then began a dual performance of a highly stylized oratory. According to several family members who were standing beside me in the room, this paralinguistic oscillation—coupled by the fact that Rufino's wife accompanied her husband with a simultaneous rapid banter of her own, also shifting back and forth between shouting and whispering—made for an overall chorus in which neither of their speeches could really be comprehended as discursive narrative events. They clearly were dramatic speech acts evoking a context of strangeness that signaled mystical communication. Although their speeches could not be understood in their entirety, family members reported catching the gist of their orations, which asked God to care for one of his children, a direct reference to Felipe, the patient.

Felipe sat still and was silent. As the patient listened intently to this eerie invocation, Mauricio, the apprentice-assistant to Rufino, went outside where the rest of the crowd was continuing the drinking party. He carried with him the gourd of *pinole*, with one of the three curing crosses stuck in it, going around the large patio cross erected on the domestic dance ground where earlier in the day Benito had opened the drinking party by offering *wiróma*, tossing libations of *tesguino* up to God and the four directions. There, gourd in hand, he methodically made three counterclockwise circuits. Meanwhile, at the behest of Rufino, the musicians began to play. Now Rufino took the other two curing crosses. One of these he placed inside Felipe's shirt, resting the stem against his chest, "the place of the heart," with the top protruding in front of his neck, the cross visible just below Felipe's chin. Telling Felipe to hold the first cross in this position, Rufino now uncovered the olla, lifting the two other gourds and removing the upside-down basket. Taking the second cross in his hand, Rufino dipped the stem into the *tesguino* and proceeded to paint three maize beer crosses on each of the four sides of the *olla*, starting with the side facing him and moving counterclockwise. He then resumed his seat, holding the cross out in front of him, with the bottom touching the *olla*'s side and the top inclined toward his body at about a sixty-degree angle.

Mauricio now reentered the room carrying the gourd of *pinole* and said loudly: "*kwíra-bá!*" ("*greetings!*"). Everyone responded, saying "*kwíra-bá*" back to him in unison. He was then told to twirl around in front of the *olla*, on the western side, and to circle around the participants, twirling around at each of the cardinal points. When he started to go the wrong way, however, he was corrected by Rufino and his wife and sent in the other direction, being told to always move "to the right," or counterclockwise. Mauricio thus made nine circuits around the participants and then sat back down beside Felipe. Periodically, the musicians played at the behest of Rufino. When they rested, Rufino and his wife resumed their dual oratory until the music began again. Now the violinist's wife was summoned inside. Replicating the procedure when Mauricio reentered the curing area, there again was the *kwíra-bá* greeting, the counterclockwise twirling before the *olla*, and nine counterclockwise circuits around the group. She then sat facing Felipe on the other side of the *olla*.

The gourd with the *pinole* and the third curing cross stuck upright in the cornmeal was placed in front of Rufino. With the second curing cross still held in his hand, Rufino made the sign of the cross in the air over the mouth of the olla and then circled the curing cross above the *tesguino*, a gesture he repeated several times, as he previously did with the tobacco. He next tossed this cross into the *tesguino*. It sank into the maize beer, hit the bottom of the *olla*, and then bobbed back to the surface. All eyes watched the silent disappearance of the cross into the sacramental liquid and its momentary reappearance, the cross jutting up above the mouth of the *olla*. Rufino began a low incantation and repeated the act of bouncing the cross in the *olla* three times.

With this sanctified cross, Rufino now began using physical techniques to cure the *okó suwába* or "all-over pain" that had gripped Felipe's entire body. Rufino would attempt to empower Felipe's aching body through a practice known as *uchémera*, which involves specialized methods for directly touching the patient's body. The verb *uchémera* has a number of related connotations. It means to apply pressure, massage, or rub; it also means to put liquid, ointment, sap, or oil on something, especially for healing purposes. Rufino was now going to *uchémera* Felipe, using tesguino as the paradigmatic medicine and the aforementioned cross as the preeminent medical instrument.

First, Rufino rose to his feet, asking Felipe to do likewise. He then turned Felipe around and around many times in place. Next, Rufino pressed the cross, still wet with *tesguino*, three times against the patient's back and then three more times against his chest. Then he anointed the crown of Felipe's head with *tesguino*, drawing a line with the stem of the cross as if it were a wand, from the nape of the neck to Felipe's forehead and then from side to side. Periodically dipping the stem of the cross into the *tesguino*, Rufino used it to paint long streaks down Felipe's right arm, hand, leg, and foot. He then pressed the wet cross to major joints along the right side of Felipe's body, specifically his shoulder, elbow, wrist, knee, and ankle. The entire procedure was then repeated on Felipe's left side.

Significantly, the *uchémera* employed nondiscursive means not only to connect, via the cross and *tesguino*, inner and outer aspects of a person's identity, but literally to draw analogies between the body of the patient and the body of the olla. The points on Felipe's body mentioned above that were anointed with *tesguino* by the curing cross are especially meaningful because, according to Merrill,[27] these correspond to places on the surface of the body where inside dwell a person's souls. Furthermore, it will be noted that the way Rufino used the cross to mark Felipe's body with *tesguino*—on his right and left sides as well as front and back—corresponded exactly to the manner in which, earlier in the ceremony, he used this same instrument to streak maize beer on all four sides of the body of the *olla*.

Then, from the olla that spatially had defined the center of the ceremony and had been the focus of so much ritual attention, Felipe finally was served a gourd brimming with *tesguino*, which he gulped down immediately. At this point, the patient was now literally coated, internally as well as externally, with the Rarámuri's quintessential medicine. Maize beer had been painted on him outside and poured down his insides. The body of the man, like the body of the *olla*, not only contained the intoxicating liquid and exhibited lustrous surfaces anointed with sacred beverage, but now Felipe himself was actually a vessel of the holy, regenerative, fluid.

From the *olla* to Felipe to the others in the room, the sacred drink now flowed to all, though it poured into the crowd along a hierarchy of structured relationships, highlighting channels of power based on principles of seniority, gender, bloodline, and social ties among the assembled. First to drink were members of the curing party, beginning with Rufino and his wife. Then people were called into the room based on their kinship distance to the patient, Felipe. A set procedure was followed for each person. Soon everyone drank their fill and the *olla* was empty.

Rufino now picked up the gourd of *pinole* and again began to chant his personal curing song, which he later told me God taught to him when he visited heaven in his dreams. Meanwhile, with his index and middle fingers he scooped up some of the *pinole* and placed it into the mouth of Felipe. Next he hand-fed *pinole* to his wife, then to his apprentice-assistant, Mauricio, and finally to the violinist's wife. This completed, the low chant that Rufino had been singing periodically throughout the ceremony now boomed forth from his lungs with great gusto. I had permission from the ritual host and the patient to record this and other chants. The shaman also gave his approval.

1. *Ech-cho-ná, we semati kúrasi atí*	Over there, such beautiful crosses standing
2. *Semati atí, suwí choná*	Beautiful is, maize beer over there
3. *Mapu nehá, asá suwí*	Where [one] gives, sits beer
4. *Echi kúrui, bahí choná*	Those boys, drink over there
5. *We semati, atí choná*	So beautiful, being over there
6. *Mi re'pá, mi rabó*	There on top, there on the ridge
7. *Ga'rá atí, nehé choná*	Well am I, over there
8. *Hiwera atí choná, seko-ri-chi*	Strength is there, in the olla
9. *Ma bahí, suwí choná*	Now drink, maize beer over there
10. *We semati, atí choná*	So beautiful, being up on the ridge
11. *We semati, kúrusi atí*	So beautiful, crosses standing
12. *We semati, rawé-ware*	So beautiful, day dawning
13. *Mi re'pá, atí choná*	There on top, over there are
14. *Wa'rú wabé, kú-ru-si*	Very large, crosses
15. *Mi re'pá, atí nehé ko*	There on top, I keep going

16. *We semati, atí rabó*	So beautiful, being up on the ridge
17. *We semati, atí choná*	So beautiful, being over there
18. *Mi re'pá, mi rabó*	There on top, there on the ridge
19. *We semati, atí choná*	So beautiful, being over there
20. *We semati, nawahí cho ko*	So beautiful, chanting going on too
21. *Mi re'pá, rabó aní*	There on top, on the ridge I say
22. *Beikiá kúrui, choná aná biré*	Three boys, over there walks one
23. *Mi re'pá, mi rabó*	There on top, there on the ridge
24. *Echiriwé, nawahí atí*	Thus, keep chanting
25. *Besá namókame, atí paní*	Third plane, being in heaven
26. *Echiriwe, nehé aní*	Thus, I say
27. *Mi're'pá, mi rabó*	There on top, there on the ridge
28. *Riósh natéterabá!*	God, thank you!

The curing party now performed a counterclockwise round dance (*awí kuríka*, literally, "dance in a circle") around the empty *olla* in the following order: the shaman, the patient, the musicians playing their instruments, the apprentice-assistant, the shaman's wife, and the violinist's wife. As elsewhere in the ceremony, this sequence again evidenced structures of symbolic classification illustrating not only the complementariness of male and female, as well as senior and junior principles, but the primacy of the former in each of these pairs.

Now that the participants were "beautifully drunk" and moving about, formality gave way to more ludic elements, a sequencing mechanism that often signals the close of rituals. At one point, Rufino took the violin (which belonged to Benito) and played it for a while before returning it to the normal violin player. As he danced, several people encouraged Felipe by calling out to him, "*iwérasa!*"—meaning "be powerful" or "have strength!" After innumerable times going round the *olla*, Rufino had everyone stop dancing as he playfully shouted out, "*kípu hú*" ("how many?"), to which Mauricio answered "*ochéch*" ("again!"), making everyone laugh as they resumed dancing. This call and response, which stopped and started the dancing, went on several more times during the next twenty minutes as people went round and round, until they visibly tired from the vigorous dance. Rufino then shouted "*Riosh natéteraba!*" ("God, thank you!"), which finally halted the circle dance.

When the round dance was over, Rufino handed the gourd of *pinole* to Felipe, saying "*kórisa, má kusawíma*" ("*take this gift, now your health will be restored*"). Felipe replied "*natéteraba*" ("thank you"), accepted the gourd with his right hand, transferred it to his left and then passed it on to Rufino's wife, saying to her "*kórisa, kuyáma*" ("take this gift, give back in return"). This was a continuous motion from the shaman to the patient to the shaman's wife, who finally emptied the *pinole* into a square of white muslin. In both word and deed it was a beautiful and graphic illustration of the Rarámuri concept of "reciprocal exchange" or *nakuríwa*, literally meaning "something that goes in a circle." Later, Rufino was additionally given five thousand pesos for his services.

Treatment Protocol

After the ceremony, Rufino took Felipe aside and the two quietly conversed for a while. Later, Felipe told me that Rufino had given him specific instructions as to how he should continue the therapeutic process on his own and how it was important for him to heed this advice if Felipe wanted to get well. Felipe said that he was supposed to continue working on his body with the curing crosses, that he should rest but also try to get back to work little by little, beginning by laboring alongside his father and brothers in the family's cornfield. Since he was now healed, he should no longer feel sad or depressed (*o'móna*), but instead feel happy (*ganire*) and be at peace (*kirí hu*). He was enjoined to be true (*bichíwame*) and giving (*neháame*) with God and other members of the community, showing these dispositions by hosting another *tesguinada* and sacrificing a goat during the fall harvest. Moreover, Rufino told Felipe that he would recover his lost *bakánawi*, which would be instrumental in his eventual recovery. Felipe was instructed to pay close attention to his dreams, for through them the *bakánawi* would reveal its magic, imparting renewed strength and vitality by showing Felipe empowering images, songs, and dances. Felipe was to learn these, being able to see, hear, and feel them even when he was not dreaming, directed to re-experience the vision and its power at will in his daily life, especially whenever he needed a boost. In general, Rufino's message to Felipe was that he could regain a working identity by normalizing his relations as a moral Rarámuri on the one hand, and by attending closely to even small signs of returning power on the other. For in recognizing that power was contingent on relationships, Felipe would slowly regain his health.

Following Rufino's advice, during this period Felipe increasingly became an active participant in his own therapeutic process. Each morning, as soft rays of sun filtered through the trees, Felipe blessed himself with the two curing crosses, by touching them to all the parts of his body that had received the *uchémera* treatment during the ceremony. He also began singing portions of Rufino's curing chant.

Eleven days after the ceremony, Felipe came to my hut at night to tell me that he had begun to have beautiful *bakánawi* dreams, filled with inspiring songs. He explained that even though his *bakánawi* was still missing, it was now calling out for him. Over the course of several nights, Felipe said that he had been taught by his *bakánawi* a personal healing song: the Chant of the White

Horse Woman. Space prohibits presentation of the complete text of this chant, but here it is sufficient to note the following. The sublime grace of the horse has impressed people worldwide, irrespective of culture, but in the Sierra Tarahumara, those who own and ride horses convey specific messages of wealth and status, power and prestige. In Mexico, equestrian prerogatives have long been associated with the elite. The animal, therefore, is particularly auspicious in this context. Described as continually singing and dancing throughout the chant, the White Horse Woman mimetically invigorates the exhausted Felipe, renewing and energizing the man through successive iterations of her beauty and stamina. Appearing again and again, standing upright, stomping backwards, dancing with high steps, her repeated presence imparts strength, confidence, and power.

Twice in the chant Felipe sang: "How frequently, she empowers here!" (*"kípu wésa, uméro enaí"*), the verb *uméro* meaning to have power or ability; to be capable of doing something; to possess might, potency, force, or capacity. In the second part of this same phrase he sang *"népi ga'rá nikú gawé rosákame!"* ("the greatest help is the white horse!"). Elsewhere in the song, the White Horse Woman shows Felipe the path of power and recovery, not only by pointing it out, but by bringing her magic towards him, chanting:

Enaí, ech aní, bowé ga'rá hú	"Here," she says, "is a good trail."
Wé simí, bayóame awí	She keeps on going, beautifully dancing,
Echi ka, gawé rosákame	Towards this way, the white horse.

In closing, she reveals that one can reevaluate apparently negative situations into positive outcomes, showing that bad luck can be transformed into good. In the end, as she disappears, the chant enjoins its listeners to believe, by employing a term (*bichí*) that is also the root for the word "true" (*bichíwame*):

Kípu wésa, mitiwá enaí-che	How frequently, misfortune is here, yet
Népi ga'rá hú, échi aní muhéri	"It is really good," so say you.
Mukí ga'rá hú, muhéri	Woman, you are good.
Má kowána, ko bichí	Now move backwards, believe
Echi gawé rosákame!	That is the white horse!

Several days later, Felipe did in fact recover his lost *bakánawi*, as Rufino had predicted. According to Felipe, it was because he was able to concentrate on the song, focusing on its words and images of constant encouragement. He also had regularized his relations with family members and others in the community, which included doing more cooperative labor and wearing a white loincloth and woolen sash over his pants, as Rufino similarly had advised. Two weeks after the curing ceremony, Felipe was telling people he had regained his power and was healed.

The Recovery of a Working Identity

The Empowering of Bodies and Embodying of Power

Heeding the call for greater specificity in anthropological discourse by writing "ethnographies of the particular,"[28] I have purposefully subordinated the project of theorizing to a microsociology of fine-grained description. Nevertheless, I do wish to point out some salient patterns. By analyzing both discursive and corporeal aspects of curing, I now draw together the major themes of the therapeutic process discussed above, a study in processual healing concerning the ironic case of the powerless body of a Rarámuri leader. The subsequent discussion examines how bodies are empowered by placing them in association with specific agents, sites, and practices held to embody power in Rarámuri ritual and world view.

Recovery is linked to the recuperation of a working identity, manifested through ethnically polarized valuations of the body linking ethics and aesthetics, goodness and beauty, Rarámuri and God. Rarámuri say their bodies are "black" (*chókame*), whereas the bodies of Mestizos are contrasted as "white" (*rosákame*), although this is not a value-neutral coding. On the contrary, the linking of body color and ethnicity is tied to a moral dimension, reflecting Rarámuri ideas about separate creations of Indians and non-Indians: the Rarámuri were made by God and fashioned from clay, hence they are the color of the earth. By contrast, the devil made non-Indians, forming their bodies from ashes, hence they are white.[29] If clothing is a kind of social skin, then Felipe's ethnically coded sartorial choices represented an inversion of the kind of dress, and implicit morality, normally associated with Rarámuri bodies. Put simply, Felipe had been acting "white" (i.e., non-Indian).

Indigenous views of the meaning of work and its relation to an ethnic division of labor are equally significant for cultural constructions of identity and well-being. Rarámuri stereotypically describe non-Indians as lazy, greedy, and stingy—regarding them as people who work inside at desks writing papers or who buy and sell as merchants. By contrast, Rarámuri typically say their work consists mainly of "planting and dancing" and of generously sharing the fruits of their energy with friends at ceremonies, drinking parties, and feasts. Noteworthy is that the Rarámuri pride themselves on the very physical labor stereotypically disparaged by town-dwelling non-Indians, saying that this strength and vitality was given to them as a gift by God and is demanded of them in their fields. In preceding the curing ceremony sequentially, the working *tesguinada* hosted by the patient Felipe's father naturally modeled a healthy

Rarámuri identity for Felipe, showing him the path to recovery. The joy of physical labor was celebrated along with togetherness and the exchange of words, laughter, and drink. A complete identity, therefore, is not only one that is whole, in both body and soul, but one that *works*, engaging a fully functioning self with the give and take of social life.

The embodiment of a working identity is accomplished by putting the patient, Felipe, directly in contact with *powerful agents*, *powerful sites*, and *practices of power*. Powerful agents are cultural entities, instruments, authorities, substances, beings, and personnel that are causative sources for transformative reactions in other beings. Powerful sites are spatiotemporal loci of ritual attention. Practices of power are varieties of performance and experience.

Powerful Agents

The first kind of powerful agent that deserves mention are the obvious objects of ritual, which constitute the medicines and instruments of curing. Here, this included certain plant substances or products, such as *tesguino*, cornmeal (*pinole*), tobacco, and *bakánawi*, as well as certain articles, such as crosses, *tesguino ollas*, and drinking gourds. Other types of powerful agents operative in the therapeutic process are not objects, but rather empowering beings or personnel, figures of authority, encouragement, or control. Key players here included God, souls, *bakánawi*, the White Horse Woman, the shaman, his wife and apprentice-assistant, the musicians and violinist's wife, as well as family, friends, and relatives of the patient. In different ways, contingent on their relationship to Felipe, each of these were actors who served as models or conduits of strength, contentment, and well-being.[30]

Powerful Sites

Powerful sites are loci for the convergence of cultural, natural, and supernatural forces. In healing rituals, the most obvious site for the inscription of power is the patient's body. Felipe's physical woes reflected that, as a prominent member of the community, the political symptoms of the region were literally embodied in him, the body politic manifesting itself through the patient. The express intention of Felipe's curing ceremony, therefore, was to empower him. This was achieved by ritually reinvigorating his souls, which in turn imparted new strength and vitality to his aching and exhausted body. Chief among these bodily reinvigorations were the procedures involving *uchémera*, or healing by touching, anointing, and pressing the *tesguino*-moistened cross to the points on Felipe's body where the souls reside.

Besides the human body, other sites are also important loci for the inscription of power. Spatially, the most salient place for the *gentiles* is the *awírachi*,[31] the household dance ground or domestic ritual patio, which in some way is involved in virtually all ceremonies conducted in the rancherías. Since *tes-*

guinadas are multipurpose occasions, a large work party may be drinking out-side, while a curing ceremony may be in progress inside the house. While these may appear to be separate functions, involving different people, places, and sets of behaviors, in fact they are integrally related and frequently overlap. Ritual performances on the dance patio outside were symbolically linked with the curing ceremony inside, further connecting the work party with the heal-ing ritual. The *tesguino* used in the curing ceremony inside the house earlier had been consecrated by Benito, the patient's father, on the dance patio out-side, just as Mauricio, the shaman's apprentice-assistant, took cornmeal from inside the house outside around the *awírachi*, as well as walking the curing cross around the patio cross three times counterclockwise. Mauricio explained that in circling the *awírachi* three times he was walking around each of the three disks of the upperworld. This connected God on the third level of heaven, to whom the cornmeal was first being offered, with the curing party on the sur-face of the earth, who would be fed the cornmeal later in the ceremony. Overall, a mundane inner room of an ordinary house was sanctified in a dou-ble sense: first, because it was the focus of the entire healing ritual, and sec-ond, because it was metonymically connected to the overt ritual area of the *awírachi* via the physical movement of sanctified food, drink, and bodies. The connection between health, strength, and beauty—associated with crosses, mountain tops, *tesguino*, the third plane of heaven, the three boys, and the dawning day—is likewise the subject of Rufino's curing chant. Agents of power thus oscillated between the two sites of power, connecting the implicit cosmology of the *awírachi* outside with the explicit beauty and vigor of the cer-emony inside.

Time, as well as space, is also a dimension where powerful sites are found, especially at points of meaningful cultural and natural conjunctures. For the Rarámuri, like many agricultural peoples, time is inextricably conjoined to the daily and annual cycles of the sun, which in turn are linked to their notions of God. The divine, for the Rarámuri, embodies opposing yet complementary aspects, consisting of the male *Onorúame* (The One Who Is Father), and the female *Iyerúame* (The One Who Is Mother). *Onorúame* is associated with the sun (*rayénari*), while *Iyerúame* is indexed by the moon (*micháka*). As the embodiment of the dominant aspect of God, and the primary marker of time, the sun is the most fundamental physical entity of order and potency in the Rarámuri uni-verse.[32] It is therefore significant that Felipe's curing ceremony took place when the sun was at an especially favorable position in the sky, representing a conver-gence of diurnal, seasonal, medicinal, and agricultural cycles of renewal.

Felipe's curing ritual began around midday. That is, a ceremony intended to impart strength to a weakened individual was performed when God, whose source of strength is embodied in the sun, was highest in the sky, at the zenith of his own radiant power. The fact that it took place on June 25 is also noteworthy, for two reasons. First, this date is during the week when the sun is also at its highest point in the annual cycle, occurring only four days after the summer solstice (June 21), and second, it is also only one day after Dia de San Juan (June 24). This period, when elders of Cuervo observe the sun setting in the same spot for about a week, is of vital importance for agricultural reasons, and Rarámuri customarily hold *tesguinadas* as offerings to God for the rains that begin at this time, inaugurating the planting season.[33]

Practices of Power

Vitally important for the restoration of Felipe's health and identity are practices of power, for it is only through these that the aforementioned agents and sites are put into action. The most basic and pervasive motif of normal Rarámuri social life is the practice of reciprocity, an ideal of dynamic balance evidenced in their economic, social, political, and religious subsystems. Besides the exchanges of prayer, offerings, and thanksgiving that occur between Rarámuri and God, there are obvious social exchanges that take place between households in alternately being hosts and guests at various *tesguinadas*. Yet reciprocity also is manifested between persons within any given ceremony in the elaborate rituals of giving and receiving described above in the work party and subsequent curing ceremony. Although elements of reciprocity are evident throughout the ritual, a microanalysis of the final moments is enough to show the principle in sharp relief.

The last line of the curing chant together with the final ritual transactions involving the cornmeal *pinole* underscore via discursive as well as bodily actions the primacy of reciprocity as a practice of power. Rufino begins his chant by singing of the giving and receiving of *tesguino* beside crosses (lines 1–4), effectively mirroring in words the exchange of maize beer that constitutes a critical part of this and virtually all other Rarámuri rituals. Yet after portraying scenes of strength and beauty (lines 5–20), he shifts rhetorically, gradually directing attention towards the zenith, the ultimate source of that power (lines 24–28). Finally, by closing his chant with the statement *"Riosh natéteraba"*—meaning "thanks be to God," or literally, "God, thank you"—Rufino was acting "as if" the petition for health already had been granted at that moment. Here, Rufino was acknowledging a cycle of reciprocity with God, persuasively communicating to Felipe that now he was healed by expressing gratitude to God for the receipt of his gift.

In this healing context saying something is also doing something.[34] Giving thanks is conventionally understood as acknowledging receipt of a gift already bestowed. That is, saying "thank you" itself performs the action of thanking. Other phrases in the chant likewise mark them as performative utterances. The words do not beseech God for health, hoping for some cure in the future, but on the contrary, actively constitute health by persuading, commanding, and

153

proclaiming wellness in the present. Note that at four key points in the chant (lines 7, 15, 21, and 26) the first person singular pronoun ("I") is conjoined with verbs that are in the active present tense. Announcing, "Well am I, over there" (line 7) or "There on top, I keep going" (line 15), the chanter creates a mood of health and vitality not only by manifesting it through the words of the song, but also because the chant itself transports us "there." The magical power of the healing song is that it cures the patient, and thus *works*, in a double sense. First, in a perlocutionary sense, it works because Felipe is persuaded by the chant, performatively demonstrating his recovered vitality by joining others in a vigorous round dance. Second, the chant works in an illocutionary sense, because when Felipe later repeated the song over the next few days, Felipe himself became the "I" of the chant. Thus, by simply uttering the words of the song, the patient gradually pronounces himself "well" and able to "keep going." Indeed, he says he is "there on top." The chant for strength is its own accomplishment.

Similarly, the *pinole* exchanges enact a ritualized performance of power and reciprocity, demonstrating an expectation that the existing exchanges between shaman and patient will continue as part of an enduring set of reciprocal relationships. The giving and receiving of *pinole* is socially significant in itself because it is the most basic of all Rarámuri foods and most common item reciprocated for favors among friends. It is also symbolically significant because, like *tesguino*, it is made from maize—the staff of life. Moreover, while in the ritual it may seem as if the patient is politely declining the *pinole* by apparently giving it back (accepting it from the shaman and passing it on to the shaman's wife), in actuality the *pinole* originated from Felipe's family yet ended up in Rufino's. In addition, at the very moment that the patient is in the act of giving, he is also asking for something to be given back at some point in the future. Since normalcy requires that an individual be part of the give and take of everyday life, the work of recovery places the patient at the point of power. To become healthy is to become an active agent in one's own recovery, accepting the responsibility of maintaining reciprocal social relations. Healthy persons are receptive as well as generative.

More generally, the Rarámuri conceive of an overarching reciprocity existing among cultural, natural, and supernatural orders. The relations of reciprocity that the Rarámuri hold as the norm among themselves also serve as the model for their relationships with supernatural entities. This reciprocity, however, often implies an asymmetry in power, which in turn is harnessed for the purposes of healing. When Rufino fed Felipe the *pinole*, the gesture modeled the feeding of a child by its parent, which similarly replicates the nourishment provided by God for his children, the Rarámuri. Correspondingly, just as God and the *bakánawi* spirits help the families of Benito and Felipe, so they are expected to reciprocate by making offerings to them. Both humans and deities are embedded in relations of cosmic balance and reciprocity. Maintaining balanced reciprocity among different dimensions of reality is the fundamental goal of Rarámuri ritual. Well-being is predicated on harmony and a sense of encompassing cosmic wholeness:

> Because there exists a dynamic equilibrium among different orders of reality, it is particularly noteworthy that plants, animals, and humans all participate in cognate idioms of health and illness through the contiguity of their relations. Since "curing" something and "caring" for something are closely allied concepts in Rarámuri world view, crops, livestock, and people all require periodic curing ceremonies and are healed in similar ways.[35]

The gathering on June 25 at Benito's household was held for three functions, which all had to do with curing. Held during the auspicious days of the summer solstice when at sunset God "dances on the same mountain" along the horizon for about a week to inaugurate the planting season, the event was: (1) the annual ceremony for assuring rain and a good crop; (2) a medical treatment for Felipe; and (3) a time for constructing a new corral on Benito's field, thereby fertilizing the plot with dung from his herd of sheep and goats. Since the Rarámuri's model of curing encompasses practices of balanced reciprocity and dynamic equilibrium among different orders of existence, Felipe's curing strategically was linked with the curing of crops and livestock. Because it occurred when human and natural cycles of regeneration converge during the summer solstice, Felipe participated in the ecological transition from dead dry season to growing wet season. This underscores not only that Rarámuri healing is postulated upon a contiguity of relations among diverse entities in the cosmos, but that the encompassing relationship between the patient and the environment upon which he and all Rarámuri depend is critically linked to the position of the sun.

The patient's assumption of responsibility in the overall therapeutic process exemplifies another practice of power in the work of recovery. Felipe's curing was linked not only to practices of reciprocity, as seen above, but also with his ability to actively identify with normative behavior that occurred before, during, and after the curing ceremony. Rarámuri healing embraces practices of power that transcend the ostensible curing event itself. During the work party that preceded the curing ritual, as well as during the treatment protocol that followed it, Felipe was presented with corporeal, visual, and auditory models of healthy bodies and right action. More importantly, he incorporated these images of power and protocol into a vision of himself as a revitalized decision maker taking steps to follow the "good trail" he had been shown by his *bakánawi* spirit guardian. Conceptualizing the embodiment of power as transtemporal recovery means recognizing the interdigitation of therapy as event and therapy as process. Overall, it means interlacing the healer's imposition of order and the patient's assumption of responsibility into a single model of wellness, not only recognizing a difference between sickness and health, but manifesting a readiness to exchange the former state for the latter.

The final practice of power that I briefly mention is the ritual conveyance of an ordered universe, integral to the patient's recovery through his involvement in the stereotyped performance of Rarámuri principles of structure and precedence, recognizing wholeness in the perception of patterns. Through a condensation of meaning, the curing ceremony shows in high relief some of the most basic axioms of Rarámuri world view: the interrelationship between cosmological and moral orders; the unity of ethics and aesthetics; health and harmony. The cross is an icon of divinity and the body is a vessel of the soul. Crosses and circles describe the geometry of sacred centers, so movements that follow these patterns summon holiness, renewal, and transformation. Community is restored by eating and acting together. Healing requires touching—and listening, speaking, twirling, dancing, and sometimes just being still. Throughout the curing process, the aforementioned powerful agents, powerful sites, and practices of power are invoked. Yet they are most eloquently drawn together, and most richly elaborated in terms of underlying principles of order, through the performance of the healing chant and subsequent communal dancing.

Rufino's song is replete with parallelism, the pairing of couplets, a characteristic of ritual language among diverse peoples both ancient and modern throughout the world. Redundant verbalizations of distance, beauty, and height in Rufino's chant combine to impart the message that splendor is above, up is an orientation of power, and the shaman knows the way to heaven. Gradually the song carries its listeners, as if climbing a mountain step by step, in the new light of the "dawning day," upwards to God, source of magnificence and strength. The curing chant is all about continually going higher and cresting a summit, directing attention "over there" away from illness and pain in the present, to the "beautiful" places in the distance, "there on top, there on the ridge." The emphasis on physical ascension towards the peaks, and from there to the third and highest realm of heaven, where God lives, effectively communicates the image of *getting over* one's illness, *surmounting* one's infirmity, and *rising above* one's pain. In sum, the chant manipulates the powerful rhetoric of *transcendence* as a persuasive language for healing.

The primacy of maleness in reference to the sun, the order for *tesguino* consumption, and participation in the dance appears in several places. At first, Rufino sings about how "those boys" are drinking *tesguino* far above. Towards the end, as the lyrics move from mountain tops into the upperworld, the chant says "three boys, over there walks one." Felipe interpreted this line to mean Benito's three sons, and the reference to the one who walks alone as signifying Felipe himself, since he was the patient. The shaman's apprentice-assistant said that it referred to God and his two helpers, conventionally represented by three crosses on the dance patio, while the other shaman attending the ceremony told me it referred to Rufino and his two spirit helpers walking in heaven. Combining the poetics and politics of healing, Rufino avoided specifics altogether when I asked him what the phrase meant. Instead, he simply kept pointing above with his index finger, telling me that the chant's images describe what he sees in heaven through his dreams. In sum, the chant indexed maleness (as well as the number three, which is ritually associated with men), allowing different people their own interpretations and the possibility, as with Felipe, of seeing themselves in the song.

Conclusion

This chapter has examined ritual healing among the Rarámuri of northern Mexico by using a case-study approach to suggest that the recovery of a working identity is contingent upon the embodiment of power in the therapeutic process. Although power may be regarded as concentrated in certain persons, places, times, or entities, it is ultimately a *relational* concept of control concerning the ability to produce an effect.

Tracing connections among therapeutic, political, and spiritual power reveals healing to be a process that transcends the discrete therapeutic event.[36] By following a case from its historical roots to a paradigmatic display of health, I have argued that the recuperation of a working identity, physically, psychologically, and socially, depends upon a patient's ability increasingly to become an active agent in his or her own recovery. Responding to findings that there may exist "links between passivity and disease,"[37] I have suggested that healing is associated with symbolic and normative activities. Among other things, this implies engaging in relations of reciprocity, assuming responsibility, and developing a growing anticipation of one's returning health. In sum, I have explored in Rarámuri ritual and world view "healing as a mode of empowerment wherein small changes can mean the difference between effective coping and defeat, between endurance and the remoralization of lived experience and the passive acceptance of despair."[38]

Notes

1. This chapter is dedicated to the memory of Isidro Roque, whose good works in this life surely mean he now farms with Onorúame on the third plane of heaven. I first thank those individuals—both Rarámuri and Mestizo—who over the years have shared so generously of their time and knowledge. This material is based on field research and writing made possible by financial support from the following institutions,

which is gratefully acknowledged: Minnesota Humanities Commission (Works in Progress Scholars' Grant); Carleton College (Faculty Development Endowment Large and Small Grants); Harvard University (Sheldon Traveling Fellowship, Department of Anthropology, Center for the Study of World Religions Senior Fellowship); Fulbright-Hays Doctoral Dissertation Abroad Fellowship; Institute International Education-ITT Fellowship; and the Tinker Foundation. I thank Evon Vogt, David Maybury-Lewis, Sally Falk Moore, Kenneth George, Stanley Tambiah, Arthur Kleinman, Byron Good, and Lawrence Sullivan for introducing me to social and symbolic analyses of culture, medicine, and religion; Thomas Csordas for generously sharing his materials on ritual healing; Don Burgess and Wes Shoemaker for their valued suggestions on the translation of Rarámuri terms and concepts, and Clifford Trafzer, Diane Weiner, Pamela Feldman-Savelsberg, the anonymous reviewers, and my students at Carleton—Joshua Rising, Rogelio Medina, and Ross Chavez—for their helpful recommendations and remarks on earlier drafts of this chapter. I am indebted to my wife, Tara AvRuskin, for her critical insights on the work of recovery, conceptions of empowerment in medical anthropology, and keen editorial eye.

2. Thomas J. Csordas and Arthur Kleinman, "The Therapeutic Process," in Carolyn F. Sargent and Thomas M. Johnson, eds., *Handbook of Medical Anthropology: Contemporary Theory and Method* (Westport, CT: Greenwood Press, 1996), 19.

3. Ibid., 19–20.

4. Nancy Scheper-Hughes and Margaret Lock, "The Mindful Body: A Prolegomenon to Future Work in Medical Anthropology," *Medical Anthropology Quarterly* 1 (1987): 6–41. Recent studies that build on the work of Scheper-Hughes and Lock include Andrew Strathern, *Body Thoughts* (Ann Arbor: University of Michigan Press, 1996), and Paul Stoller, *Sensuous Scholarship* (Philadelphia: University of Pennsylvania Press, 1997).

5. Scheper-Hughes and Lock, "The Mindful Body: A Prolegomenon to Future Work in Medical Anthropology," 31.

6. The event-centered approach to social and symbolic analysis taken in this chapter has been informed by Thomas Csordas and Elizabeth Lewton, "Practice, Performance, and Experience in Religious Healing," *Transcultural Psychiatry* (forthcoming); Victoria Bricker, *The Indian Christ, the Indian King: The Historical Substrate of Maya Myth and Ritual* (Austin: University of Texas Press, 1981); Pamela Feldman-Savelsberg, *Plundered Kitchens, Empty Wombs: Threatened Reproduction and Identity in the Camaroon Grassfields* (Ann Arbor, University of Michigan Press, 1999); Kenneth M. George, *Showing Signs of Violence: The Cultural Politics of a Twentieth-Century Headhunting Ritual* (Berkeley: University of California Press, 1996); Gary Gossen, *Telling Maya Tales: Tzotzil Identities in Modern Mexico* (New York: Routledge, 1999); Carol Laderman and Marina Roseman, eds., *The Performance of Healing* (New York: Routledge, 1996); Stanley J. Tambiah, *Culture, Thought, and Social Action: An Anthropological Perspective* (Cambridge, MA: Harvard University Press, 1985); Victor Turner, *The Forest of Symbols: Aspects of Ndembu Ritual* (Ithaca, NY: Cornell University Press, 1967); John Watanabe, *Maya Saints and Souls in a Changing World* (Austin: University of Texas Press, 1992); Evon Z. Vogt, *Tortillas for the Gods: A Symbolic Analysis of Zinacanteco Rituals* (Norman: University of Oklahoma Press, 1993).

7. Mary-Jo Del Vecchio Good, Paul E. Brodwin, Byron J. Good, and Arthur Klienman, eds., *Pain as Human Experience: An Anthropological Perspective* (Berkeley: University of California Press, 1992). For the anthropology of power, see also Lowell John Bean, "Power and Its Application in Native California," *Journal of California Anthropology* 2(1) (summer 1975): 25–33; Raymond D. Fogelson and Richard N. Adams, eds., *The Anthropology of Power: Ethnographic Studies from Asia, Oceania, and the New World* (New York: Academic Press, 1977); and W. Arens and Ivan Karp, eds., *Creativity of Power: Cosmology and Action in African Societies* (Washington, DC: Smithsonian Institution Press, 1989).

8. Richard N. Adams and Arthur J. Rubel, "Sickness and Social Relations," in Manning Nash, ed., *Social Anthropology*, vol. 6 of *Handbook of Middle American Indians*, gen. ed. Robert Wauchope (Austin: University of Texas Press, 1967), 333–56.

9. Stefani Paola and Agusto Urteaga, "La Población de la Sierra," *Ojarasca* (1993): 20–21.

10. Fieldwork was conducted in the summers of 1985 and 1986, and again from January 1988 to August 1989. Brief visits to the Sierra were also made in December 1994 and April 1997. Pseudonyms are used throughout this chapter to protect the privacy of individuals.

11. Luis González Rodríguez, "Los Tarahumares," in Luis González Rodríguez, Don Burgess, and Bob Schalkwijk, eds., *Tarahumara* (Mexico City: Chysler de Mexico, 1985), 43; Jerome M. Levi, "Pillars of the Sky: The Genealogy of Ethnic Identity among the Rarámuri-Simaroni (Tarahumara-Gentiles) of Northwest Mexico," Ph.D. diss. (Harvard University, 1993); William Merrill, "Conversion and Colonialism in Northern Mexico: The Tarahumara Response to the Jesuit Mission Program, 1601–1767," in Robert W. Hefner, ed., *Conversion to Christianity: Historical and Anthropological Perspectives on a Great Transformation* (Berkeley: University of California Press, 1993), 129–64; Thomas E. Sheridan and Thomas H. Naylor, eds., *Rarámuri: A Tarahumara Colonial Chronicle* (Flagstaff, AZ: Northland Press, 1979).

12. John G. Kennedy, "Tesguino Complex: The Role of Beer in Tarahumara Culture," *American Anthropologist* 65: 620–40.

13. John G. Kennedy, *Tarahumara of the Sierra Madre: Survivor's on the Canyon's Edge* (Pacific Grove, CA: Asilomar Press, 1996), 177–78.

14. Frances Slaney, "Death and 'Otherness' in Tarahumara Ritual," Ph.D. diss. (Université Laval, 1991); Slaney, "Double Baptism: Personhood and Ethnicity in the Sierra Tarahumara of Mexico," *American Ethnologist* 24 (1991): 279–310.

15. William L. Merrill, "Thinking and Drinking: A Rarámuri Interpretation," in Richard I. Ford, ed., *The Nature and Status of Ethnobotany, Anthropological Papers* 67 (Ann Arbor: University of Michigan, Museum of Anthropology, 1978); William L. Merrill, "The Concept of the Soul among the Rarámuri of Chihuahua, Mexico: A Study in World View," Ph.D. diss. (University of Michigan, 1981); William L. Merrill, "The Rarámuri Stereotype of Dreams," in Barbara Tedlock, ed., *Dreaming: Anthropological and Psychological Interpretations* (Santa Fe: School of American Research, 1992), 194–219.

16. William L. Merrill, *Rarámuri Souls: Knowledge and Social Processes in Northern Mexico* (Washington, DC: Smithsonian Institution Press, 1988).

17. Ibid., 112.

18. Ibid., 95.

19. In the 1890s, Carl S. Lumholtz documented several short chants with words and presented these in *Unknown Mexico: A Record of Five Years' Exploration among the Tribes of the Western Sierra Madre; in the Tierra Caliente of Tepic and Jalisco; and among the Tarascos of Michoacan*, vol. I (New York: Scribner's, 1902), 338. Thirty years later, however, Wendell C. Bennett and Robert M. Zingg suggested that the chants had degenerated into jargon: "It is a common claim that the chants possess words, but that only jargon is sung, since the real words are kept secret by the chanter. It is true that intelligible words are not sung. Monosyllables and humming comprise most of the chants" (*The Tarahumara: An Indian Tribe of Northern Mexico* [Chicago: University of Chicago Press, 1935] 272). Nevertheless, Don Burgess, working in the Baja Tarahumara area, has published several collections of songs in Spanish as well as Rarámuri, *Ralámuli Wikala (Canciones de los Tarahumaras)*, 1st ed. (1973), 2d ed. (1994). Laurent Barbier recorded an interesting healing song titled "Sixth Chant of the Scraping Stick," which was "sung during a magical cure with *bakanoa*" (i.e., *bakánowa*, a variant pronunciation of *bakánawi*). It appears in Rodríguez, Burgess, and Schalkwijk, eds., *Tarahumara*, 167. Unfortunately, the Rarámuri text is not reproduced, nor is there any accompanying discussion.

20. For the different plants identified as *bakánawi* and a discussion of how the Rarámuri substitute words for powerful subjects—especially the names of certain plants, animals, places, and people—as a way to code their world view, see Jerome M. Levi, "Hidden Transcripts among the Rarámuri: Culture, Resistance, and Interethnic Relations in Northern Mexico," *American Ethnologist* 26(1) (1999): 8–9.

21. Kennedy, "Tesguino Complex"; Merrill, "Thinking and Drinking"; Slaney, "Double Baptism," 282–83.

22. This corroborates Merrill, *Rarámuri Souls*, 71–72, although some people I spoke with said there were more, and others fewer, than seven planes. The word *namókame* is related to the verb *namoma*, which refers to things being on top of each other, further explaining why the cosmos is sometimes analogized to a stack of tortillas. That the dance patio symbolizes the three planes above in Rarámuri cosmology is also encoded in the words of a short chant recorded by Bennet and Zingg, *The Tarahumara*, 269, who transcribed *namó* as the word for the cosmic planes.

23. Gary H. Gossen, "Temporal and Spatial Equivalents in Chamula Ritual Symbolism," in William A. Lessa and Evon Z. Vogt, eds., *Reader in Comparative Religion: An Anthropological Approach* (New York: Harper & Row, 1979), 116–29.

24. Tobacco may have the body of a plant, but, according to one myth, its inner essence is that of a Rarámuri man. Moreover, the tobacco's manlike "soul" not only enjoys conversing with other anthropomorphized items comprising the men's traditional fire-making kit and leather tobacco pouch, but yearns to assume the form of smoke exhaled from human mouths and noses during drinking ceremonies. Like other Native peoples elsewhere in the Americas, the Rarámuri accord the ceremonial smoking of tobacco a special place in ritual and world view.

25. Levi, "Pillars of the Sky," 418; Merrill, "Thinking and Drinking"; Merrill, *Rarámuri Souls*, 108–11; Slaney, "Double Baptism," 286.

26. Merrill, *Rarámuri Souls*, 88.

27. Ibid.

28. Lila Abu-Lughod, "Writing against Culture," in Richard G. Fox, ed., *Recapturing Anthropology: Working in the Present* (Santa Fe: School of American Research Press, 1991), 149–57.

29. For another explanation, grounded in a different myth, of why Rarámuri have dark bodies whereas non-Indians have light ones, see Levi, "Hidden Transcripts among the Rarámuri," 6.

30. The distinction between the two subcategories of potent entities, however, should not imply a distinction between inanimate objects and animate beings. Tobacco and *bakánawi*, for example, have the physical morphology of plants, but contain an inner essence or humanlike soul that causes many Rarámuri to classify them in the same category as powerful sorts of people.

31. The *awírachi* is a small flat area outside, near the dwelling, ideally circular in shape though occasionally squarish. Depending on the ceremony, there may be anywhere from one to four crosses and/or pine saplings erected on the *awírachi*, sometimes cloaked in white muslin. *Ollas* of *tesguino* are also placed there, as well as a ritual table or "altar" to hold offerings of various foods, herbs, minerals, and other "medicines." It is also the site where all animal sacrifices and initial offerings of *tesguino* are made, as well as the most common place for chanting and dancing to occur, in both night and day. The *awírachi's* indexical relation to the sun, divinity, and Rarámuri cosmology, referencing both the creation of the world and the disks of the cosmos, already has been discussed.

32. Although balance between these two celestial bodies is necessary for cosmic harmony, the solar aspect is regarded as the stronger presence, just as maleness is accorded precedence in ritual contexts. Thus "God" is often glossed *Tata Riosh*, "Father God," or sometimes just *Riosh*, from Spanish *Dios*, as seen in the last line of Rufino's curing chant. The term for day (*rawé*), as well as times of the day (for instance, *nasipa rawé*, "noon" or "midday") linguistically derive from the word for the sun (*rayénari*). Moreover, the sun denotes both spatial and temporal equivalents; *mapu machina rayénari* can mean either "east" or "sunrise," depending on context. The idea that the sun is a primary principle in Mesoamerican views of language, ritual, and cosmology is also widespread; for example, among the Tzotzil of Chiapas, see Gary H. Gossen, "Temporal and Spatial Equivalents in Chamula Ritual Symbolism" and *Telling Maya Tales: Tzutzil Identities in Modern Mexico* (New York: Routledge, 1999).

33. In the Catholic calendar, the Dia de San Juan is associated with water symbolism, since it is the Feast of St. John the Baptist. Not surprisingly, in many parts of the Sierra, Tarahumara people regard this day as the time when the searing heat of the dry season supposedly gives way to the first rains of summer, thus initiating the growing season. At Cuervo, it is also recognized that this falls during the time of an agriculturally significant *astronomical* event, since both summer and winter solstices are carefully observed as signs of changing seasons. Male elders pointed out the two spots along the horizon where the sun stops and reverses its direction at the farthest reaches of its annual north-south trajectory across the sky.

34. For a cogent explanation of speech act theory as applied to ritual, see Tambiah, *Culture, Thought, and Social Action*, 78–79, 135.

161

35. Merrill, *Rarámuri Souls*, 137–45.

36. Csordas and Kleinman, "The Therapeutic Process."

37. David Gutman, *The Human Elder in Nature, Culture, and Society* (Boulder, CO: Westview Press, 1997), 50; Todd Dundras and Sue Fisher, eds., *The Social Organization of Doctor–Patient Communication* (Norwood, NJ: Albex, 1993).

38. Csordas and Kleinman, "The Therapeutic Process," 19.

NINE

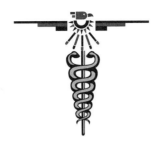

Meeting the Challenges of American Indian Diabetes

ANTHROPOLOGICAL PERSPECTIVES ON PREVENTION AND TREATMENT

American Indians have faced many challenges to survival and well-being over the last five hundred years. In terms of health, these hardships persist as Native peoples continue to cope with infectious diseases, with the added burden of burgeoning chronic diseases. Holistic and comprehensive frameworks are necessary to most effectively address the broad scope of pressing maladies like cancer, HIV/AIDS, and cardiovascular diseases. One problem that exemplifies the need for multiple strategies of solution is Type 2 diabetes, a condition that affects American Indian and Alaska Native populations at some of the highest rates in the world. A closer examination of diabetes among American Indians reveals that it is not just an ailment of the body, it is a problem that needs to be understood within the context of Native history, culture, and experience.

In reference to American Indian diabetes, the perspective of medical anthropology can aid in understanding cultural issues such as food preferences, health beliefs, the impact of acculturation, and Native healing strategies. Medical anthropologists focus on how cultural beliefs influence health and treatment choices, in addition to examining the social aspects of health, such

163

as the manner in which social inequalities can negatively impact access to health care. This perspective highlights the extent to which ethnicity, acculturation, history of prejudice, and social position affect the overall quality of health and health care among American Indians. These are essential factors to consider when trying to fully understand diabetes and why American Indians are experiencing such health problems disproportionately when compared to other populations.

In addition to providing a broader contextual framework, anthropology offers other important insights to help face the challenge of American Indian diabetes. First of all, anthropologists can act as "culture brokers" between biomedical personnel, local health planners, and members of Indian communities.[1] Within this framework of cultural dialogue, medical anthropologists can help to identify the junctures at which biomedical and American Indian discourses can be united to teach people about diabetes in ways that are culturally sensitive and respectful, and also medically helpful. In addition to this, medical anthropologists have experience with collaborative projects, not only in the sense of working on multidisciplinary academic, clinical, and policy teams, but also in the sense of collaborating with members of the community so that the needs and concerns of intended populations are best met.

Diabetes and American Indians: Scope of the Problem

Diabetes is one of the most significant health problems facing Native peoples today.[2] The most prevalent type of diabetes is referred to as "Type 2 diabetes," or what has been termed "non-insulin–dependent diabetes mellitus" (NIDDM). Diabetes has been described as "epidemic" for many American Indian tribes.[3] The Pima Indians of Arizona have the "highest recorded prevalence and incidence of NIDDM of any geographically defined population."[4] Among other Native North American groups, prevalence of Type 2 diabetes does vary, with Alaska Natives (Aleuts, Inuits, Yuits, and Indians) having the lowest prevalence rates,[5] and other groups such as the San Carlos Apache, Seminole, Choctaw, Cherokee, and Seneca Indians having high rates of the disease.[6] In American Indian tribes overall, the current Type 2 diabetes prevalence rates among adults between the ages of 30 and 64 years are between 29 percent, like the Navajo, and 50 percent, like the Pima.[7]

The challenging physical burdens of diabetes come primarily from the secondary complications, which frequently manifest among American Indians, including blindness, kidney failure, heart disease, limb amputations, circulation problems, coma, and depression. Left unchecked, these conditions can result in death.[8]

Type 2 diabetes is not a simple matter of regulating blood sugar levels—

many of these secondary complications are the result of impaired circulation that accompanies high blood sugar.[9] An analogy that may be used is to think of blood sugar particles (glucose molecules) in the circulatory system as logs going down a river—the more logs in the river, and the faster they come, the slower the river flows and the more it becomes clogged. The glucose needs to be transferred, with the help of insulin, from the bloodstream into the cells, where it will be consumed as energy. When this process becomes hampered the glucose backs up in the bloodstream and restricts circulation, which can lead to infection, gangrene (often in the feet where circulation is the poorest), and limb amputations, among other complications. These debilitating conditions can be avoided with early detection, accompanied by prevention measures and lifestyle changes.[10]

Historical, Epidemiological, and Genetic Considerations in American Indian Diabetes

History and the Role of Acculturation and Stress

Historical and epidemiological perspectives are essential in understanding the complex causal factors associated with diabetes and how to minimize these factors in education and treatment programs. One significant factor that needs to be highlighted is the role of acculturation, or the processes whereby major cultural changes are forced onto a society as a consequence of intensive firsthand contact or conquest.[11] In reference to the Navajo, Huttlinger contends that the diabetic disease process directly reflects the historical process of domination of Navajos by non-Native groups, particularly Anglos.[12] This assertion emphasizes the point that the most comprehensive understanding of American Indian diabetes will be realized when the forces of postcolonialism and acculturation are factored into an analysis of the problem of diabetes and how to most productively address it.[13]

Although acculturation has been occurring ever since the beginning of the European conquest, some lifestyle changes that promote the expression of diabetes have happened relatively recently. Before the 1940s and 1950s, diabetes was rare in Indian populations. Although cases of diabetes did begin to appear more frequently after this period, many groups did not see significant increases until after the mid-1970s,[14] a situation that reflects the continued impact of Western lifestyles on American Indians. Judkins describes how Seneca Indians with diabetes reflect on the "old days" when "Indians lived close to the earth, used herbs and plants, and didn't have 'sugar,'"[15] the term for diabetes often used by American Indians. In more recent times, American Indians have lived more urban, industrialized, and sedentary lifestyles. Since World War II, there has also been an increased reliance on machines and store-bought foods.[16] Weidman documents these accelerated lifestyle changes of American Indians over the last 50 years among the Oklahoma Cherokee.[17] He describes the rapid alteration in technology and infrastructure that led to a profound cultural change from an agricultural to an industrial economy in the space of ten years, from 1936 to 1946. This transition, accompanied by changes in diet and lifestyle, occurred simultaneously with the first appearance of Type 2 diabetes among the Cherokee.

United States governmental policies during the 1940s and 1950s were also a driving force in the continued lifestyle changes of American Indians, especially through the assimilationist agendas to end federal commitment to Indian reservations and entice Indians to the cities. The Bureau of Indian Affairs' Relocation Program of the 1950s, called by some "the largest forced migration in history," aimed to deal with "the Indian problem," through application of the "four gospels" of termination, relocation, assimilation, and acculturation.[18] While many American Indians ultimately returned to the reservations, instigated by unemployment and racism encountered in the urban areas, their assimilation to American mainstream lifestyles and food habits was promoted by the government tactics.

The processes of culture change can result in significant amounts of stress, which can create imbalances in the body. Dressler describes stress as the difficulties that can arise in the process of adjusting to the physical, social, cultural, and historically produced environment.[19] When adjustment is difficult, there is a breakdown in the system and sickness may result. The importance of this definition is that it does not reduce stress to a purely physical or mental state, but it includes cultural and social factors (e.g., perceptions of what is stressful; social relationships that may either contribute to stress or act as a buffer to stressful situations). Studies have shown that some Native peoples living a Western lifestyle (e.g., the Dogrib) may experience more stress and more difficulty in adjusting to different lifeways, thus making the body less capable of regulating blood sugar levels, a condition that if prolonged can lead to diabetes.[20]

EPIDEMIOLOGICAL CONCERNS: AGE AND GENDER. Epidemiological research supports acculturation theories of the complex etiology of American Indian diabetes. To date, studies have indicated that the triggers of diabetes include obesity, lack of exercise, high-fat/high-sugar diets, and stress, all concomitants of industrialized and Western lifestyles. Age and gender are also important epidemiological considerations. Type 2 diabetes usually afflicts non-Indian peoples when they are in middle age of the 40s and 50s, but many American Indian groups experience Type 2 diabetes in their 20s and 30s. In recent years there has been an alarming increase in diabetes in Indians under the age of 20,[21] and in the past ten years, there has been a two-fold increase in Indian diabetes for those under the age of 16 years old.[22] For instance, among

Pima adolescents, the 1996 prevalence of Type 2 diabetes aged 15–19 years was approximately 51 per 1,000.[23]

In addition to the risks associated with younger people, American Indian women face diabetes and its secondary sequelae with much greater frequency than men. A 1991 report from the Department of Health and Human Services stated that a "review of the current literature reveals that Indian women suffer disproportionately from lifestyle-related diseases and premature deaths."[24] The two most significant threats listed are cancer and diabetes. The report also asserts that the "health of Indian women is integrally tied to the overall health status of the general Indian population."[25] Consequently, an analysis of Indian diabetes needs to be placed not only in a sociocultural framework, but a gendered one as well.

GENETIC THEORIES OF AMERICAN INDIAN DIABETES: THE THRIFTY GENE. Genetic susceptibility may also play an important role in the detrimental effects of acculturation in the development of diabetes. In addition to the hereditary genetic effect of diabetes clustering in families, it has been suggested that Native peoples have what is called a "thrifty genotype,"[26] which purportedly developed as an adaptation to hunting and gathering lifestyles. In this situation, subsistence patterns that included cycles of feast and famine would have promoted the body to store fats quickly when food was available, so that the periods of food scarcity could be survived with stored body fat. Although this bodily adaptation would have been very efficient in traditional precolonial lifestyles and in some postcolonial situations, after contact with a relatively consistent food, the thrifty gene seems to have been maladaptive. During the past few centuries, many Native peoples have not only had their territories reduced or changed altogether, but they have also been given rations of lard, sugar, coffee, and have access to other such foods high in sugars and carbohydrates, which are deleterious to maintaining proper nutrition and weight and antithetical to the benefits of a "thrifty gene." Nevertheless, recent assessments of longitudinal research suggest that genetic susceptibility may "not be the important factor" in diabetes onset;[27] rather environmental factors such as obesity and levels of physical activity appear to be two key triggers that interact with familial propensity in Type 2 diabetes onset.[28]

Diabetes Health Education in Native Communities: Developing Treatment and Prevention Strategies

Education has been singled out as the most important factor in the prevention and management of diabetes.[29] Many anthropologists argue that health-education programs need to be culturally relevant and sensitive in order to achieve

the goals of improving health status in specific populations.[30] When this caution is not heeded, the possibilities of program failure are numerous. Both
overt and more implicit factors need to be considered in any diabetes programs
associated with American Indians, from the content of the educational message to how it is delivered. For example, strategies of learning may differ cross-
culturally.[31] One basic distinction that has been made is between direct and
indirect learning. Direct learning is didactic, as in a lecture style, and nonpar-
ticipatory. This happens when a doctor or nurse dictates the biomedical facts
to a patient, usually resulting in a one-way flow of information. Direct learning is associated with Western European, American, and Euro-Canadian cultures. Indirect learning is a somewhat different mode where life examples, stories, metaphors, myths, and experiences are used to teach important concepts
and ideas. This type of teaching and learning has traditionally been used in
Native cultures. Consequently, health-education programs for American
Indians that only adopt a direct learning style, just telling people the "facts,"
may not have the impact that a combination approach would have.

In addition to differences in learning styles, the culture and lifestyles of specific groups need to be assessed to develop culturally relevant diabetes-education messages.[32] American Indians have commented on the inadequacy of
existing diabetes-education campaigns in relation to their cultural beliefs and
ways of life.[33] The mitigating effects of culturally related health beliefs should
always be considered in program designs. The ways that diverse peoples learn
"depends in part on the orientation of the culture to such issues as whether
human nature is good or evil, how independent of nature humans can be,
whether the basic orientation is present, past, or future, whether an individual's cultural role is primarily active or passive, and how the individual is bound
to other individuals."[34]

The matter of including cultural considerations into health education is a
sensitive undertaking, which includes both ethical and epidemiological considerations. Any time a people's culture and belief system are involved, health
educators should reflect on the extent to which they are adapting their programs to the existing culture, or trying to supplant local belief systems with
outside ideas and values. More positive outcomes for the management of diabetes will come from adapting programs to fit in with existing beliefs and
behaviors in American Indian communities.

The Need for Ethnographic Research

The level of understanding that is needed to construct appropriate health-edu-
cation programs requires in-depth research on particular tribes and cultures.
This type of ethnographic research has heretofore been scant in the area of
American Indian diabetes, while biomedical reports of rates and incidences of
Indian diabetes have been numerous.[35] At the 1995 Third International Con-

ference" on Diabetes and Indigenous Peoples in Winnipeg, Canada, a consensus emerged that there was a dearth of descriptive research on the experiences of Native peoples living with diabetes. Previous literature has focused on sociological models of health beliefs and how such beliefs may impede or facilitate biomedical treatment of diabetes. Laudable exceptions include the work of Joycelyn Bruyere, Veronica Evaneshko, Linda Garro, Joel Gittelsohn and colleagues, Rebecca Hagey, Jennie Joe, Russell Judkins, Gretchen Lang, Cheryl Rodriguez and Derek Milne, and Diane Weiner.[36] What distinguishes the work of these scholars is the commitment to understanding the cultural context of American Indian diabetes and what ramifications this has for treatment and prevention strategies.

Many of the insights and program designs that have emerged from this handful of researchers, most of whom collaborated with community members, resulted from comprehensive explorations of how cultural beliefs affected the ways in which people conceptualized diabetes and responded to intervention programs. Following from this research, it is evident that there are some general questions and culturally influenced areas that should always be considered before diabetes education and prevention programs are implemented. For example, implicit types of cultural knowledge should be considered; many diabetes programs developed for the mainstream population (primarily whites) emphasize competition, deferred gratification, and a linear model of thinking, which may not always be appropriate models to employ in American Indian cultures.[37]

Another formative consideration should be the extent to which biomedical and scientific models will be utilized in the program, and how such perspectives can be balanced or integrated with traditional ideas and themes. One of the factors in such a balancing act is the extent of diversity in the intended population, and the degree to which people adhere to traditional cultures and lifeways. As a way of assessing the range of beliefs and behaviors that may exist, the following themes should be explored in ethnographic and participatory research: local/cultural conceptualizations of foods, health beliefs (including etiologies and metaphors of diabetes), and conceptions of the body and how it works.

FOODS. Essential questions in this area are: "What kinds of foods are eaten in this tribe/group/community?"; "When and how often are these foods eaten?"; and "How are these foods prepared?" These questions need to address not only foods currently consumed and considered typical, but also those foods that are deemed culturally important. It is hard to believe, but some diabetes educators have never thought to ask these simple questions when dealing with Indian diabetics. Among the Zuni in New Mexico, an early diabetes program advocated that people eat foods "good" for their diabetes, like tuna fish and cottage cheese—foods that the Zuni did not normally eat.[38] They ate tortillas and beans and other types of Southwestern foods, which left them wondering if their "traditional" foods were beneficial or harmful for their diabetes. More recent programs at Zuni (such as the HELP Program) have incorporated culturally relevant types of foods into comprehensive and community-based programs.[39]

Another blunder, reported by Lang,[40] occurred with the Dakota Nation where diabetes educators advocated that traditional foods were good for diabetes, but the Dakota considered commodity or store-bought foods such as lard and fry bread and the like as "traditional." The Dakota had, according to current memory, been eating these items for a long time. This was also an issue deeply intertwined with cultural identity. In the Dakota community, food has been viewed as a unifying community symbol around which Dakota gather and heartily partake. If diabetics reject foods that are viewed as traditional, they may be seen as challenging community solidarity.[41]

The idea of food as a powerful symbol of cultural identity was reiterated by the majority of Native speakers at the 1997 Fourth International Conference on Diabetes and Indigenous Peoples in San Diego. A key task in diabetes programs, highlighted by these discourses, is to have members of the community define what is meant by "traditional" food, and then incorporate these emic definitions into program designs, as initiatives among the Kahnawake, Mohawk have done.[42] There are a number of Native foods (beans, wild game, fish, roots, herbs) that are excellent for managing diabetes, but many health practitioners, including both Indians and non-Indians trained in Western medicine, are not very knowledgeable about these. Medical anthropologists, as well as ethnobotanists and nutritional anthropologists, can facilitate the identification of culturally salient and diabetic-appropriate foods, taking on the culture-broker role between biomedical practitioners, local health planners, and the community.

HEALTH BELIEFS. Investigating indigenous health beliefs is a critical endeavor in any Native diabetes program. A basic approach that can be used as a starting point in assessing health beliefs is to investigate lay etiologies and discourses on how/why people get diabetes and what they should do about it. In many Indian communities, diabetes is referred to as the "sugar disease,"[43] which may reflect and influence people's conceptions of the cause of diabetes as eating too much sugar. Elucidating such explanatory models of diabetes should be sensitive to intragroup variability and the effects of interactional dynamics, or how people may co-construct meanings about illness with others, such as friends, family, and health workers over periods of time.

What this type of analysis will likely reveal are the disjunctures between biomedical conceptions of diabetes as a disease and American Indian conceptions of diabetes as an illness and a historically and culturally situated text. For example, Huttlinger recounts the story of a colleague who had worked for the Indian Health Service among the Navajo for many years. Although diabetes did not seem to be a big problem until the 1970s,

[s]he did recall, however, that in the 1980s there was an "outbreak" of diabetes in one particular area. In fact, she related that one of the trading posts almost went out of business because it was believed that if you "stopped in Dilcon [a small community on the Navajo reservation] you would 'catch diabetes.'"[44]

Both Lang and Judkins have explored cultural conceptions about diabetes and its treatment among the Dakota and Seneca, respectively.[45] They have reported that diabetes is often viewed as a "white man's disease." The disease and biomedical treatments were viewed as yet another intrusion of white culture into their lives. There is a number of potential outcomes of these beliefs: refusal to seek biomedical treatments ("white man's medicine" may further oppress them), reluctance in seeking biomedicine (suspicions exist, but also a recognition that such medical treatments may be powerful), actively seeking Western medicine ("white man's medicine" for "white man's disease"), seeking indigenous remedies (from herbalists, shamans, and other ritual experts of healing), and any combination of these aforementioned options.

These cases indicate that in many instances, issues involving diabetes are not confined to the individual (as in the biomedical model), but must be understood from cultural, social, and historical perspectives as well. The importance of this was highlighted several years ago when I was conducting an assessment of an Indian Health Service clinic in New York state. I had interviewed some of the clinical staff members who were in charge of diabetes management and education about how well they thought Native people understood the technical/biomedical aspects of diabetes, whether they perceived any cultural issues to be at play, and what kinds of secondary complications there were. As a medical anthropologist, I was dismayed at the responses I heard, which can be summed up as: culture was not thought to be a factor, people seemed to understand the biomedical information about diabetes just fine, and there were hardly any secondary complications in the population they served. Shortly after this encounter, I was asked by a staff member in social services (not in the health department) if I could offer some assistance to a diabetic Indian woman who suffered from severe secondary complications. I gave her a ride to a specialized clinic where she was supposed to go for regular check-ups, although this was difficult for her as the clinic was an hour away. She was crippled from impaired circulation in her legs (and was tenaciously holding on to keeping her foot, although the doctors said it should be amputated), and renal dialysis was imminent in her future. Basically, what I witnessed was a major disjuncture in the health clinic staff's perception of the impact of diabetes among their American Indian patients and the experiences of the people suffering with the illness.

BODY. Central issues to be explored here include an assessment of what the beliefs about the body are, especially notions of ideal body size and perceptions of obesity and moderate overweightness. In many Native populations in the world, a large body is viewed as a sign of health, wealth, and sexual attractiveness. Being thin may represent an individual and/or communal history of poverty, hunger, and illness (including tuberculosis).[46] In rural Jamaica, cultural importance is placed on reciprocal relations with kin, which includes the sharing of food; "cultural logic has it that people firmly tied into a network of kin are always plump."[47] Once this prevalent cross-cultural norm is appreciated, it is not surprising that there may be adverse reactions to advocating that people should lose weight and be thin. The unwritten text here is that they should aspire to look like skinny white people, an understandably dubious suggestion when viewed with a cultural perspective that includes a prominent history of neocolonial and imperialist agendas for American Indians by whites.

Non-Native health educators may not be aware of these differences in such body-related issues as food consumption, health, and body beliefs, and they may wonder why some Native peoples are not more responsive to initiatives involving exercise and diet changes to reduce body weight. As Gittelsohn notes for the Ojibway-Cree of northern Ontario, "While dietary linkages to diabetes are recognized, physical activity as a means of controlling obesity and decreasing the risk for diabetes, is not part of the local ethnomedical model."[48] This attitude may be changing. A recent Phoenix Indian Medical Center client telephone survey suggests that 43 percent of females and 53 percent of males questioned had tried to lose weight during the past two years most often through diet and exercise. Their primary motivation was to avoid diabetes, heart disease, and other conditions.[49] Additionally, cultural perceptions of body ideals are changing for some groups. Weiner learned from her California Indian consultants that non-Indian celebrities are often viewed as the preeminent achievement in bodily form; in turn, overweight Indian bodies are often considered to reflect high-fat diets linked to individual and group financial and infrastructural constraints.

In my research with American Indians in New York state, I have come across some newly developed diabetes programs that need to take a deeper look at cultural issues. Aerobics classes are a good example of a health initiative that can be easily altered to better fit Native experiences and expectations. If aerobics classes targeted for Indian women are run by thin, non-Native, well-toned instructors, it may be difficult for the Indian women to identify with this ideal. Also, some of the Native health programs I have visited advertise their aerobics classes with pictures of thin white women in specialized, and expensive, exercise attire jumping up and down. Frankly, many women, Native or not, may be intimidated by super-fit aerobics instructors because the average woman usually does not live up to the idealized cultural body image that instructors often have. Programs at Pleasant Point Wellness Center (Passamaquoddy Tribe), Kahnawake Schools Diabetes Prevention Project, "All of Us

Be Well" (Hualapai-Peach Springs, Arizona), and Zuni are but a few exceptional models that are based on community knowledge and experiences.

Incorporating Traditional Wisdom Through Community Collaboration

The most successful diabetes health interventions are those that are sensitive to local cultural concerns and needs and that involve the community in their development and implementation.[50] For example, medical anthropologists, health personnel, and locals at Zuni developed a community-based diabetes program that built upon the cultural history of the Zuni as long-distance runners.[51] It was recognized that the Zuni had this cultural propensity for exercise that could be developed in ways that stressed traditional identity in diabetes management, rather than an imposed outside ideology. The program has been very successful in facilitating weight loss among the Zuni and many diabetics have decreased or even eliminated the need for insulin to control their diabetes—they are able to manage it through diet and exercise alone now.

The Zuni also started an aerobics program. At first, it was not so successful due to the ways in which it was described and promoted. The key feature of a revamped program that made a significant difference was using pictures of average women (versus thin women) exercising to promote their program, and more importantly, pictures of Zuni women. But more than this, they trained as instructors local women who often were fairly overweight, at least according to outside norms. Newer initiatives among the Zuni include incorporating traditional music into exercise programs to encourage elders to participate in wellness campaigns.

Among the Navajo in Arizona, educational materials about diabetes have been translated by Navajos into *Dine Bizzad* (Navajo language), accompanied by pictures, as part of their campaign to deal with the rapidly increasing diabetes rates.[52] Other successes in diabetes care have built on familiar traditions in Native cultures. For example, the oral traditions in many Indian groups emphasize storytelling as an important cultural activity. For Canadian Natives, this has proven to be an effective way to communicate ideas about diabetes and how to prevent and manage it, without overwhelming the listener with biomedical terminology, models, and jargon.[53] Within this context, insulin can take the guise of heroes defeating monsters and other threats to the people (i.e., diabetes).

Other innovative programs that I have heard about at conferences or while visiting various Indian Nations, included incorporating traditional ideas and wisdom into health programs.[54] This is especially important because behavior is so difficult to change that it necessitates educational messages that convey meanings relevant both personally and culturally. It is often not effective in any population when unknown doctors or nurses dictate that people change their lives—the way they eat and what they do.[55] American Indians have been subjected to a long history of being told where they are supposed to live (on reservations), what they are supposed to eat (rations supplied by the U.S. government), and how they are supposed to look and speak (especially as enforced in the tragic circumstances of Indian boarding schools). If health messages about lifestyle changes come from the perspective of that culture and have support and reinforcement from the community, or at least the family, there is a much greater chance of having an impact—of getting people to improve their eating and increase their exercise to manage or avoid diabetes.

What follows are some other areas of American Indian wisdom and tradition that tribes, nations, and health programs can consider when constructing diabetes education and prevention initiatives.

Native Games

There are many ways to incorporate Native games into different health programs for preventing diabetes and other health problems. The Haudenosaunee, or Six Nations Iroquois, support young people in lacrosse leagues, a game that is supposed to have originated with the Haudenosaunee. Canoeing among Northwest-coast groups, snowshoeing among the Inuit, shinny among the Hupa, and kickball races in the Southwest, are some other examples of traditions promoting exercise.[56] Moreover, inter- and intratribal leagues and competitions of such sports as basketball, handball, and baseball encourage physical activities within a framework of social exchange and interaction.

There are many other traditional games that are part of tribal cultural histories that could be revived to promote cultural revitalization, while at the same time encouraging exercise and activity to assist in diabetes care. As discussed previously for the Zuni in New Mexico, attempts to control diabetes through exercise have incorporated indigenous notions of physical activities, such as the traditions of long-distance running.[57] The successful outcomes for individuals with diabetes in this program has relegated the Zuni program as a model for other American Indian communities.

Native Foods

Many nations now have programs for people to get involved with learning about and growing traditional, healthy foods (such as the Three Sisters—corn, beans, and squash—programs seen in some Haudenosaunee groups[58]). Another strategy that has been used is the development of educational videos; the Native American Research and Training Center (see appendix) developed a video in conjunction with the Tohono O'odham Nation in Arizona entitled "Diabetes and Desert Foods: Examples from O'odham Traditions." This video, designed for health practitioners, O'odham people, and the interested public, explores the cultural significance of desert foods. The Indian narrator describes the transition in foodstuffs from the eighteenth century, when Spanish missionaries introduced lard, beef, and sugar, to World War II, when the O'odham diet significantly shifted to a reliance on store-bought and commodity foods. Before this diet shift, diabetes was unknown to O'odham people. The video stresses that desert foods such as cactus pads, beans, and desert fruits and seeds, are not only culturally important, but they may help to control and prevent diabetes. There is also a "how to" segment that describes how store-bought foods can be modified to make them healthier, such as draining the fat off of cooked beef and straining/rinsing canned fruits (if they are packed in a sugar syrup). What is especially important in the video are encouragements to self-empowerment in tribes—the narrator advocates that communities take more control in ordering commodity foods, growing traditional foods (through the help of organizations that promote the preservation of indigenous seeds, like Native Seeds Search), learning from elders, and revaluing and teaching each other about traditional and other types of foods that promote wellness. The "Awakening the Spirit: Pathways to Diabetes Prevention and Control 2000 Calendar" designed by the Native American Program Design Team of the American Diabetes Association (see appendix) is an effort to educate the national population about healthy foods, teas, herbs, and juices. Each month profiles a photograph of the foods, crafts, or food-preparation items of a distinct ethnic group, like the Cherokee, or a region such as the Northwest. Different tips about diabetes prevention and treatment are also profiled.

Referral Systems for Traditional/Alternative Healers

Diabetes education, treatment, and prevention programs could focus much more on collaborating with indigenous healers and other practitioners who may have a lot to offer for dealing with the many physical, psychological, spiritual, and social factors of diabetes, in addition to other chronic diseases. While referrals to traditional healers are primary, it is also important to include other nonbiomedical practitioners (often described as complementary practitioners), such as acupuncturists, herbalists, massage therapists, etc. Because stress is a factor in diabetes, and many other health problems in any population, stress-reduction techniques such as meditation, massage, acupressure, and acupuncture may be very effective means of facilitating illness management. As part of this endeavor, health-care personnel (doctors, nurses, health aides, etc.) should be educated about the important place of traditional healing for total well-being. A sense of partnership, not a hierarchy, should be developed between biomedicine and more culturally sensitive and holistic forms of medicine.

Talking Circles

Talking circles with talking sticks (to allow each person the power to express themselves) have been used in some American Indian groups as a strategy for dealing with many problems from alcoholism to chronic illnesses such as diabetes and cancer. Often, when someone is diagnosed with a chronic illness, issues of self-image, identity, and coping figure prominently.[59] Talking circles provide an excellent opportunity to encourage discussion about some difficult emotions and meet with others who are facing the same challenges. As Burhannstipanov points out, talking circles should be demarcated as nonceremonial so that educational ideas expressed in the circle can be more easily shared with others.[60] At the 1997 Fourth International Conference on Diabetes in San Diego, several presenters focused on how to incorporate the traditional talking circle into American Indian diabetes programs.[61]

Using and Adapting Local Myths, Stories, Legends, Heroes, and Heroines

As Weiner discusses in this volume, drawing upon Native myths and stories is an effective method of educating about problems such as diabetes, especially considering how easily doctors can overwhelm diabetics with unfamiliar biomedical jargon and scientific concepts. Using culturally appropriate stories can make an immense difference if it helps someone understand their disease and cope with it successfully. In southern Ontario, an innovative program developed by Rebecca Hagey and her colleagues, used Nanabush, a mythic Ojibway teacher, in a story to tell about how diabetes had come to Native peoples.[62] The story they developed is called "Nanabush and the Pale Stranger" and it has greatly facilitated understanding diabetes in more accessible ways for laypeople.[63]

Conclusion

There is, of course, no one formula for developing health education and prevention programs that will work in every American Indian nation, culture, and population. Each tribe and group will have different practices, beliefs, and stories from their culture that will be most appropriate for dealing with diabetes and the many other health problems that face Native peoples today. It should be stressed that if the goal is to promote wellness, then research and program development in this area need to be ethnographic, collaborative, and sensitive to diversity within and between populations.

Another serious issue is the nature of intratribal conflicts and the extent to which they are impeding health and wellness for group members. For example, in one study among the Navajo, Miller found that employing Navajo staff members at the local health clinics could be an impediment to health care because of people's clan affiliations, fear of local gossip by other Navajos, and potential associations of Navajo clinic personnel with witchcraft.[64] In my research with the Iroquois in New York, I have witnessed the divisions between the "progressives" (pro-gambling contingents) and the "traditionalists" as having a profound influence on not only health-care politics, but also on interactions and conflicts in day-to-day life.

As a final recommendation, there should also be an emphasis on networking to promote communication links with other Indian Nations, diabetes programs, and those working in the field of American Indian wellness (see appendix). This kind of climate has been fostered in recent years by the International Conferences on Diabetes and Indigenous Peoples, which usually draw several thousand participants in an eclectic exchange of information from Native peoples, anthropologists, nutritionists, nurses, physicians, traditional healers, and others concerned with diabetes and wellness in Native populations.

APPENDIX
References for Native Diabetes-Prevention/Education Programs

Awakening the Spirit:
Pathways to Diabetes Prevention and Control

This is the Native American Program of the American Diabetes Association. The program designs and distributes health-education brochures, calendars, literature, and newsletters. It also trains community mentors to develop local avenues of empowerment. Organization members also advocate political actions. For more information contact:

American Diabetes Association
Awakening the Spirit
1701 North Beauregard Street
Alexandria, Virginia 22311
telephone: 1-800-diabetes (342-2383)
e-mail: awakening@diabetes.org
website: <http://www.diabetes.org/>

Canadian Diabetes Association (CDA)

The CDA published a comprehensive issue in the fall of 1994 in their *Diabetes Dialogue* magazine on "The Silent Epidemic: Diabetes in the First Nations." This issue looks at the problem from a Native perspective and talks about the many innovative programs being tried to halt the rapid spread of this disease.

In this issue you will find information on the Native SUGAR group, the Northern Food Tradition and Health Kit, information on the Atlantic First Nations Diabetes Coordinator, and the "Nanabush and the Pale Stranger" story. To obtain a copy of the magazine, contact:

Canadian Diabetes Association
15 Toronto Street
Suite 1001
Toronto, Ontario M5C 2E3

Centre for Nutrition and the Environment of Indigenous Peoples (CINE)

This is an organization, begun in 1993, developed at McGill University "in response to a need expressed by Aboriginal Peoples for participatory research and education to address their concerns about the integrity of their traditional food systems. Deterioration in the environment has adverse impacts on the health and lifestyles of Indigenous Peoples, in particular health and nutrition as derived from food and food traditions. CINE is a university-based endeavor to assist Indigenous Peoples in dealing with their concerns related to traditional food systems, nutrition and the environment" (taken from the CINE Two-Year Report 1994–1996). CINE puts out a newsletter available to everyone on issues such as cancer, diabetes, environmental hazards in Native territories, comparing traditional foods to market foods, etc. CINE's governing board has representatives from the Assembly of First Nations, Council for Yukon Indians, Dene Nation, Inuit Circumpolar Conference, and Metis Nation of the Northwest Territories. To get on their mailing list, contact:

Centre for Nutrition and the Environment of Indigenous Peoples
MacDonald Campus of McGill University
21,111 Lakeshore Road
Ste-Anne-de-Bellevue, Quebec H9X 3V9
telephone: (514) 398-7544
fax: (514) 398-1020

Indian Health Promotion

This is an organization at the University of Oklahoma that sponsors conferences on Indian health, such as the Native Wellness and Women conferences. For information, contact:

Health Promotion Programs
University of Oklahoma
555 Constitution Street
Norman, Oklahoma 73037-0005

telephone: (405) 325-1790
fax: (405) 325-7126

National Aboriginal Diabetes Association (NADA)

The mission of NADA is to address diabetes among Aboriginal Peoples by creating networks and opportunities for individuals and communities in accord with their culture, traditions, and values. Some of the goals of NADA are to promote Aboriginal community-based diabetes initiatives and develop and facilitate initiatives for prevention, education, research, care, and support of diabetes among Aboriginal Peoples.

> National Aboriginal Diabetes Association
> 108, 150 Henry Avenue
> Winnipeg, Manitoba R3B 0J7
> telephone: (204) 775-3625
> e-mail: nada@escape.ca
> website: <http://www.nada.ca/about.htm>

Native American Research and Training Center (NARTC)

This is an excellent organization at the University of Arizona in Tucson that sponsors a lot of research on Native health issues, often directed and organized by Native peoples. They have many monographs and videos that can be used in education programs.

> Native American Research and Training Center
> Department of Family and Community Medicine
> University of Arizona
> Tucson, Arizona 85719
> telephone: (520) 621-5920

Internet Resources

Internet resources on American Indian health have burgeoned in the last several years. Any inquiry with a general search engine (such as Lycos, Infoseek, or Netscape) is likely to yield many references. For example, if you type in "Native American health" on Infoseek, 14,650 results come up (although not all of these actually relate to Native health). Here are some productive sites to explore Internet information:

> *Minnesota Indian Women's Resource Center* (with links to a number of different health sites)
> <http://www.nnic.com/miwrc.html>

Native American Diabetes Project
<http://www.laplaza.org/dwc/prof/nadp>

Native American Health Resources on the Internet
<http://www.hanksville.phast.umass.edu/misc/nahealth.html>

Native Web
<http://www.nativeweb.org/>

The Pima Indians: Pathfinders for Health (with a main focus on diabetes)
<http://www.niddk.nih.gov/health/diabetes/pima/index.htm>

Notes

1. Joel Gittelsohn et al., "Use of Ethnographic Methods for Applied Research on Diabetes among Ojibway-Cree Indians in Northern Ontario," unpublished manuscript, 1993; Rebecca Hagey, "The Phenomenon, the Explanations, and the Responses: Metaphors Surrounding Diabetes in Urban Canadian Indians," *Social Science and Medicine* 18:3 (1984): 265–72.

2. J. R. Gavin, "Diabetes Mellitus: An Unrelenting Threat to the Health of Minorities," testimony given in the hearing before the Select Committee on Aging, U.S. House of Representatives, 102nd Cong., 2nd Sess., 6 April 1992 (pub. no. 102-864, 1992); D. M. Gohdes, "Diabetes in North American Indians and Alaska Natives," in National Diabetes Data Group, eds., *Diabetes in America* (Rockville, MD: National Institutes of Health, 1995); D. M. Gohdes et al., "Diabetes in American Indians: An Overview," *Diabetes Care* 16:1, supplement 1 (1993): 239–44.

3. W. L. Freeman et al., "Diabetes in American Indians of Washington, Oregon, and Idaho," *Diabetes Care* 12:4 (1989): 282–88; Gavin, "Diabetes Mellitus."

4. W. Knowler et al., "Determinants of Diabetes Mellitus in Pima Indians," *Diabetes Care* 16:1, supplement 1 (1993): 216.

5. T. Kue Young, "Diabetes Mellitus among Native Americans in Canada and the United States: An Epidemiological Review," *American Journal of Human Biology* 5 (1993): 399–413.

6. Knowler et al., "Determinants of Diabetes Mellitus in Pima Indians."

7. P. Bennett, "Diabetes and its Impact in American Indian Communities: The Pima Indians." Paper presented at the annual meeting, Diabetes in American Indian Communities: Creating Partnerships for Prevention in the Twenty-First Century (October 1999, Albuquerque).

8. American Diabetes Association, "Direct and Indirect Costs of Diabetes in the United States in 1987" (Alexandria, VA: American Diabetes Association, 1988); Gohdes et al., "Diabetes in American Indians"; A. Jacobson, "Depression and Diabetes," *Diabetes Care* 16:12 (1993): 1621–23.

9. W. L. Freeman and G. M. Hosey, "Diabetic Complications among American Indians of Washington, Oregon, and Idaho: Prevalence of Retinopathy, End-Stage Renal Disease, and Amputations," *Diabetes Care* 16:1, supplement 1 (1993): 357–61.

10. Frank Vinicor, "Is Diabetes a Public-Health Disorder?" *Diabetes Care* 17:1 (1994): 22–27.

11. W. Haviland, *Cultural Anthropology*, 8th ed. (New York: Harcourt Brace Publishers, 1996).

12. Kathleen Huttlinger, "A Navajo Perspective of Diabetes," *Family and Community Health* 18:2 (1995): 9–16.

13. See also, Benjamin R. Kracht, "Diabetes among the Kiowa: An Ethnohistorical Perspective," 147–68; and Linda C. Garro and Gretchen C. Lang, "Explanations of Diabetes: Anishinaabe and Dakota Deliberate upon a New Illness," in Jennie R. Joe and Robert S. Young, eds., *Diabetes as a Disease of Civilization: The Impact of Lifestyle and Cultural Changes on the Health of Indigenous Peoples* (Berlin: Mouton de Gruyter, 1994).

14. Knowler et al., "Determinants of Diabetes Mellitus in the Pima Indians."

15. R. Judkins, "Diabetes and Perception of Diabetes among Seneca Indians," *New York State Journal of Medicine* 78 (1978): 1320–23.

16. Gretchen C. Lang, "Making Sense about Diabetes: Dakota Narratives of Illness," *Medical Anthropology* 11:3 (1989): 305–29; Jennie Joe and Robert Young, "Diabetes and Native Americans: The Impact of Lifestyle and Cultural Changes on the Health of Indigenous Peoples," *Native American Research and Training Center Monograph* (Tucson: University of Arizona, n.d.); Paul Skinner and Dana Silverman-Peach, "Diabetes and Native Americans: Sociocultural Change, Stress, and Coping," *Native American Research and Training Center Monograph* (Tucson: University of Arizona, 1991).

17. Dennis Weidman, "Type II Diabetes Mellitus, Technological Development, and the Oklahoma Cherokee," in Hans Baer, ed., *Encounters with Biomedicine: Case Studies in Medical Anthropology* (Philadelphia: Gordon & Breach, 1987), 43–73.

18. Ray Moisa, "The BIA Relocation Program," in Susan Lobo and Steve Talbot, eds., *Native American Voices* (New York: Longman, 1998), 154.

19. William Dressler, "Culture, Stress, and Disease," in Thomas Johnson and Carolyn Sargent, eds., *Medical Anthropology: Contemporary Theory and Method* (Westport, CT: Praeger, 1996), 252–71.

20. E. Szathmary and R. Ferrell, "Glucose Level, Acculturation, and Glycosylated Hemoglobin: An Example of Biocultural Interaction," *Medical Anthropology Quarterly* 4:3 (1990): 315–41.

21. Jennie R. Joe and Robert S. Young, eds., *Diabetes as a Disease of Civilization: The Impact of Lifestyle and Cultural Changes on the Health of Indigenous Peoples* (Berlin: Mouton de Gruyter, 1994).

22. Canadian Diabetes Association, "The Silent Epidemic: Diabetes in the First Nations," *Diabetes Dialogue* 41(3) (fall 1994): 23.

23. Anne Fagot-Campagna et al., "The Public Epidemiology of Type 2 Diabetes in Children and Adolescents: A Case Study of American Indian Adolescents in the Southwestern United States," *Clinica Chimica Acta* 286 (1999): 90.

24. J. Kauffman, "Indian Women's Health-Care Consensus Statement," Indian Health Service Round Table Meeting: January 1991 (Department of Health and Human Services, monograph no. 01-90-1508, 1991), 1.

25. Ibid., 1.

26. J. Neel, "The Thrifty Genotype Revisited," in J. Koberling and R. Tattersall,

eds., *The Genetics of Diabetes Mellitus* (New York: Academic Press, Serono Symposium, no. 47, 1982), 283–93.

27. Bennett, 1999.

28. David Satcher, "Keynote Address, Diabetes in American Indian Communities: Creating Partnerships for Prevention in the Twenty-First Century" (Albuquerque, October 1999); Fagot-Campagna et al., "The Public Epidemiology of Type 2 Diabetes in Children and Adolescents," 81–95.

29. Edward James Olmos, "Diabetes Mellitus: An Unrelenting Threat to the Health of Minorities," testimony given in the hearing before the Select Committee on Aging, U.S. House of Representatives, 102nd Cong., 2nd Sess., 6 April 1992 (pub. no. 102-864, 1992).

30. For example, see Mark Nichter, "Drinking Boiled Water: A Cultural Analysis of a Health Education Message," *Social Science and Medicine* 21:6 (1985): 667–69; Martha Balshem, *Cancer in the Community: Class and Medical Authority* (Washington, DC: Smithsonian Institution, 1993).

31. Barbara Redman, *The Process of Patient Education* (Boston: Mosby, 1993).

32. Gittelsohn et al., "Use of Ethnographic Methods for Applied Research on Diabetes among Ojibway-Cree Indians in Northern Ontario"; Rebecca Hagey, "The Native Diabetes Program: Rhetorical Process and Praxis," *Medical Anthropology* 12 (1989): 7–33.

33. J. Knows His Gun, "Diabetes Mellitus: An Unrelenting Threat to the Health of Minorities," testimony given in the hearing before the Select Committee on Aging, U.S. House of Representatives, 102nd Cong., 2nd Sess., 6 April 1992 (pub. no. 102-864, 1992); Native American Research and Training Center, *Living with Diabetes: A Native American Perspective* (video) (Tucson: University of Arizona, 1988).

34. Redman, *The Process of Patient Education*, 24.

35. For example, *Diabetes Care*, "Diabetes in Native Americans," 16:1, supplement 1 (1993).

36. Veronica Evaneshko, "Presenting Complaints in a Navajo Indian Diabetic Population," in Joe and Young, eds., *Diabetes as a Disease of Civilization*, 357–78; Joycelyn Bruyere, "Understandings about Type 2 Diabetes Mellitus among the Nehinaw (Cree)," paper presented at the American Anthropology Association Annual Meeting, Philadelphia, 1998; Linda Garro, "Continuity and Change: The Interpretation of Illness in an Anishinaabe (Ojibway) Community," *Culture, Medicine, and Psychiatry* 14 (1990): 417–54; Gittelsohn et al., "Use of Ethnographic Methods for Applied Research on Diabetes among Ojibway-Cree Indians in Northern Ontario"; Hagey, "The Phenomenon, the Explanations, and the Responses"; Jennie Joe, "Perceptions of Diabetes by Indian Adolescents," in Joe and Young, eds., *Diabetes as a Disease of Civilization: The Impact of Cultural Change on Indigenous Peoples* (Berlin: Mouton de Gruyter, 1994), 329–56; Judkins, "Diabetes and Perception of Diabetes among Seneca Indians"; Gretchen C. Lang, "Talking about a New Illness with the Dakota: Reflections on Diabetes, Food, and Culture," in R. Winthrop, ed., *Culture and the Anthropological Tradition* (Lanham, MD: University Press of America, 1990); Cheryl Rodriguez and Derek Milne, "The Importance of Family Support for Diabetes Self-Care among Navajos," paper presented at the American Anthropology Association

Annual Meeting, Philadelphia, 1998; Diane Weiner, "Luiseno Theory and Practice of Chronic Illness Causation, Avoidance, and Treatment," Ph.D. dissertation (Los Angeles: University of California, 1993).

37. M. Urdaneta and R. Krehbiel, "Cultural Heterogeneity of Mexican-Americans and Its Implications for the Treatment of Diabetes Mellitus Type II," *Medical Anthropology* 11:3 (1989): 269–83.

38. Native American Research and Training Center, *Living with Diabetes* (video).

39. Personal communication with Nicolette Teufel, University of Arizona, 1994.

40. Lang, "Making Sense about Diabetes."

41. See also, Weiner, 1993.

42. Ann Macaulay, "Kahnawake Schools Diabetes Prevention Project (KSDPP): Intervention and Results of a Native Community-Based Primary Diabetes-Prevention Project," paper presented at the Fourth International Conference on Diabetes and Indigenous Peoples (San Diego, October 8–11, 1997); Alex McComber et al., "Grass-Roots Participation in the Primary Prevention of Diabetes in a Mohawk Community," paper presented at the Fourth International Conference on Diabetes and Indigenous Peoples (San Diego, October 8–11, 1997).

43. M. Fox, "'Zeesbakadapenewin': Words of an Elder Grandmother about the Sugar Disease," *Diabetes Dialogue* (Canadian Diabetes Association) 41:3 (1994): 22, 24.

44. Huttlinger, "A Navajo Perspective of Diabetes," 10.

45. Lang, "Talking about a New Illness with the Dakota"; Judkins, "Diabetes and Perception of Diabetes among Seneca Indians."

46. Diane Weiner, personal communication, 1999.

47. Elisa Sobo, "The Sweetness of Fat," in N. Sault, ed., *Many Mirrors: Body Image and Social Relations* (New Brunswick, NJ: Rutgers University Press, 1994), 132.

48. Gittelsohn et al., "Use of Ethnographic Methods for Applied Research on Diabetes among Ojibway-Cree Indians in Northern Ontario," 1.

49. Yvette Sakiestewa et al., "Weight Loss Practices of American Indians," paper presented at the annual meeting, Diabetes in American Indian Communities: Creating Partnerships for Prevention in the Twenty-First Century (Albuquerque, October 1999).

50. S. Ponchillia, "The Effect of Cultural Beliefs on the Treatment of Native Peoples with Diabetes and Visual Impairment," *Journal of Visual Impairment and Blindness* (November 1993): 333–35.

51. G. Heath et al., "Community-Based Exercise Intervention: Zuni Diabetes Project," *Diabetes Care* 10:5 (1987): 579–83; Zuni Wellness Center, "Evaluation of the Zuni Diabetes Project and the Zuni Wellness Program" (Hogansburg, NY: Department of Health and Human Services, SRC, Inc., 1992).

52. Canadian Diabetes Association, "The Silent Epidemic"; Huttlinger, "A Navajo Perspective of Diabetes."

53. Hagey, "The Phenomenon, the Explanations, and the Responses" and "The Native Diabetes Program."

54. Birdena Sanchez and Stephen Poirer, "American Indian/Native American Community Intervention: Zuni Treatment and Prevention Program," paper presented at the Fourth International Conference on Diabetes and Indigenous Peoples (San

Diego, October 8–11, 1997); Macaulay, "Kahnawake Schools Diabetes Prevention Project (KSDPP)"; McComber et al., "Grass-Roots Participation in the Primary Prevention of Diabetes in a Mohawk Community."

55. Many of the issues relating to this have been discussed in the literature on compliance and adherence to therapeutic recommendations; see, for example, M. R. DiMatteo and H. Friedman, *Social Psychology and Medicine* (Cambridge, MA: Oelgeschlager, Gunn, and Hain, 1982); additionally, Freund and McGuire note that "when doctors' 'orders' involve major lifestyle changes (such as changing eating or exercise patterns), compliance is even less common" (Peter Freund and Meredith McGuire, *Health, Illness and the Social Body* [Englewood Cliffs, NJ: Prentice-Hall, 1995], 187).

56. There is a number of reference books that can be consulted to learn more about Native games, such as Allan Macfarlan and Paulette Macfarlan, *Handbook of American Indian Games* (New York: Dover Publications, 1958).

57. Heath et al., "Community-Based Exercise Intervention."

58. More information on Three Sisters programs can be obtained from Dr. Jane Mt. Pleasant, Coordinator, American Indian Agriculture Project, Cornell University, Ithaca, New York.

59. D. Kelleher, "Coming to Terms with Diabetes: Coping Strategies and Non-Compliance," in Anderson and Bury, eds., *Living with Chronic Illness: The Experience of Patients and Their Families* (Boston: Unwin Hyman, 1988), 137–56.

60. Linda Burhansstipanov, "Developing Culturally Competent Community-Based Interventions," in D. Weiner, ed., *Preventing and Controlling Cancer in North America* (Westport, CT: Praeger, 1999), 167–83.

61. Sara Boskovich, "The Healing Circle: An Urban Community Diabetes Program for Native Americans," paper presented at the Fourth International Conference on Diabetes and Indigenous Peoples (San Diego, October 8–11, 1997); Louise Sanderson, "A Holistic and Cultural Way to Wellness," paper presented at the Fourth International Conference on Diabetes and Indigenous Peoples (San Diego, October 8–11, 1997).

62. Hagey, "The Phenomenon, the Explanations, and the Responses" and "The Native Diabetes Program."

63. Canadian Diabetes Association, "The Silent Epidemic."

64. Janneli Miller (Vojta), "How Do We Do It Right? Rural Health Care on the Navajo Reservation," unpublished M.A. thesis (Flagstaff: Northern Arizona University, 1991).

TEN

FELICIA SCHANCHE HODGE
and JOHN CASKEN

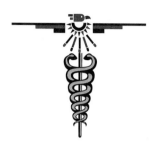

Pathways to Health
AN AMERICAN INDIAN BREAST-CANCER EDUCATION PROJECT[1]

Introduction

Many studies have demonstrated that cancer prevention works and that the earlier that a cancer is detected the more likely it is that a useful intervention can be engaged, which will lead to a longer life for the patient.[2] Breast-cancer prevention activities such as mammographies are very important to identify possible early cancers for intervention. Educating the public and those at high risk can, however, be a very challenging task for the health-care worker. This chapter demonstrates that many women do not consider themselves at risk for cancer, thus, for them, screening activities are less of a priority.[3] Many women approach the whole issue of cancer prevention from a very different perspective than the health worker. The case study in this chapter deals with one relatively small group of American Indian women. It is critical to realize that there are a wide variety of other social, economic, and cultural factors that affect a person's perspective on cancer. Even among indigenous peoples there can be considerable differences in how a person approaches the issue of cancer.[4,5]

185

FELICIA SCHANCHE HODGE and JOHN CASKEN

Focus groups have been proven to be exceptionally useful for obtaining explicit and tacit knowledge about cancer.[6] The focus-group approach is useful not merely for American Indians or other indigenous groups. Indeed, we should be aware that the massively heterogeneous nature of the population in the United States means that most people are not "mainstream" as far as health-care issues are concerned. We should note, for instance, that more visits are made to complementary or alternative-medicine practitioners than to the typical physician trained in the Western tradition.[7] In 1993, over $21 billion in out-of-pocket expenses was paid to nonclinical physicians—a sum that was greater than the out-of-pocket sum paid to Western-trained medical professionals.[8] Thus we must accept that the majority of the population does not necessarily accept standard models of Western health-care behavior. Health-care providers, policy-makers, and administrators need new approaches to reduce the burden of morbidity and mortality; we must find new ways that effectively engage the individual in meaningful approaches.

Background

The American Indian population faces many important health issues including cancer, injuries, diabetes, alcohol and substance abuse, violence, suicide, cardiovascular disease, and obesity. Cancer has become the second leading cause of death for Alaska Native women and is the third leading cause of death among American Indian women.[9,10] Due to a large Indian population residing in California,[11] and the fact that American Indian women have a high mortality and low survival rate in certain cancers,[12] California's American Indian population is an ideal target for cancer-control efforts—particularly in the early detection and treatment of breast cancer, a condition that when identified at an early stage is frequently treatable.

The Indian Health Service reports 309,238 American Indians living in California,[13] of which approximately 70,000 are women over the age of 18 years. California boasts the largest concentration of American Indians in any state according to the U.S. census. Seventy percent live in major metropolitan areas, and the remaining 30 percent reside in rural counties on or near the state's 85 reservations. Health-care services are limited, despite the size of this population. Currently, no Indian inpatient facility exists in California. The small clinics are Indian-run and operated. The Indian Health Service supplements these clinics by contracting for inpatient and specialized outpatient services. These services, however, are limited and have restricted eligibility requirements (IHS).

Cancer has recently become a major public-health concern among American Indians.[14] Although breast-cancer data specific to American Indians are difficult to obtain and interpret, current data suggests that the age-adjusted

186

breast-cancer incidence rates are much lower among Indian women than white women.[15] The Surveillance, Education, Evaluation Reports (SEER) data indicate that American Indians experience a cancer incidence rate for all sites that is half the rate of the white population (157.3 vs. 359.2).[16] Reported breast-cancer mortality rates are also lower in this population. The age-adjusted breast-cancer mortality for nine Indian Health Service Areas is 16.1 compared to the reported 26.7 rate for whites.[17] Considering the available data, which indicates low breast-cancer incidence and mortality rates, health-care providers may conclude that breast cancer is not a problem among American Indian women. American Indian women may also conclude that they need not participate in breast-cancer screening programs because breast cancer is not an "Indian problem."

These low incidence and mortality rates, however, may be misleading. First, there is no accurate database that reports cancer-related information for American Indians.[18] Second, studies have shown that current sources such as death certificates, Indian Health Service, and tumor registries have problems in racial misclassification and other reporting errors.[19] Third, there are increasing reports among Indian communities and Indian health clinics, and other trend data, which indicate that breast cancer mortality rates are increasing.[20] Although the cancer-survival rates for American Indians are very sketchy, national data reports that American Indian women have poorer survival rates from cancer of any racial group in the United States.[21] For all sites combined, American Indians appear to experience a five-year survival rate of 35.2 percent, relative to 50.3 percent for whites. The disparity is even greater for breast cancer (49 percent relative to 76 percent in whites).[22] This information supports the fact that breast cancer is a significant problem among Indian women and signals a need for the development of appropriate breast-cancer control programs for American Indians.

Developing a breast-cancer early-detection and treatment-education project for American Indians requires an understanding of the American Indian culture, illness beliefs, barriers to breast-cancer screening, and the cultural constructs that inhibit or facilitate the utilization of screening protocols and treatment recommendations. This chapter describes the steps taken in the development, implementation, and evaluation of the Pathways to Health project, a breast-cancer education program targeting American Indian women in California.

Methods

The Center for American Indian Research and Education (CAIRE) supports research, evaluation, education, policy development, planning, prevention, and community-service activities nationally. In 1994, CAIRE received a three-year training grant from the National Cancer Institute to develop, implement, and evaluate a culturally sensitive breast-cancer educational program targeting American Indian women in California. The goals of the project were to: (1) increase breast-cancer–prevention knowledge levels among primary-care physicians, other health professionals, and American Indian women; (2) increase breast-cancer early-detection knowledge among primary-care physicians, other health professionals, and American Indian women; (3) increase breast-cancer treatment knowledge among primary-care physicians, other health professionals, and American Indian women; and (4) to widely disseminate up-to-date professionally known information about prevention, early detection, and treatment of breast cancer to primary-care physicians, other health professionals, and American Indian women. This chapter reports on the portion of the Pathways to Health project that targeted American Indian women.

There were three major activities taken in the development and implementation of the Pathways to Health project targeting American Indian women and breast cancer. First, a series of six focus groups were held to identify cultural illness beliefs, to identify barriers and facilitators to breast-cancer screening, and to provide feedback on the project's educational materials. Second, breast-cancer educational materials were developed in response to the identified barriers, risk factors, illness beliefs and specific informational needs of the targeted group. And third, a series of breast-cancer educational workshops were offered to American Indian and Alaska Native women residing in California. The information obtained from the focus groups served as a framework for the development of key culturally sensitive messages and educational approaches used in the educational materials and workshops to increase knowledge and change breast-cancer screening behaviors.

Focus Groups

In an attempt to identify the cultural response and milieu of breast cancer, the barriers to care, and the cultural aspects and beliefs surrounding breast cancer, we met with six groups of American Indian women. Criteria for selection for inclusion in the focus groups were as follows: American Indian women over the age of 18 years, who were residing in the target communities. Initial contacts for focus-group participants were made at the local health clinics. A snowball technique was adopted, such that respondents were asked to provide names of other individuals in the community who fit the study criteria. The identification of American Indian was self-reported. The focus groups were held in San Francisco ($n = 15$), Oakland ($n = 18$), Santa Rosa ($n = 9$), Round Valley Reservation ($n = 8$), Berkeley ($n = 5$), and the Hupa Indian Reservation ($n = 10$) (Total: $n = 65$).

An American Indian focus-group leader conducted the sessions guided by broad topic categories. The focus-group phase used anthropological field methodologies to identify and describe knowledge, attitudes, and behaviors related to breast-cancer screening and health care. This phase provided a preliminary look at health-care beliefs and behaviors. The focus-group discussion included the following areas:

1. How important do you think breast cancer is in your community? Is it a problem among Indian women?
2. What are the barriers/facilitators to breast-cancer screening (self-breast exam, physician's exam, and mammography)?
3. What are the cultural aspects surrounding breast cancer in terms of taboos and prohibitions?
4. What beliefs do you hold about breast cancer, your risk, surgery, treatment, etc.?

The focus-group sessions were held at local Indian agency facilitates, in a setting that was familiar and comfortable to the participating women. The sessions were coordinated and facilitated by a trained American Indian member of the community. Indian women over the age of 18 years were invited by word of mouth to attend the focus-group meeting. A flyer was also distributed in each of the four communities.

An attempt was made to hold the sessions on a weekend or during evening hours to alleviate time barriers and to increase attendance. Special requests were made and approved for use of Indian-agency meeting rooms.

Food (snacks) and drinks (water, coffee, tea, and soda) were offered to participants as is the custom in many American Indian meetings. The meeting minutes were not tape-recorded in response to participant request to not tape the sessions. Project staff recorded the focus group minutes by hand. The sessions were 1 to 1½ hours in length. The meeting minutes were transcribed and the data analyzed.

The second phase of focus groups held later in the year was composed of those focus-group members available from the original group (approximately one-half of the group participated in this second phase). They responded to the educational materials in terms of (a) media preferences, (b) communication styles, (c) presentation of materials, (d) literacy levels, and (e) cultural acceptability. The materials were assessed for their cultural acceptability, relevance and message appeal, level of comprehension, accuracy of information, and degree of credibility with the target population.

Data gathered from focus-group meetings also assisted in the development of the workshop curriculum and the cultural approach used in the workshop. The curriculum included sessions on (a) breast-cancer risk factors, (b) breast-cancer screening techniques, (c) breast-cancer treatment and treatment options, (d) patient rights and second opinions, (e) communication techniques, and (f) cultural differences and strengths. Information from these focus groups was also used to develop a pre- and post-test survey instrument.

Focus-Group Results

The findings from the focus-group interviews identified several areas as important constructs to be considered in developing and implementing educational and training programs.

BELIEF IN BREAST-CANCER RISK. The American Indian women participating in the focus groups did not feel that breast cancer was of particular significance in their communities, and therefore prevention and treatment were somewhat useless. Although several participants had friends and relatives who were diagnosed with breast cancer—and some knew women who had died of breast cancer—as a whole the group felt they were at low risk of breast cancer. Indeed, many considered other problems such as poverty, alcoholism, and diabetes of greater significance. Several women noted that there are so many problems to confront in the American Indian community, breast cancer is lower on the scale of everyday concerns. This belief—that breast cancer does not happen to them and that there are so many other problems of even greater magnitude to deal with—is troublesome, but it supports the low cancer-screening rates evident in this population.

BARRIERS TO CANCER SCREENING AND TREATMENT. The focus-group results highlighted numerous barriers that interfere with cancer screening and treatment efforts. These barriers include, but are not limited to, culturally inappropriate recruitment protocols, lack of culturally appropriate cancer prevention and control materials, inaccessible science and or research educational training opportunities, language and communication problems, poverty, transportation, cancer-causation beliefs, lack of Native health providers, and unavailability of health facilities. The types and impact levels of such barriers vary among Native communities in different regions of the country.

Cultural barriers, specifically, contribute to underutilization of medical care. Modesty, taboos, and utilization of traditional healing practices are important elements of the cultural belief system among urban and rural Indians. Beliefs about modern medical procedures, such as radiation for detecting and treating cancer, may also be barriers. The female patient may also be offended by what she might consider to be an abrupt or impersonal manner. Being treated with respect and courtesy by health-care staff was identified as an important feature to successful health-care practice. This attitude included the view that providers take the time to explain procedures and not rush clients in and out of the office.

Many Indian women were frightened by the treatment for breast cancer.

Fear of surgery and of radiation and chemotherapy treatment was identified. Although there were significant fears identified with dying, fears of its repercussions were also voiced, as responsibility for surviving children and other families members were of concern. To many, a diagnosis of cancer was a diagnosis of death and would produce an overwhelming financial hardship and distress within the immediate and extended family.

Several women stated, and many agreed, that cancer was not talked about in their families. When their grandmothers, mothers, or other relatives died of cancer, it was never discussed. The word "cancer" was not openly talked about as a disease, and its treatment, or the long-term effect of the disease, was not acknowledged.

CULTURALLY SENSITIVE ISSUES. American Indians live in a bicultural world combining both indigenous and Eurocentric cultural patterns. These cultural characteristics and differences are important in understanding the influences that shape their interaction with the health-care-delivery system. To many American Indians, "health care" means more than dealing with illness and pain; it reflects the basic world view and cultural values of the group, which in turn influences health and illness behavior. It is believed that healing takes place not only in the body, but also spiritually and includes the family and community. These cultural characteristics also affect the acceptance of preventative medicine particularly with respect to breast-cancer screening, and are important factors in designing an intervention that is acceptable to the American Indian population.

Family and community are of high importance for many American Indian women, and family needs take precedence. Only after the children's and family's needs are met will they tend to their own health-care needs, especially in regards to health-screening exams. Time orientation also is different, with the focus on the present rather than the future. It is said that it is important to take care of today as tomorrow may never come. However, this does not mean that the women do not value prevention or the important role it plays in keeping healthy. Rather, it is necessary to explain the impact that actions taken today have on the health of individuals and families in the future. Health-care workers need to recognize the American Indian's orientation to the present and to short-term goals.[23] This orientation makes screening more difficult. Modesty and the value of privacy are important, particularly with discussing breast self-exams and the actual breast examination. It is important that the procedures are explained beforehand and that care is taken to keep the patient draped as much as possible. The examiner should try not to expose both of the patient's breasts at the same time. Additionally, female health-care workers should always be present during a breast examination by a male practitioner. Most importantly, American Indian patients should feel they are treated with care and courtesy and that their traditional beliefs are accepted and valued.

TABLE 10.1

AMERICAN INDIAN CULTURAL VALUES FOR DEVELOPING A BREAST-CANCER SCREENING PROGRAM

- Health beliefs linked to cultural values of religion and spirituality

- Modesty, taboos, and illness beliefs linked to tribal beliefs

- The importance of family and community

- The importance of women and their role in caring for the family

- Time orientation to the present

- The value of health for the well-being of the tribe and community

---

AMERICAN INDIAN ILLNESS BELIEFS. It is important to note that among many tribes the same beliefs about health and illness are not shared. Most health beliefs are, however, closely linked to the tribe's religious beliefs. Generally, American Indians embrace a much more holistic approach to health than do most Euramericans. Health is considered not only a physical, but also a spiritual state; a person is considered to be made up of body, mind, and spirit. Wellness is the harmony of these three components, whereas disharmony and a state of being out of balance cause sickness. Table 10.1 illustrates the cultural values held by many American Indians, which influence health behavior.

Development of Educational Materials

The focus groups described above provided important information for designing the Pathways to Health breast-cancer education materials and for implementing the breast-cancer screening workshops. First, the focus groups findings identified a common theme of the importance of family and the importance of health to the American Indian women in regards to the role they played as providers and caretakers for their immediate and extended families. Second, the focus-group results pointed out that the view toward cancer was pessimistic; early detection was not seen as meaningful, because it was felt that little could be done to prevent or treat the disease. It was also pointed out that Indian women responded well to programs that included health workers from their own communities and clinics. Thus, the Pathways to Health materials stressed the message of the importance of women to their families and how early-detection techniques were important in saving lives and keeping families together. All Pathways to Health material included Indian designs and information that was specific to the Indian women, such as how to improve communication with their health-care providers and how to involve the family in the prevention and treatment for breast cancer. Also, all Pathways to Health workshops included panel members and workshop assistants who were members of the community being targeted, and the workshops were held at American Indian community sites.

The Pathways to Health project produced three educational products for American Indian women at risk of breast cancer: a video, a treatment manual, and a resource guide. The following provides information on the development and production of these three products.

PATHWAYS TO HEALTH VIDEO. The focus-group interviews identified the preference for visual educational materials as opposed to written pamphlets or booklets. American Indians and Alaska Native peoples tend to be visually oriented—oral testimonies, oral histories, and storytelling are important aspects of the culture.

The production of the Pathways to Health video took two major steps. First came the planning stage, where the actors/participants were identified, the video theme and messages were selected, and the storyboard was created. It was important that credible American Indian actors participate in the video; thus we recruited Indian women with breast cancer or Indian women with significant experience having a relative with breast cancer, having a high personal risk for breast cancer, or having experienced a breast biopsy or other breast-cancer screening or treatment protocols to provide testimonials. Additionally, we identified an American Indian leader to narrate the much-needed information and message regarding breast-cancer screening to the American Indian women. Our video message encompassed the importance of screening, the importance of Indian women in their role of caretaker and homemakers, and the importance of health care. Techniques to survive in the medical-care arena included communication techniques with providers, obtaining needed support, record-keeping, and obtaining second opinions.

The testimonials heard from local Indian women recalling their experience with screening, their relative's experience with breast cancer, and the cultural milieu and barriers to care, supported the 15-minute video's theme of the importance of Indian women and their role in their community and family.

Upon completion, the contents were reviewed by members of the focus groups to consider the cultural acceptability, level of comprehension, length, and degree of credibility with the target population.

PATHWAYS TO HEALTH AMERICAN INDIAN WOMEN'S BREAST-CANCER GUIDE. The *Pathways to Health American Indian Women's Breast Cancer Guide* was designed to provide information to the American Indian women on breast-cancer risk and treatment, the patient–physician relationship, patient rights, Indian Health Service health care, services, and alternative resources, and breast-cancer information resources such as cancer support organizations, insurance information, physician data-query programs, and recommended readings. The appendices contained the names and addresses of California's health and welfare agencies, references, glossary, and acronyms.

The guide was printed in an attractive booklet format with American Indian art work strategically placed throughout. The authors were careful to maintain a sixth- to ninth-grade reading level (not taking into account medical terminology). A glossary of terms and a description of acronyms were placed at the end of the booklet. Each chapter was also outlined in bold letters with bulleted sentences or learning lessons. The summary at each chapter's beginning was shaded in a light beige color to highlight the points.

PATHWAYS TO HEALTH RESOURCE GUIDE. The *Pathways to Health Resource Guide* was intended to assist American Indian women at risk for breast cancer, or breast-cancer patients and their families, to easily identify such resources as treatment centers, Indian health-care clinics, screening centers, social-service agencies, and hospitals. Other resources, such as telephone numbers and various websites available to the population, were also listed. The resource guide was divided into three sections for easier review: the first section highlighted the counties in northern California above San Francisco; the second section covered the central portion of the state and listed the resources by those counties found between San Francisco and Los Angeles; and the third section contain information by counties for southern California.

The focus groups were again valuable in their review of the educational materials in terms of media preferences, communication styles and patterns of speech, presentation of materials in terms of font size, art work, and readability. Literacy levels were maintained at a sixth- to ninth-grade level. Most importantly, cultural acceptability of the materials was assessed. In summary, the educational materials developed were pilot-tested to ascertain their cultural acceptability, relevance, and message appeal, level of comprehension, accuracy of information, and degree of credibility with the target population.

Pathways to Health Workshop Curriculum

In the second year of the project, American Indian women residing at two urban and two reservation settings were invited to participate in one of four breast-cancer educational workshops offered by the Center for American Indian Research and Education (CAIRE). Formal one-day workshop session's curriculum included information on the following:

1. *Breast-cancer risk factors:* Information was provided on the risk American Indian and Alaska women face with regard to breast cancer. Current literature was presented, and panel members discussed issues regarding perceived low risk, obtaining adequate information on breast cancer,

and how to keep oneself and one's family healthy through appropriate screening.

2. *Breast-cancer screening techniques:* The hows and whys of breast-cancer–screening techniques were presented. Topics surrounding radiation, the safety of the screening techniques, and the importance of screening were presented.

3. *Communicating with providers:* The patient–provider relationship was presented in terms of the responsibility of the patient to present information to the provider about their health and to listen carefully and to follow prescribed medical protocols. The responsibility of the provider is to listen carefully to the patient and to identify and treat the aliments of the patient. Memory techniques, such as taking notes or taping conversations, and support aids, such as involving the family in major decisions and having a friend or family member accompany the patient to the office visit, were discussed.

4. *Treatment options and second opinions:* The various treatment options—from biopsies to modified and radical mastectomies—were discussed. The relationship to the stage of cancer diagnosed and the treatment option recommended was highlighted. In addition, workshop participants were encouraged to consider obtaining a second opinion with regard to their cancer diagnosis and treatment plan. How to get a second opinion, in terms of what to say to your physician, how to find an appropriate physician for a second opinion, and how to assess the recommendations were reviewed.

5. *Patient rights:* The idea that patients have well-defined rights in the medical arena was new information to many of the workshop participants. Delineating exactly what the patient has a right to expect, such as access to their records and a right to informed consent, was presented.

The Pathways to Health video for American Indian women was presented at each of the workshops along with the printed resource booklet and patient's guide. Sufficient educational materials were mailed to each Indian health-care clinic in the state for further dissemination.

Three hundred and fifty-two American Indian women residing at four targeted sites participated in the Pathways to Health workshops. Participation was limited to American Indian and Alaska Native women between the ages of 18 and 80 years old. The workshops were held in various locations: at tribal facilities, Indian-agency conference rooms, and at a local hotel meeting room. The Pathways to Health workshops highlighted American Indian panel members. The project was staffed with American Indian trainers and workshop assistants who were members of the community being targeted. In addition, the workshops were held at American Indian community sites identified as acceptable sites for the target population.

Pre- and post-test questionnaires based on data from the focus groups were administered at the beginning and at the end of the workshop. The participating women were asked to evaluate the workshop in terms of logistics, information provided, and strengths or weakness of the presenters or speakers.

Discussion

Few health-education materials exist for American Indian populations. There is also a dearth of breast-cancer materials designed specifically to promote early-detection screening and treatment for breast cancer among American Indians. For this reason, cultural adaptation and cultural sensitivity were major goals in the development of the Pathways to Health project educational materials. These materials, a video for women on the risk and treatment of breast cancer, a resource directory, and a patient breast-cancer treatment guide were designed specifically for American Indian women. A video and a booklet for American Indian health-care providers were also developed. These tools can be used to improve communication with American Indian women at risk or with breast cancer, and as a breast-cancer treatment manual and resource guide. These provider materials were disseminated separately to the Indian health-care clinics in California.

Findings from the focus-group interviews identified significant educational constructs important in designing and implementing instructional workshops in the American Indian community, including the importance of the American Indian family, orientation to the present and to short-term goals, modesty and the value of privacy, and cultural illness beliefs. The development and presentation of educational materials, and implementation of educational workshops designed to heighten awareness of breast cancer and to increase breast-cancer–screening compliance requires an understanding of the target population's illness beliefs, environmental milieu, and barriers to screening. Providing culturally appropriate educational materials heightens the acceptance of the materials and encourages the adoption of these materials.

The breast-cancer educational program was designed, developed, and implemented based on the findings from the focus groups. The Pathways to Health project differs from other breast-cancer programs by using such information as a framework for material development, therefore increasing the likelihood of meeting the needs and acceptance among American Indian women. The material also provides general knowledge regarding breast cancer. Educational material focused on the importance of family and cultural illness beliefs to encourage participation and compliance in screening, treatment, and

196

follow-up care. The project also provided women with tools to work within the current health-care-delivery system as well as skills to improve communication with health-care providers. Further long-term study is necessary to see whether the information the program presented has significantly changed behavior.

Notes

1. This research was made possible by support from NIH National Cancer Institute Grant R25CA66797.

2. Andrew Weil, *Health and Healing: Understanding Conventional and Alternative Medicine* (Boston: Houghton Mifflin, 1983).

3. Paul Starr, *The Social Transformation of American Medicine* (New York: Basic Books, 1982).

4. Ellen Corin, "The Social and Cultural Matrix of Health and Disease," in Robert G. Evens, Morris L. Barer, and Theodore Marmor, eds., *Why Are Some People Healthy and Others Not? The Determinants of the Health of Populations* (New York: Aldine de Gruyter, 1994). See also Diane Weiner, *Preventing and Controlling Cancer in North America: A Cross-Cultural Perspective* (Westport, CT: Praeger, 1999).

5. See also C. S. Glover and F. S. Hodge, eds., "Native Outreach: A Report to American Indian, Alaska Native, and Native Hawaiian Communities," NIH Publication No. 98-4341, National Institutes of Health and National Cancer Institute, 1999.

6. David W. Stewart and Prem N. Shamdasani, *Focus Groups: Theory and Practice* (Newbury Park, CA: Sage, 1990).

7. D. M. Eisenberg, R. C. Kessler, C. Foster, F. E. Norlock, D. R. Calkins, and T. L. Delbanco. "Unconventional Medicine in the United States: Prevalence, Costs, and Patterns of Use," *New England Journal of Medicine* 328 (1993): 246–52.

8. Michael Siegel and Lynne Doner, *Marketing Public Health: Strategies to Promote Social Change* (Aspen, CO: Gaithersburg, 1998).

9. Department of Health and Human Services, PHS, Indian Health Service, *IHS Trends* (Washington, DC: Government Printing Office, 1992), 34.

10. S. Valway, M. Kileen, R. Paisano, and E. Ortise, *Cancer Mortality among Native Americans in the United States: Regional Differences in Indian Health, 1984–88 and Trends over Time* (Rockville, MD: Indian Health Service, 1992).

11. Felicia Schanche Hodge, *The Health Status of American Indians in California* (Woodland Hills, CA: The California Endowment and The California HealthCare Foundation, 1997).

12. L. Burhansstipanov and C. M. Dresser, "Documentation of the Cancer Research Needs of American Indians and Alaska Natives," NIH Publication No. 94-3603, National Institutes of Health and National Cancer Institute, 1994.

13. Indian Health Service, PHS, Office of Planning, Evaluation and Information Resources Management, *California-Area Profile FY 94/95.*

14. A. M. Michalek and M. C. Mahoney, "Cancer in Native Populations: Lessons To Be Learned," *Journal of Cancer Education* 5 (1990): 243–49.

15. B. A. Miller et al., eds., "Racial/Ethnic Patterns of Cancer in the United States 1988–1992," NIH Publication No. 96-4101, National Institutes of Health and National Cancer Institute, 1996.

16. Ibid.

17. Burhansstipanov and Dresser, "Documentation of the Cancer Research Needs of American Indians and Alaska Natives."

18. Ibid.

19. See chapter 11 in this volume by Burhansstipanov, Hampton, and Tenney.

20. Angela Harras, ed., Cancer Rates and Risk (Bethesda, MD: National Institutes of Health, National Cancer Institute, Cancer Statistics Branch, Division of Cancer Prevention and Control, 1996), 36.

21. Department of Health and Human Services, PHS, NIH, NCI, Report of the Special Action Committee, 1992: Program Initiatives Related to Minorities, the Underserved and Persons Aged 65 and Over (Washington, DC: Government Printing Office, 1992).

22. Ibid.; see also note 15, above.

23. For similar attitudes among certain Asian Pacific Islander women, see M. Kagawa-Singer and A. E. Maxwell, "Breast-Cancer Screening in Asian Pacific Islander American Women," in Weiner, Preventing and Controlling Cancer in North America.

ELEVEN   LINDA BURHANSSTIPANOV,
                              JAMES W. HAMPTON,
                          and MARTHA J. TENNEY

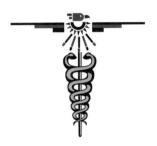

Cancer among American Indians and Alaska Natives

TROUBLE WITH NUMBERS

Cancer is a growing problem among American Indians and Alaska Natives.[1] Unfortunately, both non-Native and First Nations peoples are less aware of the growing cancer dilemma than they are of alcohol, violence, diabetes, and other well-promoted and widely dispersed conditions within Native communities. In the second half of the twentieth century, cancer has become the leading cause of death for Alaska Native women and is the second leading cause of death among Alaska Native men.[2] In fact, cancer is currently the third leading cause of death for all North American Natives[3] and is the second leading cause of death among American Indians (both sexes) over age 45.[4] The disease is the third most-cited reason for hospital stays among Indian Health Service beneficiaries served by the Alaska Area Native Indian Health Service.[5] Cancer rates, previously reported as less frequent in American Indian and Alaska Natives, have been increasing throughout the last twenty years.[6] Incidence rates among Alaska Natives have exceeded "U.S. All Races" rates for most cancer sites.[7] Rates are increasing similarly for Canadian bands.[8]

Within Native American communities, health programs continue to focus on alcoholism and diabetes, although cancer is responsible for more deaths than either of these conditions.[9] Because the word "cancer" is not indigenous, it translates into some Native languages as "the disease for which there is no cure" or "the disease that eats the body." Many tribes regard cancer as a white man's disease because of its rarity before European contact. For many Native cancer patients, the disease is not discussed and is considered a form of punishment, shame, and guilt. A few tribes consider the patient's suffering necessary in order to ensure the health of the other tribal members (they wear the pain so that their community will be spared). Some tribal members living with cancer—infected with the cancer spirit—are considered contagious and are ostracized by their communities. Other tribal members refuse cancer-treatment surgery for fear that their body and spirit will be incomplete, leaving them incapable of finding their ancestors when they move to the other side (death).[10]

National Cancer Data Limitations Affecting Native American Statistics

Accurate statistics for Alaska Natives and American Indians are critical for epidemiologic research and for the design, implementation, and evaluation of public-health interventions. Policy-makers, researchers, and health-care professionals at all levels (federal, state, and local) rely on national federal databases as accurate sources of information. Existing national databases, such as the U.S. census population figures; National Center for Health Statistics mortality data; National Cancer Institute Surveillance, Epidemiology, End Results (SEER) Program; and National Indian Health Service (IHS) are cited as reputable sources for cancer information about American Indians and Alaska Natives. However, each national cancer database has limited epidemiological information on all American Indians and Alaska Natives. This alarming deficiency needs to be acknowledged when these data sources are utilized for statistical purposes. These databases fail to describe accurately several underserved populations due to: (1) racial misclassification; (2) underreporting; (3) coding errors; (4) inclusion of insufficient population numbers; and (5) regional limitations for data collection. Cancer is underreported for American Indian and Alaska Native populations. Other ethnic groups, including Hispanics, Native Hawaiians, and Vietnamese, also have had reporting problems. Databases referred to as "good" within this document refer to those that, for the most part, have addressed at least four of the five limitations described above.

Database Quality Varies among Tumor Registries

The quality of databases varies among racial groups and among geographic regions of the country. For example, the data from the New Mexico Tumor Registry are among the more comprehensive and accurate recorders of cancer incidence among American Indians. Since its inception, the New Mexico Tumor Registry director continues to recognize the need for accurate data collection from underserved populations, including American Indians and Hispanics (race is self-reported). As a result, the data-collection protocol implemented accurately describes the ethnicity of persons living in New Mexico. Survival data are available only for these American Indian populations.

At the present time, the two states with the highest American Indian populations (Oklahoma and California) both have significant racial misclassification errors, resulting in underreporting among Native Americans living in those states.[11] Similar database undercounts of Native American cancer rates have been reported for the Northwestern states (Oregon, Washington, and Idaho) and the north-central states (Montana and Wyoming).[12] Ideally, the CDC funding of state tumor registries will help improve the data in states with a high population of American Indians.

Data Sequestration on American Indians and Alaska Natives in "Other" Category

Cancer data are available for whites and blacks but not for American Indians or Alaska Natives. This is due in part to the smaller size of Native populations in comparison to the population of these larger racial groups. Native Hawaiians and American Samoans have a similar problem. Indigenous populations are included in the "other" category when cancer data are discussed. As a result, unusual cancer patterns among specific groups of peoples are overlooked. There are cases in which data are summarized into major racial categories to permit comparisons and analyses for cancer priorities within racial groups (African Americans, Caucasians, American Indian/Alaska Natives, Asian/Pacific Islanders, etc.). However, it is difficult to develop a community-based cancer prevention and control program with such lumped data, since the American Indian community's cancer priorities are quite different from those included under the broad category of "other." When statisticians discuss cancer incidence or mortality rates, the comparisons usually are limited to blacks and whites (and occasionally Hispanics).[13] When race and ethnicity are included in statistical analyses, several disconcerting findings are discovered. For example, the racial or ethnic group with the highest breast-cancer incidence rate is Native Hawaiian. The racial or ethnic group with the highest cervical-cancer incidence rate is Alaska Native. The racial or ethnic group with the highest gallbladder incidence rate is southwestern American Indian.[14] This information could not be distinguished from "other" category data.

Heterogeneity of Native American Communities and "Masking" Variability

There is no single national database that accurately presents comprehensive cancer data for American Indians. As a result, multiple databases, including the Indian Health Services, must be relied upon to supply the overall cancer data for American Indians and Alaska Natives.

Age-adjusted cancer incidence and mortality rates vary significantly among tribes and geographic areas, and generalizations cannot be made from a single area.[15] The heterogeneity of lifestyle, culture, and traditions among Native communities prevents reporting statistics from one culture area and applying it to the entire population. Lifestyle variations may be regional. Nevertheless, the New Mexico database (mentioned earlier) is commonly used by the National Cancer Institute (NCI) for its Surveillance, Evaluation, and End Results (SEER) national database, which is reputedly representative of the total U.S. population. Regional data make it clear that the New Mexico SEER data are not representative, and thus highly misleading.

According to the Indian Health Service statistics from 1989 through 1993, the four IHS areas that continued to report significantly lower rates (Phoenix, Tucson, Navajo, and Albuquerque) are located in Arizona and New Mexico. Five of the nine IHS areas had age-adjusted breast-cancer mortality rates that were similar to other U.S. rates. When 1989–1993 IHS age-adjusted breast-cancer mortality data are compared with previously published breast data, they indicate that breast-cancer mortality rates among American Indians in geographic regions *other* than Arizona and New Mexico are actually increasing, gradually, and becoming similar to other U.S. rates for breast cancer. The "U.S. All Races" breast-cancer mortality rate was 27.1. Table 11.1 shows the 1989–1993 female age-adjusted breast-cancer mortality rates for the IHS areas with no known data problems (i.e., under-reporting Indian race on death certificates) and located in geographic regions other than the Southwest.[16]

TABLE 11.1
1989–1993 FEMALE AGE-ADJUSTED BREAST-CANCER MORTALITY RATES

IHS Areas outside AZ and NM		IHS Areas within AZ and NM	
Aberdeen IHS (ND, SD, NE, IA)	26.3	Phoenix (AZ)	11.5
Billings IHS (MT, WY)	25.6	Albuquerque (NM)	10.3
Alaska IHS (AK)	21.4	Navajo (AZ/NM)	9.4
Nashville IHS (NC, TN, MS, FL, PA, ME, GA)	20.0	Tucson (AZ)	4.2
Bemidji IHS (WI, MN, MI)	14.2		

American Indian Cancer Incidence, Mortality, and Survival Data

Historical Perspective

At the beginning of the twentieth century, cancer was considered so rare among American Indians that some authors suggested that American Indians never had cancer.[17] Although some skeletal remains found in archeological investigations of Indian burial grounds in Alaska and New York suggest that cancer occasionally was present in Native communities,[18] American Indian and Alaska Native elders have reported that cancer was not a common disease among their people. In the past 20 years, however, nearly every American Indian and Alaska Native community has experienced substantial exposure to this dreaded disease.

Being cognizant of the data limitations described earlier, examples of the cancer sites identified to be of most concern among American Indians and Alaska Natives include: lung, colorectal, breast, prostate, uterine, cervix, stomach, pancreas, and gallbladder.[19]

Age-Adjusted Cancer Incidence Rates

American Indians in the SEER database were shown to have a lower cancer incidence rate than "U.S. All Races."[20] The American Indian populations included within that database are comprised primarily of Native peoples living in Arizona and New Mexico. When compared with other racial groups, the incidence of cancer among American Indians living in Arizona and New Mexico is low. The incidence rate for "all cancer sites combined" for both sexes is less than one-half that of whites (157.3 per 100,000 person years, compared to the white rate of 359.2). However, we don't know about the data problems or the racial-classification accuracy difficulties encountered by these researchers.

Most research conducted in Arizona and New Mexico consistently indicates lower cancer incidence. These databases generally are those accepted as accurately classifying race and ethnicity. These studies include Eidson's work in New Mexico,[21] Nutting's review of screening policies among Southwestern American Indian communities,[22] Sorem's research in the Southwest among the Zuñi,[23] and Black's work with tri-ethnic populations in New Mexico.[24] In addition, SEER data from the New Mexico Tumor Registry consistently include cancer incidence rates for Native Americans lower than other racial groups, such as whites and blacks.[25] According to the New Mexico SEER Tumor Registry (an accurate database with very few racial misclassifications), American Indians living in New Mexico and Arizona have incidence rates for stomach, uterine cervix, primary liver, and gallbladder cancers that are higher than for the "U.S. All Races." American Indians have the highest gallbladder cancer incidence rate (10.9) of any racial group.[26]

Nutting's Indian Health Service–wide review of cancer incidence among American Indians and Alaska Natives (1980–1987) was known to have errors, but was the best data available at the time.[27] Based upon those data, American Indians and Alaska Natives have lower cancer incidence rates than do whites. Mahoney's work with the Seneca in New York[28] has been accepted by the tribal

TABLE 11.2

AGE-ADJUSTED (1970 U.S. STANDARD) CANCER INCIDENCE RATES PER 100,000 POPULATION BY RACE AND CANCER SITE, 1977–1983

Cancer Incidence Site	Alaska Native F	M	American Indian[a] F	M	SEER White F	M	SEER Afr. Am. F	M
Breast[b]	44.2	Unk	21.7	Unk	93.3	Unk	74.9	Unk
Cervix uteri	*28.0	NA	20.5	NA	8.6	NA	19.5	NA
Colorectal	*65.2	61.0	10.0	10.6	44.9	64.5	45.9	56.4
Gallbladder	*14.7	*6.7	*14.7	6.4	1.6	0.9	1.2	0.8
Kidney	*11.0	*11.4	7.3	8.1	4.5	10.7	4.5	9.7
Oral cavity & pharynx	*15.7	17.2	1.3	3.0	7.1	17.6	7.6	*24.0
Pancreas	9.6	10.1	4.5	7.1	7.9	11.6	*11.4	*17.0
Prostate	NA	34.5	NA	37.6	NA	73.6	NA	*126.0
Stomach[c]	8.4	22.4	13.8	22.3	5.8	13.3	8.6	22.5
Liver[d]	2.0	10.8	1.1	4.1	1.2	3.1	1.9	5.3

[a]Arizona and New Mexico only.
[b]The racial group with the highest breast-cancer incidence rate is Native Hawaiians (108.5).
[c]The racial groups with the highest stomach-cancer incidence rate for females is Native Hawaiians (28.8), and for males is Japanese (41.3).
[d]The racial group with the highest liver-cancer incidence rate is Chinese (females=3.9; males=20.8).
An asterisk indicates the highest incidence rate of any racial group.
Source: Department of Health and Human Services, PHS, NIH, NCI, 1992.

council as racially accurate. Those data indicate lower cancer rates (almost all sites) among the Seneca than among other New York–area communities.

In contrast, Lanier's work in Alaska among the Inuits, Athabaskans, and Aleuts identifies elevated cancer rates, as demonstrated by table 11.2.[29] Lanier is recognized by both Natives and non-Natives as accurately collecting and recording data. Likewise, Welty's work indicates a higher than "U.S. All Races" rate for lung cancer among the Northern Plains American Indian Nations.[30]

Cancer Mortality Rates

Native American cancer mortality rates also have been identified as lower than whites' and blacks' in multiple research studies.[31] There are major racial misclassifications and underreporting of cancer among Native people throughout the United States, and it is not known how accurate the data were in these studies. Canadian data, also questioned by several of the First Nations for multiple racial misclassifications, show similar results to those in the United States.[32] In addition to these problems, mortality statistics share with incident statistics the problem of misleading national generalization. A brief review of these data clearly illustrate the variability of cancer incidence rates among IHS areas. Examples of IHS age-adjusted incidence data (age-adjusted to 1970 U.S. population) from 1982 through 1987 follow.[33]

BREAST CANCER. See table 11.3, "Age-Adjusted (1970 Standard) Breast-Cancer (ICD Codes 174.0–174.9) Incidence Rates (top) per 100,000 Female Population and 95 Percent Confidence Intervals (bottom) for Each of the Selected Seven Nations for Whom Databases Have Few Racial Misclassification Errors," for examples of variables for breast-cancer incidence rates.

TABLE 11.3

AGE-ADJUSTED BREAST-CANCER INCIDENCE RATES

Aleut n=3,834	Apache n=12,781	Athapaskan n=4,474	Eskimo n=17,252	Navajo n=89,815	Sioux n=27,348	Tohono O'Od-ham/Pima n=14,360
40.1	26.2	106.1	50.7	28.7	57.9	18.5
(0.0–81.4)	(9.7–42.8)	(48.3–163.9)	(30.4–70.9)	(21.8–35.6)	(40.0–75.7)	(5.7–31.3)

Source: Nutting et al. (1993).

CERVICAL CANCER. It is obvious from table 11.4, "Age-Adjusted (1970 Standard) Cervical-Cancer (ICD Codes 180.0–180.8) Incidence Rates (top) per 100,000 Female Population and 95 Percent Confidence Intervals (bottom) for Each of the Selected Seven Nations for Whom Databases Have Few Racial

TABLE 11.4

AGE-ADJUSTED CERVICAL-CANCER INCIDENCE RATES

Aleut n=3,834	Apache n=12,781	Athapaskan n=4,474	Eskimo n=17,252	Navajo n=89,815	Sioux n=27,348	Tohono O'Od- ham/Pima n=14,360
29.7	31.8	39.4	33.1	26.3	29.2	41.7
(0.0–61.9)	(14.1–49.5)	(4.1–74.8)	(17.9–48.3)	(19.7–32.8)	(17.7–40.6)	(21.5–62.0)

Source: Nutting et al. (1993).

Misclassification Errors," that the data's quality is suspect, as per the large confidence intervals (the larger the confidence interval, the more questionable the data). Cervical-cancer incidence rates are comparatively high, particularly among Alaska Native populations (Aleut, Athabaskan, and Inuit). American Indian women do not appear to have a high prevalence of many of the risk factors commonly associated with cervical neoplasia among non-Native populations.[34] It is not known if genetics plays a more significant role in cervical cancer in American Indian women than it does in non-Native women. Research is needed to improve understanding of the risk factors and the determinants of cervical-cancer incidence among American Indians and Alaska Natives.

COLORECTAL CANCER. According to table 11.5, "Age-Adjusted (1970 Standard) Colorectal-Cancer (ICD Codes 153.0, 164.1, 169.0) Incidence

TABLE 11.5

AGE-ADJUSTED COLORECTAL-CANCER INCIDENCE RATES

Aleut F n=3,834	Apache F n=12,781	Athapaskan F n=4,474	Eskimo F n=17,252	Navajo F n=89,815	Sioux F n=27,348	Tohono O'Od- ham/Pima F n=14,360
89.9	13.0	96.2	116.1	10.7	19.4	9.4
(26.9–152.9)	(0.1–25.8)	(31.9–160.5)	(80.9–151.3)	(6.4–15.0)	(8.7–30.2)	(0.0–20.0)

Aleut M n=3,953	Apache M n=12,134	Athapaskan M n=4,612	Eskimo M n=17,789	Navajo M n=84,502	Sioux M n=26,144	Tohono O'Od- ham/Pima M n=13,632
114.8	9.3	40.4	53.2	9.3	24.7	1.3
(47.3–182.3)	(0.0–19.9)	(4.8–75.9)	(32.7–73.7)	(5.3–13.3)	(12.6–36.8)	(0.0–3.8)

Source: Nutting et al. (1993).

Rates (top) per 100,000 Female (F) and Male (M) Populations and 95 Percent Confidence Intervals (bottom) for Each of the Selected Seven Nations," Alaska Natives living in Alaska have the highest age-adjusted colon and rectum cancer incidence rate per 100,000 population for both sexes (Alaska, 1977–1983) compared to any other racial group. Among the Alaska Natives, unusual rates are noted both within the same subpopulation and between sexes. This unusual variability generates several questions regarding the risk-factor behaviors of these men and women.[35] As is seen in all tribal incidence data, several of the confidence intervals are exceptionally large.

GALLBLADDER CANCER. Table 11.6, "Age-Adjusted (1970 Standard) Gallbladder-Cancer (ICD Code 156.0) Incidence Rates (top) per 100,000 Female (F) and Male (M) Populations and 95 Percent Confidence Intervals (bottom) for Each of the Selected Seven Nations," indicates that gallbladder-cancer incidence rates are disproportionately high among both Native males and females. The incidence rates for whites, both sexes, is 1.3 per 100,000 people, compared with an incidence of 10.9 for American Indians living in Arizona and New Mexico and 10.6 for Alaska Natives.[36] Gallbladder cancer is 8.4 times more likely to occur in a Native person than in a white person. The incidence rates for gallbladder cancer are higher among women than men, and approximately nine times more common in American Indian or Alaska Native women than in white woman.

LUNG CANCER. A quick review of the lung-cancer incidence data in table 11.7, "Age-Adjusted (1970 Standard) Lung-Cancer (ICD Codes 162.2–162.9)

TABLE 11.6

AGE-ADJUSTED GALLBLADDER-CANCER INCIDENCE RATES

Aleut F n=3,834	Apache F n=12,781	Athapaskan F n=4,474	Eskimo F n=17,252	Navajo F n=89,815	Sioux F n=27,348	Tohono O'Od- ham/Pima F n=14,360
0	20.5	0	27.6	10.8	5.9	33.4
	(5.0–35.9)		(10.2–44.9)	(6.3–15.4)	(0.1–11.7)	(13.5–53.4)

Aleut M n=3,953	Apache M n=12,134	Athapaskan M n=4,612	Eskimo M n=17,789	Navajo M n=84,502	Sioux M n=26,144	Tohono O'Od- ham/Pima M n=13,632
0	0	9.2	3.8	3.9	4.7	5.3
		(0.0–27.2)	(0.0–9.1)	(1.3–6.4)	(0.0–10.0)	(0.0–12.8)

Source: Nutting et al. (1993).

207

TABLE 11.7
AGE-ADJUSTED LUNG-CANCER INCIDENCE RATES

Aleut F n=3,834	Apache F n=12,781	Athapaskan F n=4,474	Eskimo F n=17,252	Navajo F n=89,815	Sioux F n=27,348	Tohono O'Od- ham/Pima F n=14,360
101.7	8.3	111.3	53.2	4.6	34.1	17.9
(37.2–166.3)	(0.0–17.7)	(50.1–172.4)	(30.5–75.9)	(1.6–7.6)	(20.0–48.1)	(3.5–32.3)

Aleut M n=3,953	Apache M n=12,134	Athapaskan M n=4,612	Eskimo M n=17,789	Navajo M n=84,502	Sioux M n=26,144	Tohono O'Od- ham/Pima M n=13,632
92.3	6.1	88.4	106.1	13.1	46.2	10.5
(34.7–149.8)	(0.0–14.6)	(36.3–140.5)	(77.3–134.8)	(8.4–17.9)	(29.7–62.7)	(0.2–20.9)

Source: Nutting et al. (1993).

Incidence Rates (top) per 100,000 Female (F) and Male (M) Populations and 95 Percent Confidence Intervals (bottom) for Each of the Selected Seven Nations," clearly illustrates why it is inappropriate to use New Mexico data (which includes American Indians living in Arizona and New Mexico) to generalize about other Native population groups. In the table, those data include the Apache, Navajo, and Tohono O'Odham nations. The lung-cancer incidence among these Southwestern tribes is much lower than it is for those peoples living in Alaska and the Northern Plains.

PROSTATE CANCER. The prostate-cancer incidence rates are comparatively low among both American Indians living in Arizona and New Mexico (37.6/100,000) and Alaska Natives (34.5/100,000). In table 11.8, "Age-Adjusted (1970 Standard) Prostate-Cancer (ICD Codes 174.0–174.9) Incidence

TABLE 11.8
AGE-ADJUSTED PROSTATE-CANCER INCIDENCE RATES

Aleut n=3,953	Apache n=12,134	Athapaskan n=4,612	Eskimo n=17,789	Navajo n=84,502	Sioux n=26,144	Tohono O'Od- ham/Pima n=13,632
47.3	3.3	91.8	19.4	26.5	32.5	29.7
(5.7–89.0)	(0.0–9.7)	(37.6–146.0)	(6.7–32.1)	(19.9–33.1)	(18.6–46.6)	(12.1–47.4)

Source: Nutting et al. (1993).

208

TABLE 11.9
AGE-ADJUSTED STOMACH-CANCER INCIDENCE RATES

Aleut F n=3,834	Apache F n=12,781	Athapaskan F n=4,474	Eskimo F n=17,252	Navajo F n=89,815	Sioux F n=27,348	Tohono O'Od- ham/Pima F n=14,360
6.9	7.9	7.3	12.2	10.9	11.3	10.9
(0.0–20.5)	(0.0–17.0)	(0.0–21.5)	(0.7–23.7)	(6.5–15.4)	(2.9–19.7)	(0.0–22.1)

Aleut M n=3,953	Apache M n=12,134	Athapaskan M n=4,612	Eskimo M n=17,789	Navajo M n=84,502	Sioux M n=26,144	Tohono O'Od- ham/Pima M n=13,632
37.4	13.4	15.3	28.9	10.8	11.3	12.2
(4.1–70.7)	(1.3–25.5)	(0.0–37.0)	(13.9–43.9)	(6.5–15.1)	(3.3–19.2)	(1.1–23.3)

Source: Nutting et al. (1993).

Rates (top) per 100,000 Male Population and 95 Percent Confidence Intervals (bottom) for Each of the Selected Seven Nations," tribal data show a range of incidence rates from 3.3 to 91.8, the lowest being those for the Apache.

STOMACH CANCER. Stomach-cancer incidence rates as shown in table 11.9, "Age-Adjusted (1970 Standard) Stomach-Cancer (ICD Codes 151.0–150.9) Incidence Rates (top) per 100,000 Female (F) and Male (M) Populations and 95 Percent Confidence Intervals (bottom) for Each of the Selected Seven Nations," are high among American Indians when compared with whites, and higher among males than females.

AGE-ADJUSTED CANCER MORTALITY RATES. The annual age-adjusted cancer death rates (156/100,000) for the Alaska Indian Health Service (IHS) area also exceed those of the "U.S. All Races" (132/100,000).[37] Alaska Natives again have excessive mortality from cancers of the uterine, cervix, colorectal, esophagus, gallbladder, kidney, nasopharynx, and salivary glands (see table 11.10, "Age-Adjusted [1970 U.S. Standard] Cancer Mortality Rates per 100,000 Population by Race and Cancer Site, 1977–1983"). Colorectal, breast, pancreas, and cervical cancers are the most frequent causes of cancer death among Alaska Native women, and stomach cancer mortality rates are excessive for Alaska Native males when compared with white males.

Five-Year Relative Survival from Cancer

Unsurprisingly, given the above-mentioned data problems, the relative five-year survival data for American Indians are among the poorest for all cancer sites

L. BURHANSSTIPANOV, J.W. HAMPTON, and M.J. TENNEY

TABLE 11.10

AGE-ADJUSTED CANCER MORTALITY RATES BY RACE AND CANCER SITE, 1977–1983

Cancer Mortality Site	Alaska Native F	Alaska Native M	American Indian F	American Indian M	SEER White F	SEER White M	SEER Afr. Am. F	SEER Afr. Am. M
Breast[a]	12.8	Unk	9.0	Unk	26.7	Unk	26.9	Unk
Cervix uteri	★12.5	NA	5.5	NA	3.2	NA	8.7	NA
Colorectal	★27.2	22.1	8.0	10.1	18.4	★25.6	20.3	25.4
Gallbladder	★6.3	1.4	3.6	★1.5	1.2	0.6	0.9	0.5
Kidney	★4.4	★6.7	2.0	3.5	2.1	4.6	1.8	3.9
Oral cavity & pharynx	★6.3	★10.2	1.3	2.3	1.8	5.1	2.4	9.9
Pancreas	★10.3	9.3	4.2	5.3	6.8	10.4	9.3	★13.9
Prostate	NA	11.4	NA	11.8	NA	21.1	NA	★44.0
Stomach[b]	7.0	17.2	4.3	7.6	3.6	7.6	6.5	14.9
Liver[c]	2.6	15.2	1.1	3.1	1.3	2.7	2.1	5.6

[a]The racial group with the highest breast-cancer incidence rate is Native Hawaiians (37.8).
[b]The racial group with the highest stomach-cancer incidence rate for females is Native Hawaiians (14.5), and for males is Native Hawaiians (32.1).
[c]The racial group with the highest liver-cancer incidence rate is Chinese (females=3.8; males=16.6).
An asterisk indicates the highest incidence rate of any racial group.
Source: Department of Health and Human Services, PHS, NIH, NCI, 1992.

combined of any racial group in the United States. When compared to non-Indian peoples in the Southwest, American Indians' cancer diagnosis—even in its early stages—results in poorer survival.[38] Again based only on American Indian residents in New Mexico and Arizona, data indicate that American Indians are less likely to be alive five years after diagnosis than are whites.

Table 11.11 ("Five-Year Cancer Relative Survival [%] by Race and Cancer Site, 1975–1984") summarizes survival data for American Indians and whites. The zero survival from pancreatic cancer is true for people of all races. In about one-half of the diagnosed cases of pancreatic cancer, the cancer already has spread to other organs. This results in an overall five-year survival of just 3.2 percent for all races. Little improvement has been seen in five-year relative survival for liver cancer since the mid-1970s. The overall five-year relative survival for stomach cancer in all races is only 17 percent, but improves to 55 percent for cancers detected at the localized stage.[39]

Published survival data are unavailable for Alaska Natives, but as of July 1995 were in the process of being organized into a summary report. An Alaska Native Tumor Registry collected data from 1969 to 1983. Due to the low

TABLE I I . I I

FIVE-YEAR CANCER RELATIVE SURVIVAL (%) BY RACE AND CANCER SITE, 1975–1984

Survival and Cancer Site	Alaska Native F	M	American Indian[a] F	M	SEER White F	M	SEER Afr. Am. F	M
Breast	NA	NA	★49.7	Unk	75.7	Unk	62.8	Unk
Cervix uteri	NA	NA	65.1	NA	67.2	NA	★61.3	NA
Colorectal	NA	NA	★42.3	★33.0	53.6	52.8	47.6	42.8
Gallbladder	NA	NA	★6.4	★3.0	9.4	9.4	8.6	8.9
Kidney	NA	NA	★36.2	★39.2	51.8	51.9	55.6	49.4
Oral cavity & pharynx[b]	NA	NA	Unk	★28.0	54.6	47.2	45.8	★28.0
Pancreas	NA	NA	★0.0	★0.0	2.7	3.0	4.8	3.3
Prostate	NA	NA	NA	★51.4	NA	69.8	NA	62.0
Stomach[c]	NA	NA	12.0	★4.7	18.7	15.1	18.6	17.2
Liver[d]	NA	NA	Unk	Unk	6.5	2.8	6.7	2.1

[a]Arizona and New Mexico only.
[b]The racial group with the poorest survival from oral cavity and pharynx cancer for females is Native Hawaiians (36.4).
[c]The racial group with the poorest survival from stomach cancer for females is Filipino (8.4).
[d]The racial group with the poorest survival from liver cancer for both sexes is Japanese (females = 3.7; males = 1.2).
An asterisk indicates the poorest survival rate of any racial group.
Source: Department of Health and Human Services, PHS, NIH, NCI, 1992.

number of cancer cases (less than a hundred per year), however, the registry lost its funding for several years. The Alaska Native Tumor Registry was re-established through funding by the National Cancer Institute from 1989 through 1993 and was in the process of collecting information on incidence, follow-up, stage at diagnosis, and treatment. Unfortunately, the registry lost its funding again in 1993. It is not known how these invaluable data will be attained in the future.[40]

The low survival from cancer of American Indians reported by the National Cancer Institute (NCI) SEER data suggest that American Indian cancer patients experience the disease differently than other ethnic populations. More investigation needs to be done to explore the causative factors such as genetic risk factors, late detection of cancer, poor compliance with recommended treatment, presence of concomitant disease, or lack of timely access to state-of-the-art diagnostic and/or treatment methods.[41] Some types of cancer (uterine, cervix) may act differently within Native peoples and Native cultures, which may affect the way people respond to cancer and cancer programs. By

studying specific cancer sites that are elevated among Native peoples, information may be acquired to help people of all races. In addition, data reflecting
American Indian communities that have effectively avoided specific cancers
might shed some light on some protective factors of health behavior, diet, or
environment.

Influences on Participation in Early-Detection Screening Programs

Lack of Access to Culturally Acceptable Cancer Services

The Indian Health Service (IHS) plays the primary role in providing services
for American Indians and Alaska Natives, and is perceived by many Natives as
a culturally acceptable health-care provider. However, the IHS lacks sufficient
budget, personnel, facilities, and resources to provide quality comprehensive
cancer-screening services to all urban and reservation Indians without collaboration from other agencies such as CDC and state health departments. Medical services are not always available to the consumer and are among the more
common reasons for not using their services. For example, breast-cancer
screening has been assessed through the 1989 Survey of American Indians and
Alaska Natives (SAIAN), which was a subset of the National Medical Expenditure Survey. The SAIAN found that only 23 percent of the women reported
ever having had a mammogram.[42] When last reported in May of 1993, the IHS
had a nationwide total of only fourteen dedicated mammography machines.
Only two IHS areas had contracts for mobile mammography services.[43]
Clearly, the majority of American Indian women belong in the medically
underserved category, and are underscreened for breast cancer.

Another common complaint regarding IHS services is its inaccessibility.
For example, American Indians living in the rural New York area (for instance,
on the Seneca Reservation) must travel more than 500 miles one way to access
IHS services in Cherokee, North Carolina. American Indians living in Denver
must travel 390 miles one way to Ignacio to obtain IHS services.[44] Some
American Indians choose convenience over culturally acceptable services and
those who have access to private health insurance are also likely to use this service instead.

Changes in Lifestyle

Through assimilation over time, American Indians have adopted Western
lifestyles, which are conducive to cancer, and many forms of behavior-related
cancer have increased throughout Indian country (lung, colorectal, and stomach). For this reason, the foci of several ongoing cancer prevention and con-

212

trol programs, in collaboration with American Indian communities, are to assist those communities in undertaking lifestyle changes that may help halt the increased rates and prevent cancer.

Risk Factors

Risk factors for each of the more-common cancer-incidence sites have been identified by national organizations; agencies are based on white or black populations, and may not apply to American Indians and Alaska Natives. For example, preliminary research indicates that risk factors for cervical dysplasia in American Indian women differ from those identified for the same cancer site in Southwestern Hispanic and non-Hispanic white women (for example, presence of HPV infection, multiple sexual partners throughout lifetime). Such research emphasizes the need to investigate ethnic differences in uterine- and cervical-cancer development.[45]

Thus, it is not yet possible to distinguish risks to biological, cultural, socioeconomic, or other factors. As cited earlier, a comparatively larger proportion of First Nations peoples live in poverty than do non-Natives.[46] Furthermore, risk factors may be regional and may depend on particular lifestyles prominent in that area. Welty has shown that the high rate of smoking (56 percent for men and 48 percent for women) among the Sioux living in North and South Dakota is related closely to their high lung-cancer mortality rates. Intensive smoking cessation and prevention programs are likely to have the greatest impact on reducing such preventable cancer deaths within their community.[47] Similar programs in New Mexico—where incidence is less frequent and risk factors are lower—may not fare as well.

Barriers to Participation in Cancer Prevention and Control Programs

In comparison to other ethnic groups, American Indians and Alaska Natives seldom utilize early–cancer-detection screening programs. They also are rarely recruited to participate in clinical trials or state-of-the-art treatment programs. When recruited, they typically are not retained throughout the duration of the study, but withdraw and cannot be evaluated. There are numerous barriers that explain these low utilization and participation rates.[48]

Barriers affecting American Indian and Alaska Native participation in cancer early-detection and screening programs include poverty and psychosocial, sociocultural, and policy barriers. There are numerous policy barriers specific to Indian country. While American Indian nations have a unique, sovereign relationship to the federal government, state governments have not been tolerant of American Indian sovereignty issues. These federal government–to–tribal-government relations often are strained by bureaucratic budget cuts by the Office of Management and Budget, which have significant and devastating

213

impacts on American Indians' health care through the IHS hospitals, traditional Indian medicine, and tribal health services. These policy barriers can only be addressed through the successful implementation of culturally competent cancer prevention and control programs. When the projects are completed, modifications and outcome recommendations can be prepared as policies and submitted to the tribal communities for their approval. Only if the community can be brought into the planning will a program be successful.

Poverty has multiple, confounding effects on life priorities, from health problems other than cancer (such as alcohol/substance abuse, violence, suicide, and diabetes) to a lack of medical insurance to a need for transportation to a medical facility. Obviously, these barriers affect people of all colors who live in poverty and are not racially or ethnically specific. Psychosocial factors also affect people of all colors and include, but are not limited to, education level, knowledge about health and disease, language or nonverbal communication styles, and fear of using health services based on cultural practices or unpleasant past medical experiences. Examples of psychosocial barriers among American Indian women are related to misconceptions about breast cancer and/or the lack of breast-cancer education. Some of the identified misconceptions might be a result of dispersed cancer-education materials that are written at a very high literacy level (most National Cancer Institute materials are written for persons with an average of grade eleven or higher reading skills), whereas the average reading comprehension of large segments of the target population (within all ethnic groups) may be as low as grade five.

Sociocultural barriers include culturally irrelevant cancer education and recruitment materials, culturally specific beliefs about cancer (for example, to discuss the disease is to invite the cancer spirit into one's body), and other such misconceptions.

Culturally competent interventions are needed to find acceptable strategies of addressing these barriers. For example, the Native American Women's Wellness through Awareness (NAWWA) project, being implemented in Denver and Los Angeles, provides "Native Sisters" who assist in personalizing the cancer-screening process.[49] For example, one woman requested that she be accompanied to a sweat on the evening of her mammography screening so that she could participate in a cleansing and spiritual ceremony to help eradicate evil cancer spirits that may have been introduced during screening. The Los Angeles site also has had clients who requested that a female medicine woman be present to smudge and bless the woman both prior to and following early-detection breast-cancer screening.

Behavioral Cancer Risk Factors

Most cancers have external causes and to a great extent are preventable by practicing a healthy lifestyle. Likewise, other factors and behaviors are associated strongly with increased risk for developing cancer, such as a high-fat/calorie and low-fiber diet, habitual tobacco use, poverty, and so on. Unfortunately, the factors and behaviors that are associated with increased risk have escalated among First Nations peoples since World War II.

Thirty-five percent of all cancer fatalities in the United States are attributed to diet.[50] Dietary behaviors such as consuming chemo-preventive foods like fresh fruits and vegetables assist in preventing many forms of cancer. A 1990 report evaluating the USDA's Food Distribution Program stated that approximately 65–70 percent of the Native Americans living on reservation received either food commodities or food stamps. A typical household included an average of 3.2 persons; 40 percent of the families were one- or two-person households; and 8.5 percent were single-parent homes. The households generally included children and older adults ages 60 and over. The average level of education attained was the tenth grade. More than 50 percent of the adults worked, were looking for work, or were laid off and were looking for work. Most of the households were poor by any conventional standard and had transportation difficulties.[51] With the advent of the Indian Health Service (since 1955) and the USDA program, access to nutritional foods on reservations has improved.[52] However, Indian people who subsist on the USDA commodities programs frequently have access to five servings of fruits and vegetables a week, which is insufficient to provide protective benefits to the body, according to biomedical models and National Institutes of Health dietary guidelines.

Habitual tobacco use is estimated to be responsible for about 30 percent of cancer in people of all races and is responsible for causing 90 percent of all lung cancer.[53] Based upon Behavioral Risk Factor Surveillance System data from 1985 through 1989, Native communities in the Northern states and in urban areas are more likely to be habitual tobacco users than are people of other races (50–80 percent of individuals from selected American Indian communities in Montana are habitual tobacco users).[54]

These are just a few examples of factors, lifestyles, and behaviors related to cancer risks. Obviously, if such behaviors and conditions continue, the cancer incidence and mortality rates will continue to rise among First Nations.

Why the Lack of Awareness about Native American Cancer?

A general lack of awareness is clearly due partially to racial misclassification in statistical data collection, which subsequently has underestimated the number of cancer incidence and mortality cases. As a result, providers are misinformed about the significance of cancer within specific Native communities and are less aggressive in their efforts to identify and refer cancer symptoms. Federal agencies, such as the National Cancer Institute (NCI), until recent years were more likely to discount cancer as a problem. Since their primary data sources are from Arizona and New Mexico (where Native American cancer incidence and mortality rates are lower than for Indian communities from other parts of the United States), the institute was less apt to publicize this health problem. Unfortunately, only one-third of the 50 state health departments directly support or sponsor cancer prevention and control services for American Indians and Alaska Natives, reinforcing the misconception that cancer is not a health problem.[55] There have been very effective health-education campaigns that have raised awareness and concern within a community. These campaigns include, but are not limited to, alcohol and substance abuse, domestic violence, diabetes prevention, and education. Other health problems, such as alcoholism and domestic violence, are very visible, and effects of these behaviors are widely dispersed among Native communities; consequently, cancer is not considered particularly problematic.

These issues, along with many others affecting cancer prevention and control efforts within First Nations communities, are discussed and prioritized within the 1992 National Strategic Plan for Cancer Prevention and Control to benefit the overall health of American Indians and Alaska Natives, developed by the Network for Cancer Control Research among American Indian and Alaska Native Populations and published in a special National Cancer Institute Monograph.[56] The plan warned this special population that cancer was a major public-health problem in their community and that steps should be taken to inform them of this change in cancer epidemiology.

Network for Cancer-Control Research among Native Americans

The Special Populations Studies Branch (SPSB) of the National Cancer Institute (NCI) supported the initiative and development of a Network for Cancer Control Research among American Indian and Alaska Native Populations. The mission of this network was to "improve the health of American Indian and Alaska Native peoples by reducing cancer morbidity and mortality to the lowest possible levels and to improve cancer survival through cancer control research." The Network functioned as an empowered, independent organization and assisted the NCI in achieving its Year 2000 objectives for American Indians and Alaska Natives. From the latter part of 1991 through 1992, the Network for Cancer Control Research among American Indian and Alaska Native Populations prepared and wrote a National Strategic Cancer Plan to control cancer in this special population. The purpose of this plan was to enhance the awareness of federal agencies, other funding organizations, the Indian Health Service, health-care deliverers, and researchers about the special problems of cancer in American Indian and Alaska Native populations. The plan's focus was to recommend actions and outcomes to assist federal agencies in formulating special initiatives to address the increasing incidence of cancer in American Indians and Alaska Natives. The federal plan was presented to the director of NCI, the director of IHS, and the national board of directors of the American Cancer Society, and was published in a National Cancer Institute monograph.

During 1993 and 1994, as part of its continuing efforts to reduce cancer morbidity and mortality, the Network for Cancer Control Research among American Indian and Alaska Native Populations completed a modified strategic plan for cancer control for state health departments. This achieved greater significance as the Congress moved to shift federally controlled funding to the states in the form of block grants. State agencies need to be better informed of strategies of collaboration with tribes and nations within their boundaries and how to address the cancer prevention and control needs of this special population.[57]

Conclusions

Regional cancer data, as opposed to aggregate or generalized data, show a great diversity in the cancer incidence rates among Native American nations. This chapter highlights seven tribal nations and specific cancer sites, indicating incidence and survival rates, and major flaws in the available statistics. Although the Native American cancer databases have many quality problems, those data are the best available to communities to plan and develop culturally competent cancer prevention and control programs.

Notes

1. The National Cancer Institute has released incidence and mortality data that are more recent that those published in this chapter (see B. A. Miller et al., *Racial/Ethnic Patterns of Cancer in the United States 1988–1992* [Bethesda, MD: National Cancer Institute, NIH Pub. No. 96-4104]). However, due to fewer than 25 cancer cases of American Indians from Arizona and New Mexico, as cited by Miller et al. the majority of the tables for specific cancer sites (e.g., prostate, lung, breast) in the book have no data for Native peoples. Earlier data about Natives are used so that some numbers and rates can be reviewed by the reader.

217

2. N. Cobb and R. E. Paisano, *Cancer Mortality among American Indians and Alaska Natives in the United States: Regional Differences in Indian Health, 1989–1993* (Rockville, MD: Indian Health Service, IHS Pub. No. 97-615-23, 1997); S. Valway, M. Kileen, R. Paisano, and E. Ortiz, *Cancer Mortality among Native Americans in the United States: Regional Differences in Indian Health, 1984–88 and Trends Over Time* (Rockville, MD: Indian Health Service, 1992).

3. Office of Planning, Evaluation and Legislation, *Regional Differences in Indian Health: 1996* (Rockville, MD: Indian Health Service, 1996).

4. Department of Health and Human Services, Indian Health Services, *Trends in Indian Health: 1995* (Rockville, MD: Indian Health Service, 1995).

5. Office of Planning, Evaluation and Legislation, *Regional Differences in Indian Health: 1996* (Rockville, MD: Indian Health Service, 1996).

6. Department of Health and Human Services, Indian Health Services, *Trends in Indian Health: 1995* (Rockville, MD: Indian Health Service, 1995).

7. A. P. Lanier et al., *Cancer in the Alaska Native Population: Eskimo, Aleut, and Indian Incidence and Trends 1969–1988* (Anchorage: Alaska Area Native Health Service, 1993).

8. A. P. Lanier, L. R. Bulkow, and B. Ireland, "Cancer in Alaskan Indians, Eskimos, and Aleuts, 1969–1983: Implications for Etiology and Control," *Public Health Reports* 104 (1989): 658–64.

9. A. M. Michalek et al., "Tribal-based Cancer Control Activities: Services and Perceptions," *Cancer Supplement* 78 (October 1996): 7.

10. L. Burhansstipanov, *Cancer among Elder Native Americans* (Denver: University of Colorado National Center for American Indian and Alaska Native Mental Health Research, 1997).

11. R. A. Hahn, "The State of Federal Health Statistics on Racial and Ethnic Groups," *Journal of the American Medical Association* 267:2 (1992): 270; R. A. Hahn, "Differential Classification of American Indian Race on Birth and Death Certificates, U.S. Reservation States, 1983–1985," *Provider* (Phoenix: Indian Health Service, 1993).

12. F. Frost, V. Taylor, and E. Fires, "Racial Misclassification of Native Americans in a Surveillance, Epidemiology and End Results Cancer Registry," *Journal of the National Cancer Institute* 84:12 (1992): 957; J. R. Sugarman, R. Soderberg, J. E. Gordon, and F. P. Rivara, "Racial Misclassification of American Indians: Its Effect on Injury Rates in Oregon, 1989 through 1990," *American Journal of Public Health* 83:5 (1993): 681–84.

13. American Cancer Society, *Cancer Facts* (Atlanta: American Cancer Society, 1995).

14. Department of Health and Human Services, PHS, NIH, NCI, *Report of the Special Action Committee, 1992: Program Initiatives Related to Minorities, the Underserved and Persons Aged 65 and Over* (Washington, DC: Government Printing Office, 1992), appendix A.

15. P. A. Nutting et al., "Cancer Incidence among American Indians and Alaska Natives, 1980 through 1987," *American Journal of Public Health* 83:11 (1993): 1589.

16. N. Cobb and R. E. Paisano, *Cancer Mortality among American Indians and Alaska Natives in the United States: Regional Differences in Indian Health, 1989–1993* (Rockville, MD: Indian Health Service, IHS Pub. No. 97-615-23, 1997).

17. A. Hrdlicka, "Diseases of the Indians, More Especially of the Southwest United States and Northern Mexico," *Washington Medical Annals* 6 (3/72–3/94, 1905).

18. W. A. Ritchie and S. L. Warren, "The Occurrence of Multiple Bone Lesions Suggesting Myeloma in the Skeleton of a Pre-Columbian Indian," *American Journal of Roentgenology* 28 (1932): 622–28.

19. L. Burhansstipanov and M. Tenney, "Native American Public Health Issues," *Current Issues in Public Health* 1:1 (February 1995).

20. J. Horm, S. S. De Vesa, and L. Burhansstipanov, "Cancer Incidence, Survival and Mortality among Racial and Ethnic Groups in the United States," in Schottenfeld and Fraumeni, eds., *Cancer Epidemiology and Prevention* (Philadelphia: W. B. Saunders Company, 1997); B. A. Miller et al., eds., *Cancer Statistics Review: 1973–1989*, National Cancer Institute, Pub. No. (NIH) 92-2789 (1992), I.3–I.7; R. D. Horner, "Cancer Mortality in Native Americans in North Carolina," *American Journal of Public Health* 80 (1990): 940–44; Y. Mao, H. Morrison, R. Semenciw, and D. Wigle, "Mortality on Canadian Indian Reserves 1977–1982," *Canadian Journal of Public Health* 77 (1986): 263–68; E. T. Creagan and J. F. Fraumeni, "Cancer Mortality among American Indians, 1950–1967," *Journal of the National Cancer Institute* 49 (1972): 956–67.

21. M. Eidson et al., "Breast Cancer among Hispanics, American Indians and Non-Hispanic Whites in New Mexico," *International Journal of Epidemiology* 4:23(2) (1994): 231–37.

22. P. A. Nutting, B. N. Calonge, D. C. Iverson, and L. A. Green, "The Danger of Applying Uniform Clinical Policies across Populations: The Case of Breast Cancer in American Indians," *American Journal of Public Health* 10:84 (1994): 1631–36.

23. K. A. Sorem, "Cancer Incidence in the Zuni Indians of New Mexico," *Yale Journal of Biological Medicine* 58 (1985): 489–96.

24. W. C. Black and C. R. Key, "Epidemiologic Pathology of Cancer in New Mexico's Tri-Ethnic Population," *Pathology Annals* 15 (1980): 181–94.

25. B. A. Miller et al., eds., *Cancer Statistics Review: 1973–1989*, National Cancer Institute. Pub. No. (NIH) 92-2789 (1992), I.3–I.7.

26. Department of Health and Human Services, PHS, NIH, NCI, *Report of the Special Action Committee, 1992: Program Initiatives Related to Minorities, the Underserved and Persons Aged 65 and Over* (Washington, DC: Government Printing Office, 1992), appendix A.

27. P. A. Nutting et al., "Cancer Incidence among American Indians and Alaska Natives, 1980 through 1987," *American Journal of Public Health* 83:11 (1993): 1589.

28. M. C. Mahoney et al., "Cancer Surveillance in a Northeastern Native American Population," *Cancer* 64 (1989): 191–95.

29. A. P. Lanier, L. R. Bulkow, and B. Ireland, "Cancer in Alaskan Indians, Eskimos, and Aleuts, 1969–1983: Implications for Etiology and Control," *Public Health Reports* 104 (1989): 658–64.

30. T. K. Welty et al., "Cancer Risk Factors in Three Sioux Tribes: Use of the Indian-Specific Health-Risk Appraisal for Data Collection and Analysis," *Alaska Medicine* 35:4 (1993): 265.

31. R. D. Horner, "Cancer Mortality in Native Americans in North Carolina," *American Journal of Public Health* 80 (1990): 940–44; M. C. Mahoney et al., "Cancer

Mortality in a Northeastern Native Population," *Cancer* 64 (1989): 187–90; E. T. Creagan and J. F. Fraumeni, "Cancer Mortality among American Indians, 1950–1967," *Journal of the National Cancer Institute* 49 (1972): 956–67.

32. Y. Mao, H. Morrison, R. Semenciw, and D. Wigle, "Mortality on Canadian Indian Reserves 1977–1982," *Canadian Journal of Public Health* 77 (1986): 263–68.

33. P. A. Nutting et al., "Cancer Incidence among American Indians and Alaska Natives, 1980 through 1987," *American Journal of Public Health* 83:11 (1993): 1589.

34. T. M. Becker et al., "Risk Factors for Cervical Dysplasia in Southwestern American Indian Women: A Pilot Study," *Alaska Medicine* 35:4 (1993): 255.

35. P. A. Nutting et al., "Cancer Incidence among American Indians and Alaska Natives, 1980 through 1987," *American Journal of Public Health* 83:11 (1993): 1589.

36. American Cancer Society, *Cancer Facts* (Atlanta: American Cancer Society, 1995).

37. A. P. Lanier et al., *Cancer in the Alaska Native Population: Eskimo, Aleut, and Indian Incidence and Trends 1969–1988* (Anchorage: Alaska Area Native Health Service, 1993).

38. J. M. Samet, C. R. Key, W. C. Hunt, and J. S. Goodwin, "Survival of American Indian and Hispanic Cancer Patients in New Mexico and Arizona, 1969–1982," *Journal of the National Cancer Institute* 79:3 (1987): 457–63.

39. W. C. Black and C. R. Key, "Epidemiologie Pathology of Cancer in New Mexico's Tri-Ethnic Population," *Pathology Annals* 15 (1980): 181–94.

40. J. W. Horm and L. Burhansstipanov, "Cancer Incidence, Survival, and Mortality among American Indians and Alaska Natives," *American Indian Culture and Research Journal* 16:3 (1992): 27–28.

41. L. Burhansstipanov, *Cancer among Elder Native Americans* (Denver: University of Colorado National Center for American Indian and Alaska Native Mental Health Research, 1997).

42. Agency for Health-Care Policy and Research, *National Medical Expenditure Survey, Access to Health Care: Findings from the Survey of American Indians and Alaska Natives*, Pub. No. (DHHS) 91-0028 (Washington, DC: Government Printing Office, 1991).

43. R. C. Gwilt, May 10th letter in response to NCI queries regarding availability of breast-cancer screening services from IHS, 1993.

44. L. Burhansstipanov and M. Tenney, "Native American Public Health Issues," *Current Issues in Public Health* 1:1 (February 1995).

45. T. M. Becker et al., "Risk Factors for Cervical Dysplasia in Southwestern American Indian Women: A Pilot Study," *Alaska Medicine* 35:4 (1993): 255.

46. B. A. Miller et al., *Racial/Ethnic Patterns of Cancer in the United States 1988–1992* (Bethesda, MD: National Cancer Institute, NIH Pub. No. 96-4104).

47. T. K. Welty et al., "Cancer Risk Factors in Three Sioux Tribes: Use of the Indian-Specific Health Risk Appraisal for Data Collection and Analysis," *Alaska Medicine* 35:4 (1993): 265.

48. L. Burhansstipanov, "Developing Culturally Competent Community-Based Interventions," in D. Weiner, ed., *Preventing and Controlling Cancer in North America: A Cross-Cultural Perspective* (Westport, CT: Praeger, 1999), 167–83.

49. L. Burhansstipanov et al., "Native Sister Culturally Relevant 'Navigator' Patient-Support: The Native Sisters," *Cancer Practice* 6:3 (1998): 191–94.

50. R. Doll and R. Peto, "The Causes of Cancer: Quantitative Estimates of Avoidable Risks of Cancer in the United States Today," *Journal of the National Cancer Institute* 66 (1981): 1191–1309.

51. L. Burhansstipanov and C. M. Dresser, *Native American Monograph #1: Documentation of the Cancer Research Needs of American Indians and Alaska Natives*, NIH Pub. No. 93-3603 (Bethesda, MD: National Cancer Institute, 1993).

52. C. L. Usher, D. S. Shanklin, and J. B. Wildfire, U.S. Department of Agriculture, Research Triangle Institute, *Evaluation of the Food Distribution Program on Indian Reservations*, vol. 1, *Final Report*, prepared for the Food and Nutrition Service, USDA, Control No. 53-3198-8-96(1) (Washington, DC: Government Printing Office, 1990).

53. Department of Health and Human Services, *Healthy People 2000: National Health Promotion and Disease Prevention Objectives*, Pub. No. (DHHS) 91-50212 (Washington, DC: Government Printing Office, 1991).

54. H. I. Goldberg et al., "Prevalence of Behavioral Risk Factors in Two American Populations in Montana," *Preventative Medicine* 7:3 (1991): 155–60; J. R. Sugarman, C. W. Warren, L. L. Oge, and S. D. Helgerson, "Using the Behavioral Risk Factor Surveillance System to Monitor Year 2000 Objectives among American Indians," *Public Health Reports* 107:4 (1992): 451, 454.

55. A. M. Michalek and M. C. Mahoney, "Provision of Cancer Control Services to Native Americans by State Health Departments," *Journal of Cancer Education* 9 (1994): 145–47.

56. L. Burhansstipanov and C. M. Dresser, *Native American Monograph #1: Documentation of the Cancer Research Needs of American Indians and Alaska Natives*, NIH Pub. No. 93-3603 (Bethesda, MD: National Cancer Institute, 1993), chap. 12.

57. J. A. Hampton, J. Keala, and P. H. Luce-Aoelua, "Overview of National Cancer Institute Networks for Cancer Control Research in Native American Populations," *Cancer* 78:7 (1996): 1545–52.

TWELVE

ERIC HENDERSON,
STEPHEN J. KUNITZ,
and JERROLD E. LEVY

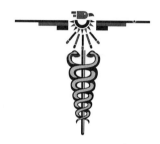

The Origins of Navajo Youth Gangs[1]

Navajo tribal members and officials have concerns about the recent prolifera-
tion of male youth gangs and perceive them as contributing to growing violence.[2] The concern is reasonable, because "injury mortality" is "the single
most important health problem of the Navajo" with accidents, suicide, homi-
cide, and "alcoholism" among the top-ten causes of death for males. Mortality
from injuries and alcohol "occur most frequently in young adult males."[3]

Gang formation has implications for both law enforcement and public-
health policy because gang activity involving risky behavior poses a danger to
individual gang members and to others. According to Terrie Moffitt, delinquency increases with "modernization" because "[t]eens are less well-inte-
grated with adults than ever before. What has emerged is an age-bound ghetto
. . . from within which it seems advantageous to mimic deviant behavior."[4]

Some of the changes in Navajo culture may fit with this view of "modernization." Although male youths in Navajo Country have forged partying
groups at ceremonies or other events for over a hundred years, increased participation in the boarding-school system during the 1950s isolated youths
from parents and community. This intensified peer-group identification and
the formation of loosely structured male groups seeking "a good time." Also,
Navajo males often have subordinate positions in a wage economy. Combined

222

with Moffitt's view that youths engage in delinquent acts to attain the desirable resource of "mature status," the frustrating socioeconomic conditions faced by males contributed to the emergence of Navajo youth gangs in the 1970s.

The data for this chapter are drawn from extensive interviews with about 50 Navajo men between ages 21 and 45 who reside on a single reservation. These men constitute a subsample of over a thousand individuals who participated in a case-control study of Navajo alcohol use.[5] During the field interviews, persons who mentioned the importance of their "gang" in their youthful drinking experiences were questioned at length about gang involvement. A larger number of individuals were asked about gangs in schools and communities during their adolescence. These men provided data concerning the emergence of gangs in two areas of Navajo Country: gang activities and gang structure (or lack of structure).

In general, former members were open about their involvement in the gang. Since only about a dozen self-identified members were encountered, the data presented provide only a preliminary sketch of the early gangs. Four members of one gang were interviewed[6] and provided relatively extensive, and basically consistent, information. Four other individuals reared in the same community also provided information regarding this gang and its members.

Navajo Culture Change and Navajo Male Youth Groups

Several historical factors are significant for understanding the emergence of Navajo gangs: (1) an end to raiding with the establishment of the reservation, (2) the waning of the livestock-based economy, (3) participation in the formal educational system, (4) the growth of the agency towns, and (5) increasing linkages of Navajos with urban areas (both border towns and distant cities). Changes in economic strategies, settlement patterns and extended-family residence arrangements have affected the extent and nature of kinship obligations—with whom individuals cooperate, how they behave towards different categories of kin, and how they conceive of and label these kin.[7] For younger males, intergenerational cooperation declined as the livestock economy waned and participation in schooling increased. In densely settled areas, there was daily contact with a greater number of peers and diminished opportunities for adolescents to share the in daily lives of older relatives.

Navajos are Athapaskan-speaking people, primarily relying on horticulture and livestock pastoralism for subsistence. Navajos are matrilineal and matrilocal. In the nineteenth century, young men could establish the nucleus of a flock through raiding, but older and wealthier individuals generally disapproved of raiding.[8] Pressure from the United States military and the establishment of the Navajo reservation (in 1868) brought an end to raiding, which created social tensions.

In the pastoral economy of the early reservation years, the ideal behavior for a young Navajo man was to marry and reside with, and work for, his in-laws.[9] Some Navajo youths, of course, did not conform to the "ideal," but traveled about, usually alone, seeking women, gambling, and drinking.[10] In the course of these travels young men often congregated at ceremonies to form ephemeral groups that sometimes engaged in gambling, drinking, and fighting at ceremonies.[11] Although often composed of individuals from a single area who were related through matrilineal kin and clan ties, the youths did not "hang around" together after the occasions passed.[12] They were not members of an enduring group.

Nevertheless, the roots of Navajo gangs may have some connection to these male associations at ceremonies. Some older interviewees refer to young men acting "like a gang" at Enemyway ceremonies. One man grew up in a rural pastoral community in the 1940s, herding sheep and playing with "cousins" and other relatives of his own age. He recalled Enemyways where his "group" fought with rocks, sticks, and fists against unrelated boys from an adjacent community.

The behavior of groups of young males at Enemyways and other ceremonies, or, more recently, tribal fairs, is often described as "ganglike" because groups of related youthful males consort together. However, the groups were not "ganglike" in the sense of having continuity and cohesion. There was little opportunity for enduring male youth "gangs" to develop in the rural areas because youths worked for their families, herding sheep or farming. Often these were solitary chores. There were few schools or other institutions where youths could congregate away from adult supervision.

In the 1950s, as the livestock economy declined, three factors promoted the development of male youth groups. School enrollments (especially in boarding schools) increased dramatically,[13] agency towns (administrative and educational centers)[14] grew in size and importance, and federal policy encouraged the relocation of younger Navajos to distant urban areas. Each of these changes altered social ties and patterns of cooperation. Males who attended off-reservation boarding schools recall the experience as regimented and disciplined. Sometimes there were fights between Navajo students and students from other tribes.

On-reservation boarding schools also spawned "ganglike" groups among Navajos from different communities. In one central reservation high school, day students banded together to fight boarding students from a rural community. Greater peer-group cohesion resulted from boarding-school rivalries. When students came home there was often less need to provide help to the family because families generally had fewer sheep to tend. Other students resided with relatives in towns, but visited relatives in rural communities, joining school friends at rodeos, ceremonies, fairs, or to "party in the boonies." A youthful male drinking "cohort" (often with a common boarding-school or kinship ties) could form "more or less spontaneously at various events and places," especially in agency and border towns.[15]

Since 1960 increasing numbers of Navajo students have attended on-reservation schools rather than off-reservation boarding institutions. Along the eastern edge of the Navajo reservation, many youths attended nearby off-reservation public schools with a predominately non-Navajo student body. Navajo "gangs" emerged in the early 1970s within these school environments in agency towns and border towns.

While most Navajos continue to live in rural communities, about a quarter of the reservation's population resides in agency towns. Others live in non-Indian border towns. Moreover, both the Indian and non-Indian populations of towns bordering the reservation also increased.[16] In these locations of dense settlement, nuclear families predominate and adults tend to work for wages. Children have fewer chores related to family subsistence and spend more time with one another in and out of school.

The changing social conditions and an emerging youth culture are reflected in a change in kinship terminology. Today, Navajo youths often use the English term "cousin-brother" to designate a set of relatives. The diffusion of this term appears to follow from the complex changes in education, residential arrangements, and networks of cooperating kin. "Cousin-brother" seems to be an informal expression of the solidarity of age-mates.[17] Gang members often referred to one another as "cousin-brothers."

The Origin and Distribution of Youth Gangs

Early Gangs on the Eastern Edge of the Reservation

The earliest references to self-identified gangs appear about 1970 in an agency town on the eastern boundary of the reservation. In that year, one interviewee claims to have formed a gang called the Cruisers[18] with about a dozen other schoolmates between the ages of 13 and 15. They drank together on weekends at the town's drive-in theater and shoplifted items "a bunch of times" to pay for liquor.

Other agency-town interviewees of the same age cohort engaged in similar behavior, but did not identify with a named "gang." Yet group violence at the agency-town drive-in figured in several accounts given for the late 1960s through the 1970s. While the use of weapons, as well as the targets of violence, differentiated the Cruisers from the more informal group, the main difference between the report of the Cruiser and a "non-gang" interviewee is self-identification with a *named* group.

During the 1970s several gangs were present in and near this agency town. Those named were the Farm Boys, Spikes, Skulls and Black Knights, Metallics (at an adjacent farm community), and Dead Boys (in a nearby rural community). These gangs had 15 to 35 members. They used guns, knives, chains, clubs, and other weapons in fights with rival gangs.

The Skulls gang was reportedly formed by agency-town high school students who were "from the reservation" (meaning rural reservation communities). There were only 15 or 20 Skulls and they did not have a leader. "They argued about that and nobody knew who the leader was," according to one individual. This young man did not consider himself a member of the Skulls, but would "just party [and] party with them." Parties, usually on the periphery of the town, primarily involved drinking beer and smoking marijuana. There was little or no violence at Skulls parties, but sometimes gang members ended up in the agency-town jail for public intoxication.

Navajo gangs of the 1970s emerged in and around the densely populated agency towns. They were small and loosely structured. Although associated primarily with "areas" in the minds of many interviewees, some noted that the core of the gang consisted of kin living in proximity to one another.

Gangs at an Interior Agency Town

Data from the interior agency town reveal patterns similar to those of the eastern agency town. A former core gang member, Paddy Lefty, described these gangs in the early 1980s. He identified six named, and two unnamed, groups.[19] These were rival groups that sometimes fought each other with bats, two by fours, chains, and knives. These gangs consisted mostly of relatives—especially cousins and brothers—who referred to each other as "Bros." The gangs were relatively small and lacked internal organizational structure. He could not identify anyone who clearly acted as leader in any of these gangs.

The gang activities Lefty described primarily involved "hang[ing] around," drinking, and vandalism. Often they would break glass bottles on the highway, to see what would happen. They spray-painted buildings, broke windows, and slashed car tires. Lefty assumed the role of "shanker" because "I wouldn't mind stabbing somebody" (and because he was one of the youngest gang members). He claimed he had stabbed several people. Mostly, however, the gang would "roll winos." Sometimes they would shoot dogs, "kill them just for the hell of it." Gang members earned money by "bootlegging" alcohol and selling marijuana. The gang disintegrated by the late 1980s as members were incarcerated (including Lefty), left town to seek work (or excitement), or took on family responsibilities.

The interior agency-town gangs apparently emerged slightly later in the 1970s than did the eastern agency-town gangs. Gangs in both areas were small and composed mostly of relatives within an age cohort. Gangs associated with adjacent rural communities were generally active only in the school and town.

Characteristics of Core Gang Members

The extent of gang membership in the two areas during the 1970s can be estimated in a rough fashion. Information from interviews indicates that, at most, 15 percent of Navajo male youths in the two areas were affiliated, peripherally or minimally, with gangs. The actual proportion was likely to have been significantly less than half this figure.[20] A number of individuals identified as gang members during this period had died (most frequently in drinking-related accidents or incidents of violence) or were in prison. Life histories of four former "core" gang members and comparisons with more peripheral members and hangers-on provide important clues about gang dynamics.

All four core gang members were from troubled families. All had fathers who were heavy drinkers and three of the fathers were physically abusive to their wives and children. One father forced his sons to fight each other because he "didn't want us to be chickenshits, he didn't want us to be pussies." Another core gang member was severely punished by his father, but it was his older brothers who were most abusive—they used to drink and "beat the shit out of me." The fourth said his father was not violent but he had abandoned his family, leaving "my mom [to] grow me up." His mother punished her son "for anything I might do . . . every evening, every day" with "a big belt" or by "twist[ing] my ears." The parents of three of the gang members divorced. The father of the fourth had a second wife and children in a distant community.

None of the families of core members were well integrated into their communities. While only one individual came from an extremely poor family, the families of the other three resided away from their home communities (two off the reservation) for several years before the boys reached adolescence. Two of the boys lived for a time with aunts and one was placed in off-reservation foster care for two years. Navajo was the predominant language in the homes of all these youths. Attitudes about abilities in both Navajo and English were ambivalent. One expressed concern about his English-language abilities, and another noted, with some disdain, that his younger siblings did not speak Navajo well but were more competent English speakers than he. Although none of the families maintained flocks of sheep, two of the youths sometimes herded sheep for grandparents. In sum, these youths were reared on the "margins" of Navajo and Anglo communities.

Prior to joining a gang, all of these youths reported delinquent behaviors. Prior to age 12, all had taken items from stores and two had run away from home. By age 13 all were frequently skipping school, three had their first sexual experience, and all but one were gang members. With gang involvement, delinquent behaviors increased. By age 14 all had smoked marijuana and had used at least one other mind-altering substance (usually glue, gas, or paint). Three reported frequently starting fights and having been arrested (the fourth was not arrested until age 16). By age 16 all reported engaging in acts of vandalism and using weapons in fights. The self-reports show early antisocial behaviors that deepened with age and gang involvement.

The "Metallics": A Case of Gang Formation

The origins of the Metallics highlight the interplay of community, marginality, and personality. The Nance family returned to Mrs. Nance's home community, a reservation farming area, in the late 1960s after over a decade in southern California. Mr. Nance was a heavy drinker who abused his wife and sons. He was frequently away from home, working, drinking, and engaging in extramarital affairs.

The three eldest sons were day students at a border-town high school after the family returned from California, where they established a reputation for violence and toughness. They were familiar with southern California gangs and self-consciously set out to create a "gang," the Metallics. One of the first individuals to join was a "clan-brother" who eventually became a core member.

At home, the three brothers frequently fought their father and younger siblings. One younger brother, Marlin, recalls that when his older brothers drank they "beat the shit out of me." Marlin began shoplifting when he was eight. At 13 he and some friends burglarized a trading post, taking jewelry and knives. They were drinking and sniffing glue under a nearby bridge when apprehended. The next year Marlin and some of these boys joined his older brothers' gang. He helped his older brothers and other gang members grow and sell marijuana. Marlin also sold peyote stolen from his father's ceremonial supply. When Marlin was 16, his father died suddenly of a stroke. "I had what I wanted," Marlin recalled, referring to an end to his father's abuse. Marlin began engaging in acts of vandalism, drinking with other gang members, and fighting members of rival gangs.

The Metallics included between 20 and 35 members. The first "members" (in the early 1970s) were of approximately the same age. They incorporated a younger group in the late 1970s. The gang lacked cohesion. The Nance brothers seem to have fought each other as much as they fought rival gangs. They partied with one another and with their "cousin-brothers," but they also partied with strangers and occasionally with members of rival gangs. Individual members drank with almost anyone, and the interest in any "party" involving alcohol seemed to prevail over group solidarity.

In the late 1970s several Metallic leaders killed a rival gang member from the agency town and were sent to prison. As a result, the gang began to dissolve. By the early 1980s, Marlin's two eldest brothers had full-time jobs. Another member and relative drifted away from the gang, joined the Job

Corps, and then worked at temporary jobs. He continued to drink heavily, but with less-aggressive groups.

Discussion

During the late nineteenth and early twentieth centuries, Navajos lived in scattered rural family settlements where males sometimes gathered at ceremonies to meet women, gamble, and drink. Such groups were ephemeral, dissolving with the termination of the ceremony. Young men spent most of their days within the extended families of their mother or in-laws. The growth of agency and border towns as well as boarding schools altered this. With frequent peer contacts and the lack of adult supervision, a youth culture of cousin-brothers emerged.

Navajo gangs first appeared in agency and border towns. In agency towns, hundreds of families lived and continue to live in relative proximity, some in housing projects. Navajo families living in agency towns were surrounded by networks of vaguely defined kin, often unaware of the precise nature of these relations. Weekend partying among informal groups of agency-town youths became commonplace in the 1960s and 1970s. Adolescent males emphasized connections to peers ("cousin-brothers") rather than location in the intricate multigenerational kinship structures.

Although contemporary Navajo gangs may have a connection to the ephemeral drinking groups long associated with ceremonies and partying, in the 1970s named gangs coalesced around core members from marginal families. Violence was not a distinguishing element of gang identity or activity. Drinking parties that turn violent are not limited to Navajo gangs, since fights, knifings, and occasional shootings occur among spontaneous partying groups. No one described a well-organized "gang fight," and only a few cases of explicitly gang-related retaliatory attacks were reported.

What then allows one, following the local use of the term "gang," to describe groups such as the Metallics as gangs? It appears to be limited to self-identification and self-ascription. Indeed, gang members of the 1970s and early 1980s had moved only a small step beyond the spontaneous party group by providing a name to a set of age-mates related through clan and community and who partied frequently with one another. Some sets of cousin-brothers called themselves a gang to set themselves apart from "rivals," while other sets of cousin-brothers never labeled themselves in this way.[21]

The transition from youth to man is difficult for many Navajos, given the paucity of local jobs, low-income families, and concerns about the need to maintain Navajo tradition while at the same time gaining skills and education necessary to transcend poverty. While a number of Navajo youths may become temporary "hell raisers," only a very few—those from abusive or disrupted families living in densely settled communities and attending local schools—become core "gang" members. The gangs attracted a somewhat larger set of peripheral members who modeled the behavior of core members.

Many core members reportedly continue antisocial acts. Two of the four core gang members who were interviewed had served prison terms, while the other two had been arrested within the two years prior to the interview for spousal abuse or disorderly conduct. Other reputed core members had died in accidents or fights, usually involving alcohol. But most former gang members, especially those peripherally involved, "aged out" of the gang. They follow the life-course pattern of "hell-raiser" to "family man" that Thomas Hill described for young Indian men in Sioux City, Iowa, in the 1970s.[22]

Peripheral gang members differed little in their antisocial behaviors from males who, prior to the 1970s, frequented ceremonies and other events in dispersed rural communities. However, in the more densely settled communities of the 1970s these youths were consistently exposed to more "deviant" and marginal youths at the core of the gangs. These core gang members apparently looked to off-reservation models, especially southern California Chicano gangs, to construct loosely organized named gangs. Although the core members were few, they attracted satellite members among peers who were neighbors and kin.

In Navajo Country, "crude mortality is highest in the[se] least remote, most densely settled areas."[23] The social dynamics that have led to the formation of youth gangs in Navajo Country help in understanding why this may be so. Gang behaviors provide an extreme example of the behaviors that generally contribute to leading causes of mortality among young Navajo men.

Since the 1970s, Navajo gangs have reputedly become more common, more institutionalized, and more closely connected with non-Indian gangs off the reservation[24] as agency towns have continued to grow and as migration to off-reservation locales has increased. Moreover, the antisocial behavior of gang members may be increasingly "imitated" by other youth[25] in the most densely settled and rapidly growing Navajo communities. Thus, gangs have been added to the repertoire of behavior for some youths making the difficult transition to adulthood within the subordinate socioeconomic conditions that prevail in Navajo Country.

Despite the limited nature of the data, there may be some implications for gang-prevention policy within the Navajo Nation. First, not all self-identifying gang members are alike. The degree of antisocial personality disorder may distinguish core and peripheral members. This distinction may aid in developing different types of intervention for different types of gang members. Second, some "gangs" may still be little more than "street-corner" groups, while others have "hardened." The former may be more amenable to the "traditional" peacemaking interventions. Third, the sociodemographic conditions should be addressed as an element in gang prevention. It may be that a small number of antisocial individuals will emerge in any community. Given contemporary circumstances, young males with such problems seem to provide the core in the process of gang formation. To the degree that conditions for youths can be improved generally, mimicry of core members should diminish. Thus, "gang prevention" is not simply, or even fundamentally, a law-enforcement issue. It is a public-health issue in the broadest sense.

Notes

1. This chapter is based on research supported by the United States Public Health Service, National Institute of Alcoholism and Alcohol Abuse (PHS Grant No. RO1 AA09420). We have benefited from the comments on earlier drafts by Jim Zion, Wilson Howard, Marlene Jasperse, Barbara Mendenhall, Amy Henderson, and Drs. Cliff Trafzer, Diane Weiner, Thomas Hill, Clemens Bartollas, Jeffrey Eighmy, and Troy Armstrong.

2. Martin Avery, "Prepared Written Statement" on Behalf of the Navajo Nation before the House Committee on Appropriations, Subcommittee on Appropriations, *Federal News Service* (April 17, 1997).

3. Cheryl Howard, *Navajo Tribal Demography, 1983–1986: A Comparative and Historical Perspective* (New York: Garland Publishing, 1993), 116; Stephen J. Kunitz, *Disease Change and the Role of Medicine: The Navajo Experience* (Berkeley: University of California Press, 1983), 111. Injuries accounted for 85 percent of all deaths for Navajo males between ages 15 and 24 during the 1980s; Howard, *Navajo Tribal Demography*, 131. Navajo injury mortality has exceeded national levels throughout the century, with young males having higher rates of accidental deaths, suicides, and homicides than women; Kunitz, *Disease Change and the Role of Medicine*, 66, 99–111; Howard, *Navajo Tribal Demography*, 128–35.

4. Terrie Moffitt, "Adolescence-Limited and Life-Course-Persistent Antisocial Behavior: A Developmental Taxonomy," *Psychological Review* 100 (1993): 674–701.

5. Stephen J. Kunitz and Jerrold E. Levy, *Drinking, Conduct Disorder, and Social Change: Navajo Experiences* (New York: Oxford University Press, 2000).

6. The "Metallics," described in some detail below.

7. "The first and most important lessons which the [Navajo] child learns about human relationships are the approved ways of dealing with various classes of relatives"; Dorothea Leighton and Clyde Kluckhohn, *Children of the People: The Navaho Individual and his Development* (Cambridge, MA: Harvard University Press, 1947), 44. In the early 1940s, the biological (nuclear) family was emphasized at Shiprock, an agency town. In rural communities, the extended family was emphasized; ibid., 126.

8. Evon Vogt, "The Navaho," in E. H. Spicer, ed., *Perspectives in American Indian Culture Change* (Chicago: University of Chicago Press, 1961), 306; W. W. Hill, *Navaho Warfare* (New Haven, CT: Yale University Publications in Anthropology, no. 5, 1936), 4.

9. David F. Aberle, "Navaho," in David M. Schneider and Kathleen Gough, eds., *Matrilineal Kinship* (Berkeley: University of California Press, 1961), 101, 146–48, 163.

10. Miller viewed such behaviors as forms of street-gang activities. Walter B. Miller, "Lower Class Culture as a Generating Milieu of Gang Delinquency," *Journal of Social Issues* 14 (1958): 5, 11.

11. Walter Dyk, ed., *Son of Old Man Hat* (Lincoln: University of Nebraska Press, 1967 [1938]), 140–42; Walter Dyk, ed., *A Navaho Autobiography* (New York: Viking Fund, Viking Fund Publications in Anthropology, no. 8, 1947), 44–45, 54; Left Handed, *Left Handed: A Navajo Autobiography*, Walter and Ruth Dyk, eds. (New York: Columbia University Press, 1980), 306.

12. Compare Malcolm W. Klein, *The American Street Gang: Its Nature, Prevalence, and Control* (New York: Oxford University Press, 1995), 21.

13. As late as 1950, less than half the school-age population attended school. Denis F. Johnston, "An Analysis of Sources of Information on the Population of the Navaho," *Bureau of American Ethnology Bulletin* 197 (Washington, DC: Government Printing Office, 1966), 48–51. By the late 1950s, nearly 90 percent of Navajo children attended school, many in federal boarding schools; Hildegard Thompson, *The Navajos' Long Walk for Education* (Tsaile: Navajo Community College Press, 1975), 127, 137.

14. These towns were places "through which federal money flowed for expenditure and as the seat of administrative authority and operations they were sources of jobs for Indians. Consequently they attracted Indians who built houses at the edges of the areas where governmental buildings were placed"; Edward H. Spicer, *Cycles of Conquest* (Tucson: University of Arizona Press, 1962), 468.

15. Martin Topper, "Navajo 'Alcoholism': Drinking, Alcohol Abuse, and Treatment in a Changing Cultural Environment," in Linda A. Bennett and Genevieve M. Ames, eds., *The American Experience with Alcohol: Contrasting Cultural Perspectives* (New York: Plenum Press, 1985), 236.

16. Data on the growth of agency towns and border towns are drawn from U.S. decennial census volumes for Arizona, New Mexico, and Utah.

17. The term may be a means of reconciling Navajo cousin terms (which, as an "Iroquoian" terminology, classifies parallel cousins with siblings but distinguishes cross-cousins by another term) with the American kinship system (an "Eskimoan" system refers to all cousins by one term and siblings by another). Kinship terminology generally responds to changes in the sexual division of labor, residence arrangements, and, more directly, descent systems; George Peter Murdock, *Social Structure* (New York: Free Press, 1949), 182–83; Harold Driver, *Indians of North America*, 2d rev. ed. (Chicago: University of Chicago Press, 1969), 259–68. Forty years ago, Aberle showed that changes in Navajo economic adaptations "required significant modifications in kinship structure" and suggested "a shift toward Hawaiian cousin terms . . . may be under way"; David F. Aberle, "Navaho," in *Matrilineal Kinship*, 101, 172–75. In Hawaiian kinship terminologies, siblings and all cousins are classified under the same term. Before the 1980s we had not heard the term "cousin-brother." The kin covered by the rubric "cousin-brother" vary depending upon the individual using the term. Some Navajos seem to include all male cousins and siblings. Others limit the term to siblings and par-

allel cousins (consistent with the Iroquoian terminology). Still others extend the term to clan members of similar age, or to any age mate who is "somehow" related. A Navajo educator commented, "I just hate it" (the term "cousin-brother"). She thought those using the term didn't know to whom they referred.

18. This is a pseudonym. We use pseudonyms for all individuals and for gangs discussed in detail. We retain actual gang names for gangs mentioned in passing. The actual gang names reflect, to some degree, what the youths consider appropriate monikers. Few gang names seem to have had off-reservation sources. This situation has changed in recent years; Barbara Mendenhall, "Identity, Acculturation and the Emergence of Youth Gangs on the Navajo Nation," M.A. thesis, California State University, Sacramento, 1999, pp. 232–36.

19. He identified the gangs as his gang, the D.T.s (a pseudonym), the Southsiders (SSRs), the LRs (who lived at "low-rent" housing), the "Bloods" (a gang name cognate with an off-reservation gang but not affiliated with that well-known southern California gang), the M—— (a clan name) Boys, and the J—— (a family surname) Boys (both from an adjacent rural community), and two gangs without names (one composed of "northsiders" and another of "westsiders" in the agency town). A second interviewee from this town mentioned only the SSRs and LRs. He "ran with" (as a peripheral member) the LRs while in high school in the late 1970s. They would party, drinking whiskey and Budweiser, pass out, wake up, and party some more. He noted that they never drank wine "because of the stigma." His sister belonged to a small, all-girl gang at the high school in the mid-1970s, but he knew little about it. The more-limited interior agency-town data on the gang scene are consistent with data from the eastern agency town.

20. If interviewees provided a relatively complete inventory of 1970s and 1980s gangs in the two communities and if the rather consistent estimates of gang-member numbers are accurate (i.e., about 15 to 35 members), then there were fewer than 350 gang members in the two communities. It is probable that the number was much lower in any single year. In 1980 the total Navajo population of the two areas was over 18,000. Males between 10 and 19, the ages that span the age range of the gang members, account for about 12 to 13 percent of the Navajo population. Thus, perhaps 10 to 15 percent of Navajo male youths was affiliated to some degree with gangs in the 1970s.

21. Gary F. Jensen and Dean G. Rojek (*Delinquency and Youth Crime*, 3d ed. [Prospect Heights, IL: Waveland Press, 1998], 286–92) provide a good introduction to the variegated definitions of gangs and other delinquent youth groups.

22. Thomas W. Hill, "From Hell-Raiser to Family Man," in James P. Spradley and David W. McCurdy, eds., *Conformity and Conflict: Readings in Cultural Anthropology*, 2d ed. (Boston: Little, Brown, 1974). These men were not affiliated with gangs.

23. Stephen J. Kunitz, *Disease and Social Diversity* (New York: Oxford University Press, 1994), 156.

24. Mendenhall, "Identity, Acculturation and the Emergence of Youth Gangs on the Navajo Nation."

25. Moffitt, "Adolescence-Limited and Life-Course-Persistent Antisocial Behavior."

THIRTEEN

TROY JOHNSON
and HOLLY TOMREN

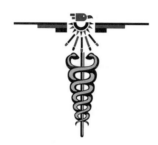

Helplessness, Hopelessness, and Despair
IDENTIFYING THE PRECURSORS TO INDIAN YOUTH SUICIDE

Suicide among American Indian youth is a matter of grave concern to members of all Indian tribal organizations across the nation and is an important issue confronting the human-service professions today. Suicide is the second leading cause of death among American Indian youth ages 15 through 24, with a rate 2.4 times (91.9 per 100,000) that of youth of all races in the United States. Suicide is the fourth leading cause of death among American Indian youth ages 5 through 14, with a rate of 1.9 per 100,000, which is 2.1 times higher than youth of all races in the United States.[1] Within the Indian-youth suicide group, American Indian children placed in non-Indian homes for adoptive or foster care suffer a rate of 70 suicides per 100,000, 6 times higher than other youth in the United States.[2] While suicide rates for youth 15 through 19 have decreased somewhat, rates for 10- and 14-year-olds are approximately 4 times higher than that for the general U.S. population and have continued to increase steadily.[3] A host of issues are germane to suicide trends. These include data vital to the planning of intervention programs such as age groups most at risk, pattern variations among tribes,[4] and common associate factors that include alcoholism, arrest careers, and interpersonal distress such as anomie, helplessness, hopelessness, and despair.[5]

American Indian suicide first came to public attention in 1968 when Senator Robert F. Kennedy visited an intermountain Indian reservation. On the particular day that he visited the reservation, the community had recently suffered the loss of an Indian youth by suicide, and thus Indian suicide became a major topic of conversation during Senator Kennedy's visit. This intermountain reservation became the focus of government attention and research that revealed a suicide rate that was approximately 100 per 100,000, nearly 10 times the national average. This number became widely publicized as the "Indian suicide rate," while it only represented the rate of one small reservation at one particular time. From this emerged the stereotype of "The Suicidal Indian."[6] On the other hand, large tribes with low suicide rates received little public attention.[7] It should be noted that this same intermountain tribe was successfully able to lower the suicide rate and improve tribal self-image.[8]

It is dangerous to generalize, oversimplify, and to overemphasize American Indian suicide. The stereotype of the suicidal Indian can lead to low self-esteem and low self-image, which may actually perpetuate American Indian suicides. According to James Shore, the major misconceptions that result from the suicidal Indian stereotype are: (1) an assumption that all American Indians have the same health problems and subsequently the same suicide pattern and rates; (2) a failure to recognize the importance of tribal differences; and (3) a danger that public-health personnel will not individualize their approach in developing tribal programs for suicide prevention and intervention.[9]

While the American Indian youth suicide rate is on average double the rate of the non-Indian population, it must be borne in mind that this rate is distorted. First, it implies a homogeneous Indian population, ignoring the differences between tribes. Some tribes have suicide rates that are much lower than the average U.S. rate, some tribes have rates similar to the U.S. rate, and some tribes have rates significantly higher than the U.S. rate. In some tribes, suicide is a relatively recent phenomenon, while in some tribes suicide was present, whether positively or negatively sanctioned, before European contact. Since written records of suicide were not kept before European contact or during the early reservation period, a true history of American Indian suicide is not possible.[10] Second, since American Indian populations are so small in comparison to the non-Indian population, small localized suicide occurrences can significantly affect the national comparison rate.[11] Third, the American Indian suicide rate most likely does not include urban American Indian people, who now represent the majority of the American Indian population; urban American Indians are often not identified as American Indian, do not use Indian Health Service facilities, and statistics are not kept regarding them. Also, several studies of American Indian adolescent suicides have been conducted with subgroups of American Indian youth, such as those in boarding schools or those who are incarcerated; these populations may have pre-existing mental-health issues and do not reflect an accurate cross-section of their community. In addition, although not unique to American Indians, many suicides are disguised or unintentionally certified as accidents on official records.[12]

Though he acknowledges that there is tribal diversity in American Indian suicide patterns, Philip May identifies several general characteristics of American Indian suicides that have emerged from over forty studies on suicide among various Indian groups[13]:

1. Suicide among American Indians is primarily among the young. This is the opposite of the general U.S. trend in which suicidal behavior increases with age. It should be noted, however, that the American Indian population is significantly younger on the whole than the U.S. population.
2. Indian suicide in most tribes is predominantly male. American Indian females tend to have lower suicide rates than the dominant population. However, Indian females attempt suicide more often than Indian males. It is important not to neglect American Indian female suicidal behavior, despite the lower completed suicide rates. Teresa D. LaFramboise and Beth Howard-Pitney's article, "Suicidal Behavior in American Indian Female Adolescents," points out that young American Indian women are much more prone to depression than young American Indian men.[14] This depression is often the result of victimization associated with racism and sexual abuse.
3. Indian males tend to use highly violent or lethal methods to commit suicide, such as guns and hanging, more so than other groups in the United States. Indian females on the other hand, tend to attempt suicide by drug overdose, which usually does not result in the completion of the suicide.
4. Tribes with loose social integration and that emphasize a high degree of individuality generally have higher suicide rates than those with tight integration and that emphasize conformity. In May's study of New Mexico Indian tribes, he found that the acculturated tribes had the highest rates, the traditional had the lowest, and the transitional had intermediates rates.[15]
5. Tribes who are undergoing rapid change in their social and economic conditions have higher rates than those who are not.

In attempting to develop a pattern of suicide behavior, researchers in suicidology have investigated medical records, suicide notes, personal diaries, police records, and clinical records of persons at risk of suicide or clients who have attempted suicide without success.[16] In addition, the issue of detecting a suicide is difficult. In his article, "Suicide among American Indian Youth: A

236

Look at the Issues," Philip May suggests another at-risk group that has not been researched, stating that "accidental death from motor vehicle crashes is higher among most tribes than the general population." He asks, how many accidents are self-inflicted? May feels that suicide attempts and single-vehicle crashes overlap, and that the single-vehicle crash among Indian youth may hide forms of self-destruction and/or suicide.[17]

The work of these scholars points to important aspects of human behavior believed to be common to individuals with suicidal tendencies, which can be applied to Indian youth. This set of relationships is composed of underlying causes that are generally circumstances in the individual's environment, precipitating stress events, with personal feelings such as alienation, anomie, helplessness, hopelessness, and despair. These personal feelings are placed into motion by stressful events, which are manifested by the development of suicidal thoughts and gestures, the culmination being the successful suicide act. Additionally, circumstances in the environment represent underlying factors such as economic and social conditions that contribute to suicide rates among Indian youth. American Indians in general have high rates of depression. According to Shore et al., one-third to one-half of all patients visiting Indian Health Service mental-health outpatient clinics have been treated for symptoms of depression. Overwhelming stress from rapid acculturation and loss of traditional identity leads to a state of chronic depression.[18] The unemployment rate for Indians continues to be higher than national averages, and on some reservations unemployment is over 60 percent. According to Census Bureau data for 1990, the median income of Indian families in the United States was $21,750—considerably lower than the national average of $35,225, and more than twice as many Indian people (31%) were living below the poverty level.[19] The educational attainment of Indians is below national averages. While 20 percent of those 25 years and older in the general population have completed four years of college, only 9 percent of American Indians have done so.[20] Finally, alcoholism is a major threat to the survival of Indian culture as fewer traditional values and lifestyles are passed on to the youth in the society.

Stress Events Leading to Self-Destruction

Environmental circumstances and coupled stress events place Indian youth on a dangerous path toward suicidal behavior. Stress events may include a death among the immediate or extended family members, failure in school or job, or conflict between white social values and deep-seated cultural beliefs. While most youth in America are faced with the problems associated with making the transition into adulthood, Indian youth face even greater conflicts, particularly due to their minority status, fewer economic and educational advantages, and cultural differences. Indian adolescents often must choose from at least two distinct cultures. Faced with this pressure, some—particularly those with little support who have suffered the consequences of prejudice, discrimination, and hostility by non-Indians—turn to various forms of self-destructive behavior, including suicide.

Alienation appears as an early symptom of fear and confusion, resulting from stress. This is often accompanied by dramatic changes in behavior patterns such as self-destructive acts of alcohol or drug abuse or a decline in school performance. Helplessness is a furtherance of the feelings of alienation and has been defined as a desire to escape from what one considers to be an insoluble problem with no hope that relief is possible in the future. It is at this point that Indian youth begin to visualize thoughts of powerlessness over his or her environment. Events seem insurmountable, and individuals feel alone. These feelings often overshadow all others and quickly lead to a feeling of hopelessness. Alcohol use among American Indian adolescents is strongly associated with feelings of hopelessness and despair. Socioeconomic factors as well as alcoholism can have an impact on family discord and dysfunction, which also contributes to the feeling of hopelessness and self-destructive behavior. At this point the Indian youth is most vulnerable. Often human resources are few and Indian youth have a limited number of people with whom to consult.

Many schools that serve American Indian students are unsupportive of the academic, social, cultural, and spiritual needs of students.[21] Indian youth may face racism from their fellow students and inaccurate portrayals of Native Americans and U.S. history, which may lower their self-esteem. According to the Group for the Advancement of Psychiatry, pathways to assimilation to dominant society are often blocked due to racism, and Indian youth slip into cultural marginalization. They have lost many essential values of traditional culture and have not been able to replace them by active participation in American society in ways that are conducive to enhanced cultural and psychological self-esteem.[22]

Without the help of friends and relatives, or if those are removed or fail, finality is near. Anomie is the next step, when the Indian youth loses his or her sense of purpose in life and personal identity. Anomie is followed rapidly by despair.

When the youth enters the final stage of despair, he or she falters between thoughts of life and death; this is usually accompanied by severe withdrawal symptoms. Often subtle clues to suicide are given, while behavior usually changes dramatically. Talking about wanting to join dead relatives or having an experience of being visited by the dead may provide a clue to an impending suicide attempt.[23] The individual seemingly will break the depression cycle, which may appear promising. However, it may simply mean that all options have been exhausted and that a plan for suicide has been developed. Intervention and planning are critical at this point, because counseling may generate thinking around activities of life to detract from thoughts about death. Planned intervention must reconnect the at-risk person with a human resource that fits his or her particular need. This reconnection is often with members of the extended family, peers, or teachers. Another critical point of reconnection is with the Indian culture from which the Indian people often draw their strength.

Intervention plans must prompt this network to reach out and reenter the life of the potential suicide victim. Thus, suicide intervention must take an active, critical approach. The intervention designs addressed in this chapter are intended to provide action guidelines for human-service professionals, family members, and other members of the support network, which will enable them to intervene and break the suicide pattern for Indian youth "at-risk" and to provide ongoing interventions that will prevent other Indian youth from starting on a self-destructive path.

The conceptual framework for designing action guidelines must mitigate impacts among factors associated with suicide rather than simply reacting to a suicide event itself. This approach anticipates a likelihood that suicide, suicide attempts, and suicidal manifestations will occur within a given population impacted by selected circumstances. The empirical literature concerning suicide among American Indian youth illuminates several specific life circumstances, or events that provide clues for planning in primary prevention. These include events that occur as a result of institutional services planned in the best interest of children and as a result of personal lifestyles. Specific predictors that can be utilized have been identified[24]:

1. Seventy percent of the American Indian adolescent suicides had more than one significant caretaker or parental figure before age 15, as compared to 15 percent of the adolescents in a cohort control group.
2. Forty percent of the primary caretakers or parent figures of the suicide group had five or more arrests, compared to 7.5 percent of the comparison group's caretakers.
3. Fifty percent of the suicide group had experienced two or more parental losses by divorce, or desertion, compared to 10 percent of the comparison group.
4. Eighty percent of the suicides had one or more arrests in the twelve months before their suicide, compared to 25.5 percent of the comparison adolescents.
5. By age 15, 70 percent of suicides had been arrested, compared to 20 percent of the control group.
6. Sixty percent of the suicides attended boarding school before ninth grade, compared to 27.5 percent of the control group.

Self-Destructive Acts

The suicide rate among American Indian youth for the age group 15 through 19 is approximately 2.1 times that of their cohorts in the dominant population. One area that has not been addressed in the empirical literature and thus is not reflected in these statistics is that of equivocal death of Indian youth by means of unexplained single-car accidents, particularly within the boundaries of Indian reservations. Philip May, in his article, "Suicide among American Indian Youth: A Look at the Issues," addresses this type of suicide and self-destructive behavior. His research indicates that suicide attempts and single-vehicle crashes overlap and that single-vehicle crashes among Indian youth hide forms of self-destruction and suicide. May maintains that "[s]elf-destructive behavior manifests itself in several other ways in American Indian society. For example, accidental death from motor vehicle crashes is higher among most tribes that the general U.S. population; 36.6 per 100,000, which is 3.4 times the U.S. rate of 39.8. Over half of these accidental deaths are from motor vehicle crashes."[25] Clearly, an intervention is needed in order to reach this unaddressed group of Indian youth. Prior to design of the intervention it is necessary, however, to identify characteristics of this group and to identify areas where an intervention might be most effective. In this regard, the use of the psychological autopsy may prove beneficial.

Intervention Teams

Psychological autopsy can be used to retrace life's events immediately prior to the suicide. The procedure is one aimed at revealing the state of mind of a deceased person prior to his or her death. The procedure itself consists essentially of interviews with survivors and examination of public and private documents that reveal the personality of the deceased party. These survivors include both the immediate and extended family members. Documents include those related to medical, hospital, adoptive, and foster-home placement. Most importantly, records would include those revealing violations of tribal, state, and federal laws. There is considerable evidence to show that as many as 80 percent of Indian youth suicide victims had experienced one or more arrests in the twelve months prior to their suicide. Data on Indian youth suggests that these early arrest careers may in fact be symptomatic behaviors akin to "cries for help."[26] Since psychological autopsy has never been utilized for the purposes considered here, a procedure has not been established for use specifically with American Indian youth. Recommendations can however be taken from the works of Selkin, Weisman, and Shneidman, who recommend the establishment of a team consisting of psychiatrists, psychologists, social workers, and nurse-clinicians.[27] A team investigating suicide among Indian youth should be headed by a person who is from the same Indian tribe as the suicide victim, and all other members of the team must be extremely sensitive to the tribal, cultural, and religious beliefs of the survivors. Selkin points out that the psychological autopsy is a multidisciplinary casework conference designed to draw together and correlate medical, social, and psychiatric information about a patient during the final period of his life. This multidisciplinary approach would be used to identify areas where intervention could have been introduced, concentrating on "cries for help" arrests. For example, since May suggests that single-car accidental deaths may in fact be suicides, arrest records could be monitored and used to identify and target this potential suicide group.

The best intervention technique is a team approach, but the requisites for a team, particularly from a financial and personnel standpoint, seem overwhelming. Operational funds are obviously necessary. Creative arrangements are possible to offset this problem. The Indian Health Service and Indian tribes are two logical and available sources for limited funding. With proper presentation of the seriousness of suicide, an issue that is not unknown to these two entities, a modest shift of 1 or 2 percent of funds into mental health is possible. Tribes could be approached using a similar strategy to set aside an amount of tribal funds for alcohol, juvenile justice, and child-welfare programs. These amounts of money would not be enormous, but would provide seed funds to launch a primary intervention program.

Hiring additional personnel could be offset by recasting existing work assignments. Through the utilization of flex-time schedules, the services of selected professionals and paraprofessionals presently employed in programs associated with high-risk factors in suicide could be arranged. This central staff could be drawn from child-welfare and alcoholism programs. The team could also include teachers, community-health nurses, and other volunteers interested in tutorial and health-education services. The work schedules of this staff should coincide with critical periods during which youth are most likely to be in crisis. The primary point of contact of this central staff would be through tribal and off-reservation courts, police, and juvenile-justice systems. Through this effort alone, large numbers of potential suicide victims could be identified, reached, and counseled.[28]

This central team might be augmented through a volunteer network of tribal elders, teachers, parents, health, and social-service personnel. These volunteers would serve three key roles: First, they could provide personal and telephone counseling as a follow up to the efforts of the central team. Second, they could canvas the community and serve as early observers of other youth in distress. Third, they could assist with efforts in community education and awareness. This would include "risk-behavior education" of members of both the nuclear and extended family. One member of this support team would be designated to serve as coordinator for training volunteers around clinical issues and for assigning work schedules. While the use of volunteers is questionable from the standpoint of availability and commitment, a selected number of parents and community residents is genuinely concerned in preventing youth suicide and would be available to provide emergency shelter and youth supervision on an as-needed basis.

Physical settings to house prevention services revolve around the question of availability. In actuality, potential sites abound in most communities. One simply needs to put idle space to work during time periods that are critical for youth services, such as early evenings and weekends. Possible sites include schools, tribal offices, churches, Head Start centers, or dining centers. Key to securing space is creating a climate that is tolerant of youth behavior. Given time for trial and error, space for permanent operations is generally available. It involves surveying the community and communicating the seriousness of the situation.

Cultural Intervention

Over the past two decades a number of investigators have examined important cultural issues that appear to be associated with youth suicide among American Indians. A common finding was that the more traditional the tribe and the more stable the Native religious traditions, clan, and extended family, the fewer the mental-health problems and the smaller the number of suicides. As might be expected, in the less-traditional tribes where pressures to acculturate have been great and extensive tribal conflict exists concerning traditional religion, governmental structure, clans, societies, and the extended families, the suicide rate in the adolescent and young-adult population is high. Examples of disruptive pressures are chaotic families with a great number of divorces, separations, single-parent families, alcoholism, and child neglect. The Indian adolescent feels pressured to "make it" in the non-Indian world because few are "making it" in the reservation setting. Further exacerbating the cultural dilemma, the Indian youth feels the pressure to abandon the old ways, resulting in serious conflict between contradictory values.

Many Indian tribes have been displaced from their traditional lands, and their ways of maintaining economic stability have been greatly altered. People who were once agriculturists and hunters are now involved in a variety of economic pursuits. For almost a hundred years, Native religious leaders played little or no role in Indian society because American Indian religions were banned by the federal government in 1890. The Indian Religious Freedom Act was passed on August 11, 1978, and restored the right for Native people to protect, preserve, and practice their traditional religions. This includes the possession and use of sacred objects and the freedom to worship through ceremonials and traditional rite. As a result, Native religious leaders once again play a significant role in traditional healing and should be included as an integral part of the suicide-prevention process.

Extended families have become fragmented and alcoholism is prevalent throughout most reservations. It should be noted that the extended family has always been of critical importance to the maintenance of culture in most Indian communities. Traditionally, grandparents, aunts, or uncles raised children, with parents providing the economic sustenance. When extended families were intact, there was usually admiration and respect for elders within the family. Elders provide role models of effective and valued male and female adult behavior. Hunters, tribal chiefs, and medicine people now have decreased functions within the Indian community, and the extended family has been dispersed. Often few, if any, traditional role models exist on many Indian reservations. What remains for the Indian youth is a cultural vacuum, which when combined with a stress event often results in suicide.

The lack of Indian role models has led to various innovative approaches by American Indian groups to reach Indian youth. The Association of American Indian Affairs, Inc., in New York City, and the Black Hawk Dancers from the Chitimacha Tribe of Louisiana are two groups that have been involved in providing cultural approaches to youth who have exhibited self-destructive behavior, primarily through drug and alcohol abuse. The Association on American Indian Affairs supports a traditional Indian musical group known as "Project Dream." The Indian youth who started the project were former substance abusers who tried to reach out to other teenagers in trouble. In one year, Project Dream performed before 336 Indian youth who identified themselves as substance abuses or as having self-destructive behavior. The group made a video for other Indian teenagers in order to show that what they are feeling and doing are happening to many Indian youth. Most importantly, they wanted to communicate to their peers that there are other choices available. As a result of the formation of the initial Project Dream musical group, numerous traditional Indian musical groups have been formed on and off reservations across the United States.

With a home base on their reservation in Charenton, Louisiana, the Chitimacha Black Hawk Dancers, dressed in their traditional clothing, performed North American Indian dancing for Indians schools and tribal organizations in the Southeastern part of the country. Each member of the group was a former substance abuser and gave testimony of his or her experience with each performance. All members were required to have been "dry" or "clean" since joining the dance group and served as role models for the youth before which they appeared.

The formation of American Indian youth musical and dance groups such as Project Dream and the Black Hawk Dancers can provide the physical and cultural reconnection necessary to eliminate substance abuse and reduce suicide on reservations throughout the United States. The elders could once again be used as role models for these youth. It is in the memories of these elders that the traditional music and dances reside. Remy Ordoyne stated that the music and dances utilized by the Black Hawk Dancers were learned from elder American Indian men and women.[29]

The cost of implementation of the programs mentioned above would be minimal. Musical instruments utilized in American Indian music and dance ceremonies vary, but for the most part have been handmade by the user. Drums, rattles, flutes, and bells are made from material found in nature, or are available for minimal costs. Native dress, or regalia, is also custom-made by the performer, with great pride and with great care. While this can become expensive, the regalia is simple at first and becomes more elaborate and sophisticated over time as resources become available. Native musical and dance groups would, in most instances, consist of members of the local reservation and would perform on the reservation. In instances where travel to another reservation might take place, honor dances (traditional dances used to reimburse performers) where donations are solicited could be conducted to reimburse for travel expenses While these approaches to intervention may appear to be overly simple, it is the simple that is often the most effective. Both Project Dream and the Black Hawk Dancers have excellent records in reaching and halting youth substance-abusers. These youth suffered from the loss of Indian culture and the lack of role-modeling just as do the youth who become suicide victims. Project Dream members have counseled youth who have attempted suicide. In one summer, nine Indian girls who had attempted suicide joined the project and subsequently become suicide counselors. American Indian youth music and dance groups can also function as effective intervention/prevention approaches in urban areas. The Southern California Indian Center Education Component runs an intertribal dance workshop for urban Indian youth in Los Angeles and Orange Counties. Those involved with the dance workshop have seen youth diverted from gangs and other self-destructive behaviors as a result of the cultural reconnection and improved self-image that came from participation in these programs. Urban programs, however, face additional issues of tribal diversity, transportation, and communication problems inherent in an urban environment.

The utilization of traditional American Indian song and dance groups will help this extremely vulnerable group to regain touch with important cultural traditions. Indian elders can once again teach their traditional songs and dances and be revered as cultural role-models. If the "at-risk" group of Indian youth can be reached through this intervention, be reconnected with their tribal culture through traditional song and dance, and tribal elders can once again function as role models, then the substance abuse and suicide rate among American Indian youth can be reduced.

Intervention for Indian Youth in Non-Indian Care

Another high-risk group for suicide is Indian youth in non-Indian foster and adoptive homes. With a rate of 70 per 100,000, this group represents the highest suicide rate of any group in America—six times higher than youth in the U.S. general society. Between 1969 and 1974, 25 to 35 percent of all Indian children were separated from their families and placed in non-Indian foster homes or other placements.[30] In 1978, one of the most sweeping statues in the field of Indian law was enacted, the Indian Child Welfare Act (ICWA). This act provided for the welfare of Indian children by providing guidelines for placement that would ensure that they were separated from their family or tribal setting only as a last resort.[31] The ICWA authorized any recognized Indian tribe to establish group foster homes on their reservation, to be staffed by Indian people from their reservation, for the purpose of placement of Indian children when Indian families are unavailable. While the duration (or time limit) of the placement is not specified in the act, the ideal situation would be one of placement for a short period, while permanent foster-care or adoption arrangements are made. Not only would this protect the Indian child, but it would additionally employ tribal people who, on most reservations, suffer an extremely high unemployment rate.

In the 20 years since the enactment of the ICWA, the number and percentage of Indian children being placed in non-Indian foster homes have increased, rather than decreased as might be expected. A study completed in April 1988 produced some dramatic new findings concerning the numbers, placement, and care of these children. Most importantly, this study revealed that twice as many Indian children were in substitute care as previously expected, with 51 percent of them being in non-Indian homes. In 1969 this figure had been placed at between 25 and 35 percent. The number of children in tribal and off-reservation care has increased dramatically. In comparison to foster children of all ethnic groups, Indians are greatly overrepresented in the substitute-care population. Clearly, it is evident that a serious problem exists in the placement of this vulnerable suicide group, which represents the youngest American Indians and the American Indians most likely to take their own lives.

One intervention that is supported by the empirical literature is the establishment of additional Indian foster homes, or the establishment of tribal-group foster homes in which to place American Indian children, rather than allowing them to be placed in "at risk" situations in non-Indian homes.

The first of these two, the establishment of additional Indian foster homes, may be more a matter of identification of Indian homes that are available rather than the establishment of additional foster homes. The Indian people themselves are largely unaware of the high rate of placement of Indian children in non-Indian homes and the link to the extremely high rate of suicide among this group. An on-reservation and urban educational program is needed to make the seriousness of the suicide problem and the critical need for additional foster homes known to Indian people. This can be approached in two ways: First, most Indian reservations have a tribal council where council members are elected tribal members and council meetings are open to the tribal population; for the most part these meetings are well-attended. This forum, while designed primarily to conduct tribal business, also provides for the promulgation of general information to tribal members. Announcements, presentations, and printed literature could be distributed at these meetings soliciting families who would be amenable to operate a foster home on a short- or long-term basis.

Approximately 65 percent of all Indian reservations have their own tribal newspapers, published on the reservation; several have articles written in the Native language. Information concerning youth suicide and the need for identification and recruitment of foster homes could reach a wide audience through this media. Another avenue for recruitment of Indian foster homes is through local radio stations. While only a limited number of reservations have radio stations of their own, many Indian people are reached by stations from nearby towns and feature weekly programs presented by tribal representatives. Announcements through this media would reach a wide audience. Taken together, most tribal members could be reached and made aware of the importance of this issue through the tribal council meetings, the tribal newspaper, and the radio broadcasts. Such communication can also be extended to Native people in urban areas. Local and national Indian media, such as newspapers, magazines, radio and cable-TV programs, public-service announcements on radio and television, announcements at urban Indian churches, service organizations, and political organization meetings can all be used to spread this information. The urban powwow has also become an important way to communicate with the diverse Indian population found in the urban area. Effective communication in urban Indian communities is a problem that deserves greater attention.

The second approach, that of establishing tribal-group foster homes, is authorized under the provisions of the ICWA; however, it is rarely utilized. Under the ICWA the federal government will provide funding for the construction and establishment of group foster homes, on reservations, for the placement of Indian children. The federal government will also pay for the training and salaries of Indian foster-home workers. Review of the empirical literature available and the consultation with American Indians familiar with tribal compliance with the ICWA have revealed only rare utilization of this option. The 1996 study funded by the Advocates for American Indian Children found that in 1990, Los Angeles, had 250 foster children and only 12 foster homes.[32]

The link between child welfare, child placement, mental health, and suicide among American Indians in urban areas needs to be studied. To date, no formal studies have been conducted of American Indian suicides in urban areas. Most studies on suicide have been reservation-based. However, according to the 1990 U.S. Census, more than 60 percent of Indian people now live off-reservation, primarily in cities. A recent Arizona coronary study found that a major factor in American Indian suicides on reservations was the impact of the surrounding urban communities and associated social, cultural, economic, and political pressures.[33]

Risk factors for American Indian suicide, including stress, rapid socioeconomic and cultural change, acculturation and loss of culture, isolation, and lack of strong identity, are increased among American Indian youth in urban areas in comparison to those in reservation areas. Many of these youth are raised by parents who are not traditional, thus the youth do not develop a strong cultural identity, which is strongly linked with high self-esteem. Often Indian youth may be turned over to a grandparent who is traditional, resulting in not only a generational but a cultural gap. American Indian youth in cities such as Los Angeles tend to be geographically dispersed, few in number, and from many diverse tribes, which lead to a feeling of isolation. In the schools, American Indians are faced with racism, cultural insensitivity, and stereotypes, and because they are small in number they are ignored, misidentified, and/or lumped in with other ethnic groups, creating further isolation.[34] Native children may feel like they do not fit in anywhere, and they can develop low self-images and low self-esteem. These feelings of isolation and low self-esteem can lead to depression and high-risk behavior such as drug/alcohol abuse and gang-related behavior. In Los Angeles, Indian youth were diagnosed with major depression at higher rates than other ethnic youth who sought help at county facilities.[35]

Facilities such as the Indian Health Service (IHS) do not adequately serve all urban areas. According to the Los Angeles City/County Native American Indian Commission, only about 5 percent of IHS funds support the urban Indian population.[36] The IHS also funds approximately 35 urban-Indian health programs, but these do not provide comprehensive care and are only funded at 1 percent of the total IHS budget.[37] As a result, many urban Indians do not or cannot use IHS facilities, and thus their health statistics are not tracked. Non-Indian service providers tend to believe that Indians are "someone else's problem" and are not sensitive to the Indian community's needs.[38]

Identification of urban Indians is a major problem, especially in a multi-ethnic community such as Los Angeles where American Indians become invisible in the system. The *American Journal of Public Health* reported that between 1979 and 1993 California death certificates identified less than one-third of the deaths among American Indian children, and that misclassification of race is more likely to occur in urban areas.[39] When Indian people use non-Indian services, they may not self-identify as American Indian, or they may not be asked their ethnicity. Intake clerks and school teachers often assume ethnicity without asking, resulting in many American Indians being classified in another ethnic groups, usually Hispanic. In addition, Indian people in cities do not live in geographically defined areas and do not necessarily use common services or attend common events, which adds to the problem of proper identification. Many American Indians live in mixed-race homes, and children may be identified with the race of the non-Indian parent.

A Los Angeles County Department of Mental Health employee attempted to research American Indian suicide rates for Los Angeles County. The worker found that the Los Angeles County Department of Health does not keep any data on American Indians (including emergency-room data) as it does for other ethnic groups. The worker also found that the coroner's office had only been keeping data on American Indians since 1994. Further complicating the study, the coroner's office does not declare a death as a suicide unless there is a suicide note. Therefore, to draw a more accurate picture of American Indian suicides, one must also look at violent-death data. The coroner's office only reported ten suicides in a year, while a local Indian health agency was aware of several hundred American Indian suicides in the same period. The Department of Mental Health does keep American Indian data; however, identification remains a problem. There is no legal requirement to identify American Indians within the health systems.

Clearly, a comprehensive study of American Indian youth suicide in the urban environment is needed if we are to obtain an accurate picture of overall Indian youth health and suicide in this country and to design appropriate interventions. It is hoped that this chapter will in some way encourage such a study.

Notes

1. U.S. Department of Health and Human Services, Public Health Service, Indian Health Service, *Trends in Indian Health* (Washington, DC: Government Printing Office, 1996), 67.

2. Philip A. May, "Suicide and Self-Destruction among American Indian Youths." *American Indian and Alaska Native Mental Health Research* 1(1) (June 1987): 52–69.

3. Irving N. Berlin, "Suicide among American Indian Adolescents: An Overview." *Suicide and Life-Threatening Behavior* 17(3) (fall 1987): 218–32.

4. Candace M. Fleming, Spero M. Manson, and Lois Bergeisen, "American Indian Adolescent Health," in Marjorie Kagawa-Singer, Phyllis A. Katz, Dalmas A. Taylor, and Judith H. M. Vanderryn, eds., *Health Issues for Minority Adolescents* (Lincoln: University of Nebraska Press, 1996), 116–41.

5. L. H. Dizmang, J. Watson, and J. Bopp, "Adolescent Suicide at an Indian Reservation," *American Journal of Orthopsychiatry* 33(1) (1974): 43–49.

6. May, "Suicide and Self-Destruction among American Indian Youths."

7. James H. Shore, "American Indian Suicide: Fact and Fantasy." *Psychiatry* 38 (February 1975): 3886–91.

8. May, "Suicide and Self-Destruction among American Indian Youths."

9. Shore, "American Indian Suicide: Fact and Fantasy."

10. John P. Webb and William Willard, "Six American Indian Patterns of Suicide," in Norman L. Farberow, ed., *Suicide in Different Cultures* (Baltimore: University Park Press, 1975), 17–33.

11. Ibid.

12. Mary Miller, "Suicides on a Southwestern American Indian Reservation." *White Cloud Journal* 1(1) (1979): 14–18.

13. May, "Suicide and Self-Destruction among American Indian Youths."

14. Teresa D. LaFramboise and Beth Howard-Pitney, "Suicidal Behavior in American Indian Female Adolescents," in Silvia Sara Canetto and David Lestor, eds., *Women and Suicidal Behavior* (New York: Springer Publishing, 1995), 157–73.

15. May, "Suicide and Self-Destruction among American Indian Youths."

16. Ibid.; for a more in-depth study of suicide attempts, see Darryl Zitzow and Fred Desjarlait, "A Study of Suicide Attempts Comparing Adolescents to Adults on a Northern Plains American Indian Reservation," in Spero M. Manson, ed., *Calling from the Rim: Suicidal Behavior among American Indian and Alaska Native Adolescents* (Denver: National Center for American Indian and Alaska Native Mental Health Research, 1993), 35–69.

17. Philip A. May, "Suicide among American Indian Youth: A Look at the Issues." *Children Today* 18(4) (July–August 1987): 199–214.

18. James H. Shore et al., "A Pilot Study of Depression among American Indian Patients with Research Diagnostic Criteria." *American Indian and Alaska Native Mental Health Research* 1(2) (1987): 4–15.

19. U.S. Government, Bureau of the Census (Washington, DC: Government Printing Office, 1990).

20. Ibid.

21. May, "Suicide and Self-Destruction among American Indian Youths."

22. Group for the Advancement of Psychiatry, "Suicide Among American Indians and Alaskan Natives," in *Suicide and Ethnicity in the United States* (New York: Brunner/ Mazel, 1989), 30–57.

23. Donald Johnson, "Stress, Depression, Substance Abuse, and Racism." *American Indian and Alaskan Native Mental Health Research* 6(1) (1994): 29–33.

24. May, "Suicide and Self-Destruction among American Indian Youths," 199–214; James H. Shore and Spero M. Manson, "Cross-Cultural Studies of Depression among American Indians and Alaska Natives." *White Cloud Journal* 2(2) (1981): 5–12; Berlin, "Suicide among American Indian Adolescents," 218–32.

25. I. H. Dizmang, J. Watson, and J. Bopp, "Adolescent Suicide at an Indian Reservation." *American Journal of Orthopsychiatry* 33(1) (1974): 43–49.

26. May, "Suicide among American Indian Youth."

27. J. Selkin, *The Psychological Autopsy in the Courtroom: Contributions of the Social Sciences to Resolving Issues Surrounding Equivocal Deaths* (Denver, 1976), 18.

28. J. F. Levy and S. J. Kunitz, "A Suicide Prevention Program for Hopi Youth." *Social Science and Medicine* 25(8) (1987): 931–40.

29. Interview with Remy Ordoyne by Troy Johnson, November 1990.

30. Levy and Kunitz, "A Suicide Prevention Program for Hopi Youth."

31. U.S. Congress, Senate, Public Law 95-608, *The Indian Child Welfare Act*, 95th Cong., 2d Sess., 25 U.S.C. Section 1901 et. seq. 1978.

32. Quoted in Los Angeles County Department of Mental Health, "American Indians, Urban Indians, and Rural and Reservation Indians; Los Angeles County," 1995.

33. Interview with Glenda Ahhaitty, Department of Mental Health, Los Angeles, by Holly Tomren, October 1997.

34. Duane Champagne et al., *Service Delivery for Native American Children in Los Angeles County* (Los Angeles: Advocates for American Indian Children, 1996), 38.

35. Los Angeles County of Department of Mental Health, *American Indians, Urban Indians, Los Angeles County, Rural and Reservation Indians* (1995), 9.

36. Statement by Los Angeles City/County Native American Indian Commission, 1994.

37. Champagne et al., *Service Delivery for Native American Children in Los Angeles County*.

38. Ibid.

39. Myrna Epsen et al., "The Underreporting of Deaths of American Indian Children, 1974 through 1993." *American Journal of Public Health* 87(18) (1997): 1363–66.

FOURTEEN   JEANETTE HASSIN
                        and ROBERT S. YOUNG

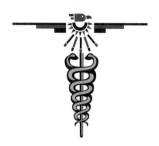

Self-Sufficiency and Community Revitalization among American Indians in the Southwest

AMERICAN INDIAN LEADERSHIP TRAINING[1]

Introduction

American Indians have been subjected to colonial domination by European nations for five centuries, resulting in a radical destabilization of their socio-cultural and economic systems, a general deterioration of mental and physical health, and rapid depopulation.[2] This domination and destruction of American Indians and their cultures began with the genocidal actions of the European invaders[3] and continues today through depressed socioeconomic structures and overarching unemployment. It is manifest in the epidemic-like incidence of diabetes and alcohol-related problems; in the mental-health issues experienced by American Indians, ranging from depression to posttraumatic stress disorder; and through ineffectual, imposed governmental institutions (e.g., Bureau of

Indian Affairs) and problematic tribal governments. Visions of economic pros-
perity outside of the boundaries of the reservation too often contrast with the
Third World situation that exists within many reservations. The exploitation
of resources within the reservation is staggering. For example, corporations
frequently lease land for mining operations that strip the earth and do little to
assist the economic activities of Native communities. All of these factors, taken
separately and together, are the anathema of self-sufficiency and feelings of
self-worth.

Broadly, the root of this sociocultural and economic devastation can be
attributed not just to warfare and oppression, but also to efforts by the dominant society to control and suppress Native peoples.[4] Once people are stigma-
tized because of their differences, they become targets for social, political, and
economic control. The dominant society uses statistics to create "truths" and
feed popular stereotypes. Additionally, by prohibiting certain topics from being
voiced and by setting up a division between what is "sanity" and "madness,"
authorities can reject from discourse all that which they classify as irrelevant or
irrational.[5] For American Indians, an example is repression of certain traditional dances. This domination goes to the heart of the disruption and destruction of cultural identity and well-being of subjugated people. Frantz Fanon
observed that within this domination process, particularly among those living
as colonized peoples, there is a continual self-questioning of identity, values,
and traditions.[6] This observation is applicable to American Indians who live in
a neocolonialist state in which all aspects of their lives and cultural identity,
including economic and political processes,[7] traumatically conflict with the
values and social perceptions of the dominant society.[8]

The resulting effects of these cultural differences and conflicts are learned
dependency, poverty, prejudice, and feelings of powerlessness and low self-
regard, which dramatically impact the health and quality of life of Native peoples. American Indians in the United States today face diabetes, substance
abuse, poor nutrition and obesity, vehicular accidents, and suicides. Alcohol
abuse is implicated in four of the ten leading causes of death among American
Indians.[9] For people seeking treatment for substance abuse, there is also a high
prevalence of co-morbid mental-health issues.[10] Entire communities are crippled by health problems, which feed into a cycle of despair, cultural disloca-
tion, and lack of self-sufficiency based in part on the usurpation of traditional
roles, imposition of an alien form of government, the removal of children from
homes for "education" and de-culturalization, and the destruction of the traditional subsistence base. Given the confluence of these health, social, political, and economic problems, concepts such as self-sufficiency and self-determination are merely meaningless abstractions.

This chapter explores how participants in a self-empowerment program
have understood and translated leadership training into self-sufficiency both at

the personal and at the community level. In analyzing this process, we present participants' own voices to detail their experiences and uses of the programs.

Aim of the Program

The self-empowerment leadership focus (S.E.L.F.) and community-revitalization program was designed to empower American Indians to identify, develop, and implement solutions to community problems. This model program consists of three interactive components: (1) a self-empowerment leadership training program; (2) a Walking-in-Two-Worlds seminar; and (3) an intensive instruction in developing community projects. The cornerstone of this leadership-training project is a "Self-Empowerment" program that emphasizes cognitive, motivational, and behavioral processes toward a goal of enhanced quality of life.[11] During the process, the individual becomes aware that there are two "minds," or ways, of perceiving, which are described as the "conditional mind" and the "unconditional mind."[12] Conditional mind is externally dependent—that is, the individual with conditional mind projects blame, anger, and guilt onto others in interactions, relationships, life situations, sickness, etc. In choosing the unconditional mind, the individual learns to accept her or his self as both observer and decision-maker, accepting responsibility for how she or he perceives and interacts with others. Exercising this process for the self also enables the individual to exercise leadership skills and interact with others in a constructive manner, which is empowering them to strive to accomplish their goals.

The Walking-in-Two-Worlds seminar engages the participants in a directed self-discovery of differing American Indian beliefs and practices, health issues, and cultural commonalties and differences, providing the participants with ancient, historical, and contemporary perspectives for understanding themselves.

The community project-development component is primarily focused on work in the areas of health and social issues. All participants in the program are required to develop a community-based project as part of their involvement. Participants define the scope of the project, the goals and the objectives, the resources they have available to conduct the project, the resources they need, and the obstacles to accomplishing the program. The participants then transfer what they have written into a grant proposal.

All workshop activities are "hands-on" experiences. A metacognitive approach is used in which participants are taught how writing can be used as a tool to help them clarify their ideas and develop practical solutions to problems.

JEANETTE HASSIN and ROBERT S. YOUNG

The Development of Self-Sufficiency

While the problems facing Indians are complicated, the solutions to these problems are even more complex because of the trauma that the populations have experienced. Unfortunately, while scholars are able to define the problems, they often fail to offer viable solutions, in part because of the extent of the sociocultural destruction and complexity of such solutions.

Key elements of any solution include culturally compatible programs that promote self-sufficiency, self-empowerment, and commitment to one's community. Most importantly, such programs must allow change to come from within. Individuals involved must take ownership if the programs are to be successful. As Pablo Freire[13] notes, it does little good to look to the oppressor for answers to the problems of the oppressed. Rather, Indian people and Indian communities need to look first to themselves for their release from oppression. The empowerment program in this study is designed to provide individuals with a process for dealing with life's challenges, both personally in terms of health and relationships and as part of a group developing a community project. From this perspective, self-empowerment is a continuous process, the operationalized outcome of which is self-sufficiency in the personal and social spheres.

Empowerment is traditionally defined in an individual context and/or as part of a group dynamic, as, for instance, collective political power.[14] Some authorities include in their definition the importance of motivation in expressing feelings, ideas, and self-worth.[15] The definition of self-empowerment differs as defined by the theoretical perspective offered in the S.E.L.F. program, providing a new way to understand the self and the individual's internal strengths. What is absent is the traditional focus on external success and power. The role of motivation is also significant because participants who come strongly motivated and committed to change are most successful in all aspects. The program provides an empowerment process and related skills to help participants sublimate their motivation into achieving self-sufficiency.

"Self-sufficiency," a term often connoting economic independence at the individual and community level and/or resilience of character, is examined here as a measure of personal and communal empowerment, and how that empowerment extends to personal and communal health. At the individual level, self-sufficiency is manifested in the reduction of factors that lead to destructive behaviors in relationships and in how individuals take claim of their own experiences. In terms of the individual, self-sufficiency is the consequence or action of the empowerment process measured in terms of personal health, attitudes, changes in personal relationships, and empowerment of others. On the communal level, it can be seen in the development and execution of community-centered programs designed for the health and survival of the community. It is also evident in their perceived sense of self-efficacy in suc-

254

cessfully motivating others to participate in the project, and, in some situations, obtaining formal tribal support to accomplish their goals.

The definition of self-sufficiency is still constrained, because it does not allow for the changes in thought processes that precede the behavioral changes and outcomes. Therefore, to analyze how participants see themselves and the impact of their efforts on others, we must expand our view of self-sufficiency to encompass behavioral outcomes and the perseverance necessary to maintain and cultivate viable options for self-improvement and nondependence.

To examine how individuals used the instruction they received in the self-empowerment and project-development training, we are taking a two-tiered approach to this analysis, examining: (1) how the participants expressed their changed perception of their health, activities, obstacles, future, and skills, and (2) how effective they were in using the training for the benefit of others and their community.

Program Participants

During the period 1995 to 1997, three generations of participants completed the self-empowerment program. All participants were American Indians from the Southwest, 21 years or older; able to articulate a community problem they would like to address; possessing basic reading and writing skills; possessing a strong desire to participate in the program; and if employed, having employer permission to attend the entire workshop. Forty-four participants—79 percent of the original number—from 14 tribes completed the two-week workshop. Twelve individuals did not complete the program because of job and personal obligations.

Tools of Analysis

Forty-two of the 44 participants who successfully completed the project were interviewed face-to-face using a semistructured format. Several months later, we conducted semistructured telephone interviews with 27 of the participants (including one of the two who were originally not interviewed). Of the remaining 17 who were not interviewed a second time, 7 did not attend any follow-up project workshops or were no longer involved in their projects. Eight participants moved and left no forwarding address or could not be reached. All but 4 interviews were tape recorded.

A discourse analysis of the narratives was used to grasp the nuances of individuals' understanding of the program and how they expressed their own self-sufficiency. Because people convey their ideas broadly through language, this chapter analyzes how program participants expressed their thoughts. It looks at issues ranging from embedded, conflicted ideas to metaphorical messages used by the person to convey their thoughts and ideas.

At the personal level, self-sufficiency included several aspects by which participants could choose to make changes in their lives. They reexamined their body, mind, and spiritual health and how they were going to take action to implement the knowledge they obtained in the training. Self-sufficiency was evident in the person's realization and ability to make choices and transfer empowerment to others.

Health: A Measure of Personal Harmony and Empowerment

Health is inextricably tied to self-sufficiency, regardless of whether the person looks at health as the measure of physical prowess or as the ability to work a full day. But health and self-sufficiency are also tied at a more basic level. For most American Indians, to be healthy is to have a harmonious balance of body, mind, and spirit. It is a sense of being complete within themselves, their family, and their community[16]:

> Healthy? Well before I would have said healthy is just physical; if you're not sick, if you don't have any illnesses, I would have considered that healthy. Now to me health is mind, body, and spirit. . . . I felt good about myself when I came, but I feel even better now. I mean I feel good because I tried to learn.
>
> . . . I want my children to have better, or how would I say, I want my kids to be healthy, to have better opportunities than, how would I say, go above me. . . . [To achieve this] I have to take care of myself. That would enable me to reach my goals and take care of the other things [the children having better].

The young man[17] who expresses these comments sees improved health as a metaphor for personal renewal and growth, a marker of personal well-being, and the vehicle for the transference of that well-being to his children. His multiple references to health, the need to take care of himself, and the beneficial feeling of learning provide the groundwork for the development of a new, proactive notion of health.

THE BODY: A CHANGE IN PERSPECTIVE, A CHANGE IN IMPORTANCE. The body is probably the most frequently used framework by which health is discussed and is often used as a measure of the presence or absence of robustness and the potential to thrive. The following narrative excerpts reflect this physical perspective and a reinterpretation of well-being through a changing perception of health. All participants relate a change of perception as they dealt with their new understanding of themselves and the role of the body and mind in health.

One man went back and forth, contrasting his behaviors and thoughts

before and after. His comments, rich in his description of his heightened interaction with his family, eventually lead him first to reflect and then to realize
his choices:

> My family said it made a difference. They saw. I felt I had more energy. . . . I
> would just apply these things to it; it's my choice. . . . Some of the other lit-
> tle things, I used to get peeved, now I just let it slide. . . . I feel like I have
> more energy. Before I was a semi-couch potato. Now I go for walks. My son
> . . . he always wants to crawl all over me. I always say, "wait, a little later."
> Now, I'm grabbing and throwing him around. . . . I felt I had more energy.
> I wanted to do things.

A woman with a major disability focused on the mind and its role in the
process of healing. She saw her new awareness and knowledge of herself leading to a new perception of her own health:

> I think that something I'm learning is that as long as you can understand
> what you're dealing with, then you're able to heal yourself. . . . If you're
> mentally intact as far as what your needs are and what you can and what you
> can't do, then you're healthy. If you're mentally healthy, then you're physically
> healthy too, even though if you have a disability.

Neither of the individuals in the two examples changed their actual physical
abilities. What they changed was their ability to make choices, "to understand
what you're dealing with," and to change inaction to action. The participants
report these behavioral changes as observable. The use of the "energy" metaphor
to describe a state of well-being was the basis of a mood change and perceptual
changes for the first person. He now saw himself as a person who could make
choices, and his first choice was to perceive his health and potential differently.
The second alteration was his ability to change himself and those around him.

THE MIND: CHANGES IN PERCEPTION AND A MOVEMENT FROM CON-
FLICT TO PEACE. Whereas some people addressed, or metaphorically expressed, their change in thinking through altered physical activity, others
focused on this cognitive change as it was manifested in an observable reduction of such behaviors, emotions, and thinking as blame, anger, and guilt. They
talked about how they were able to use the method they were given to think
about their lives differently. By using the learning process provided in the self-
empowerment training, participants changed their focus from blaming others
and expressing anger to an inward focus for healing and peace. They saw their
own actions through a new perspective, and from that perspective took
responsibility for their experiences. One man's new perceptual awareness
caused him to reflect on his past actions, his guilt over those actions, and how
his current healing had to come from within. This person describes how he

blamed events and people for his own behaviors. In the course of a day's work, he would have to stop at multiple villages. Sometimes things would come up and he would be late for his first stop and because of that he was late for all subsequent ones. The people expecting him at a particular time would get angry because he was late, and because they were elders he felt he could not answer back and explain the situation. Instead, he kept the problem to himself. Finally, after a day full of frustration, he would react: "When I get to the third reservation, all it takes is for someone to call me an ugly dog or something and I'll pounce that guy . . . [which] gave me the opportunity to take my anger out." In recounting this story, he demonstrated his awareness of his actions and how his thinking rather than the behaviors of others had caused him to lose his peace. Several months later, he articulated the core elements of empowerment and self-sufficiency:

> I found myself coming back home thinking about it [the self-empowerment process], and I realized what it was all about. It finally dawned on me. Heal yourself. This self-empowerment stuff is working. Instead of getting upset about others not doing things, I feel like I can do it myself, now.

SPIRITUALITY: EXPRESSIONS OF HEALING AND ONENESS. It was not uncommon for participants to compare what they were learning about empowerment and its impact on their health to what they had been traditionally taught by their elders and their healers. Since the teacher and developer of the self-empowerment program was non-Indian, some participants initially greeted him with skepticism. Yet it became clear through comments made during the workshop and in subsequent interviews that the self-empowerment instruction appeared to resonate with traditional teachings. Comments included, "I've heard it before at home" and "it's part of our tradition, our religion, our upbringing." The instruction was seen as a "reminder" or as being in agreement with the person's spirituality and faith:

> You have to step out there and believe. You really have to go on your faith and your belief. And the non-Indian world, they really don't get into it. I think "P" is the only one I've ever heard, non-Indian, speak about stepping out there just on faith and belief alone. And yet, that's what it's all about.

One person describes the self-empowerment process as a third way (after his biblical and Alcoholics Anonymous teachings) to practice healing.

A couple of individuals took the training to the level of healing, balance, and spiritual oneness. They talked about how the process helped them reaffirm and strengthen their culture's traditional teachings. While one person framed his discussion around the interrelated nature of health, the other related how the training reinforces her beliefs:

Well, when I really think about it, this is something that the Indians have been practicing all their lives. . . . For instance, this medicine man he only works with snakebites. He walked off, he got bitten by a snake so he was mad and said, "go ahead bite the other foot," and the snake just wandered off. And he turned around and walked back and by the time he got home he was healed because he was singing songs and healing songs. That's something like what these guys are presenting, but it's an old thing. I think, but I'm glad that they do realize that it works.

It [self-empowerment] just reinforced my beliefs. . . . I know that it works but I never knew the other side. When I say the other side I mean white people would understand it and teach it back to us. I mean I believe it and everything. It's just that nobody sat down and presented it in this fashion, so yeah, it really reinforced my beliefs. . . . I was trying to explain it to my son and he goes, oh yeah, I know what you're talking about, and he started explaining to me about it . . . they're already teaching him about blaming people. If you do something and try to blame people, you know it's you projecting your own thoughts.

This person addressed her healing through three levels of interaction: (1) traditional healing; (2) her son's awareness of healing; and (3) her own awareness of her actions and subsequent healing. The statement illustrates her awareness of self, of others, and of overall healing. This new approach brought her to an acceptance of what her own behavior was and her need to change that behavior in order to heal. Yet another person is focused more on the interconnected, harmonious aspect of health:

To me to be healthy is healthy physically, emotionally, mentally, and spiritually, they all connect. . . . So for me to be healthy all these has to be like in harmony with one another. . . . It's like . . . to be in harmony, to have a balance of all these, to be healthy.

Yet when asked how he saw his own health, there was hesitation, reflection, and reassessment of himself and his situations:

[pause] Not so good, everything's not in balance, and I have stepped away from my spirituality. . . . Now going through this program has given me some ideas, some direction. I guess that's why I say it's exciting because the tools that I have now I can go out and experience some of the tools that has been given to me, so to get healthy.

In analyzing his present situation, he reflected on what was ideal—namely, balance and harmony. "[E]verything's not in balance" resulted from the absence of spirituality. Unlike before, he felt motivated to change. He examined what he received from the program—cognitive "tools," "ideas," and "direction"—and the impact these perceptions can have on his health.

259

Action and Direction

Perseverance is a key component to the implementation of knowledge and the use of cognitive processes such as the self-empowerment training. It can be seen in the interest, motivation, and commitment of the person or of the community. Perseverance provides the impetus and the sustaining force for successful change to occur.

REALIZATION OF CHOICES. Choice is one of the key teachings of the self-empowerment process. Choice is defined as the ability to understand that reactive thinking (e.g., anger, blame, guilt) comes not from external causes but from a way of thinking and from the decisions made through that thinking, which result in the loss of personal power. To retake that power, or more precisely, to release oneself from external dependency, the person must make the conscious decision to think creatively about problems and situations and to approach these events with peace and not conflict. For many participants in this program, the tools they received provided a new way of thinking about old hurts, present difficulties, and future plans. The recognition was voiced through self-examination of their options for themselves, their families, and their communities.

"Choice," viewed at the personal level, was seen as the realization that everyone caused his or her own feelings. As one participant noted: "[It] is how we go within ourselves and learn why we behave the way we behave. And that we choose our feelings; we even choose our own thoughts. Nobody causes them." Reflecting on this notion of choice, one young man illustrated this view in his description of a potentially contentious situation that occurred during the workshop:

> A lot of people brought up a lot of things about the white man. Everybody expressed hatred. I thought, "my gosh, this is a part of our whole upbringing. No wonder we can't function in this type of world and expect to survive." A lot of these people forget what they really are; they forget what they really have in their minds and in their hearts. I was upset with "P" when he said, "don't think you're a unique person just because you're Indian." I wanted to grab that pitcher of water and dump it on him personal. I said, "wait a minute, he wouldn't have done that just to piss us off. There was something in there. What does he mean?" . . . I thought this guy has a lot of guts to say that to me. Right off the bat. But then thinking like that, and then thinking about what he said: "Wake up, you're Indian, you'll always be Indian no matter what. You just got to learn how to survive and be at peace with yourself, have oneness in yourself and go on. You have to go on." . . . People haven't thought about it. They want to carry that monkey on their back instead of taking the monkey and looking at the monkey and finding what's different about the monkey among all the other ones that they have on their back.

In the above excerpt, the person walked through his reactions and levels of understanding as he moved through his process of making choices: (1) about the message being given; (2) how to incorporate it personally; and (3) how the awareness he has discovered could help others. The narrative illustrates the compelling force of the person's thinking as he uncovers his levels of realization about himself and his choices. He talked about his awareness that choices, even the choice to listen in peace, can be liberating from the addiction to certain concepts and behaviors; for example, the hatreds people hold on to that ultimately hurt and inhibit them. He expressed this change from his own feelings of anger, to an understanding and self-awareness, to a realization of the need for others to rid themselves of their burdens.

TRANSFER OF EMPOWERMENT TO OTHERS. The process of transferring one's own sense of empowerment to others by sharing the information directly or by empowering people by letting them take responsibility for their own experiences was evident from many of the narratives. Participants used and extended the self-empowerment process to others through sharing and explanation, modeling, and enabling others to realize the consequences of their own experiences.

The following two narratives illustrate how two participants understood empowerment, manifested it, and transferred it to others. In so doing, they illustrate their own self-sufficiency as they release themselves from their reliance on external dependencies, while at the same time enabling others to experience self-sufficiency.

One man recounted his confrontation with a lifelong hostility he had for another person and how he resolved it while releasing himself and the "hated" person:

> This woman she said, "Hey, how you doing?" And this is one lady I never
> did like because she took me out of my home and put me in a foster home.
> I said, "I'm doing fine, how are you doing?" And she was shot to hell. It was
> the first time you said something, in her mind I knew she was thinking that.
> I said, "I forgive you, you were doing your job." She just started crying. I've
> learnt to open a lot of doors. Instead of putting Band-Aids over them, let the
> wound open and dry itself out. Let the tears take over. Or let it bleed till it
> stops bleeding. It's an exhilarating experience, top of the cake with a cherry.

His act of forgiveness not only healed his wounds, but also those of the other person.

Discovering "patience" became the focal point for another participant who talked about his reaction to learning that his oldest daughter had dented his new truck. His analysis of the situation emphasized the importance of his own conscious awareness as he describes his reaction to receiving the news, his handling of this situation, and his daughter's response to his "new reaction":

261

So I guess she made a sharp turn . . . and she dented the side of the truck. . . . They came in and my youngest daughter was saying, "L's in trouble, L's in trouble." . . . Then my oldest daughter came down and she just laid down on the bed on her stomach, and she just laid down there. Because I guess before, I would get mad at every little thing. And then I asked them what happened, and she told me, then I didn't say anything, I just like smiled. I just accepted it right there, even though it was a new truck. . . . I didn't say anything, I just accepted it; then I just told them that it was an accident. And I noticed right away that she changed . . . the way she was feeling before, like she was scared or she was like, how I would react. Then she right away, she just got happy. And then we just kind of like compared [it with another dented truck] and it was really nothing, because it was just a small dent. Compared to what she would have went through if I didn't accept her, I had done something else. It was good.

In this situation he chose to look at the event and not react, a departure from his normal response to these kinds of situations. Removing the elements of anger and reciprocal fear from his relationship with his daughter liberated him, and they were both able to look at the dent in the truck without condemnation, anger, guilt, or fear.

Sometimes people were able to see how being self-empowered actually encouraged others to be responsible for themselves. One participant recounted how he found himself dominating a staff meeting. When he realized he was doing this, he decided to "shut up and let the staff take over." In a different situation, a woman allowed her son, on trial for a DUI charge, to experience the repercussions of his actions. She used the self-empowerment process to help her realize that letting her son experience the repercussions of his own actions enabled both of them to become self-sufficient. She became a decision-maker and saw herself released from the co-dependent relationship. When she was re-interviewed two years later, this person noted that what she learned from her involvement in the program gave her courage and a greater understanding of herself. While not all had such long-term retention of the principles of the program, over 60 percent of those reinterviewed stated that they were still using what they had learned.

Many participants attributed changes in their behavior to the new way they chose to perceive events and people. Each person noted a change in at least one behavior: anger, impatience, or guilt. As a result of their decisions and choices, they saw themselves capable of decoupling another person from his or her dependency and themselves from guilt or the past. The end results were described in terms of contentment, calm, satisfaction, and increased productivity for themselves and others.

While these examples support the notion that one individual's self-sufficiency can also enable another to be self-sufficient, it is another question as to whether that empowerment can be translated into self-sufficiency at the community level. Such a process would involve a greater effort and commitment on the part of the individual.

Transferring a Personal Vision to the Community

The goal of transferring personal strengths and one's vision to a larger community forum could be a daunting task, and it was not a goal that everyone in the program felt ready to pursue. Although the ideal goal was for each participant to produce self-sustaining community programs, the real meta-goal was to see progress in the transfer of the self-empowerment process into this next level of self-sufficiency. Of the 44 participants who completed the self-empowerment leadership program, over half of the participants (25) developed a clear project plan; of that number, 15 have completed at least preliminary work on developing their projects either by assessing support or through preliminary meetings of interested community members. Seven of the 15 have also performed need-assessments and are holding regular community meetings in their project areas. These individuals are also in the process of procuring funding or obtaining final tribal approval to move forward on their projects. Six additional participants have successfully instituted or completed their projects. Although not all have realized their final goals, many have moved themselves and their communities toward greater self-sufficiency within their chosen areas. The following discussion will look at how participants pursued their goal as measured by their ability to transfer their increased personal self-sufficiency to initiate, develop, and accomplish their community project.

CREATIVITY. A key aspect of the self-empowerment leadership program is to teach participants to reduce reactive conditioned thinking that can inhibit their ability to move beyond obstacles, both personal—time, family, and work obligations—or community—apathy, politics, lack of funds. Creativity—the ability to look at situations, events, and people's capabilities in innovative ways that are consistent with their own culture's beliefs and practices—is expressed in their use of knowledge, awareness of community needs, and development and implementation of strategies. It is this effort in combination with the skills obtained in the project-development and grants-writing workshops that show how far the participants were able to take their skills and knowledge towards community-level self-sufficiency.

Transforming Individual Self-Sufficiency into Community Action and Change

Developing skills to design projects and to write grants were integral components of the leadership program. Although most participants sought these skills and were motivated to obtain this knowledge, not everyone shared that interest.

LEVELS OF REALIZATION. The following discussion focuses on the efforts of the 21 program participants representing 19 different programs, who took their goals and objectives for their programs and either realized them or made significant steps towards attaining them. All were able to express clearly the issues they wanted to address and the strategies they would pursue. Yet not all were able to realize their goals equally. For many, having enough time was an impediment to their completion or persistence with their project. Others felt that staff follow-up was not as involved as they would have liked, and for this reason they did not complete their project work. A couple of individuals admitted to having "lost track" of their project. The questions nevertheless remain: Why was time an issue for some and not for others? Why did some individuals call and work with staff and others did not? And finally, why did some people lose track of their projects while others stayed with their projects to completion?

In analyzing how participants viewed their projects, their roles in them, and their responses to possible and real setbacks, we looked at how much progress people made on their projects based on: (1) preparatory steps for the project (e.g., organizational meetings); (2) level and frequency of contact with others concerning the project, including lobbying efforts; (3) implementation of the project; and (4) structural stability of the project in the community. The projects reflected several community-level concerns:

a. *Youth:* Three language and culture programs (two for young children), a Girls and Boys Clubs program, a youth resource center, and a community theater group.
b. *Community:* Community-needs assessment, park-beautification project, alternative-housing project, and a historical video of the community.
c. *Family:* Two parenting-skills programs (one for parents of children with special needs), and a domestic violence center.
d. *Disability:* A vocational rehabilitation program, an Intertribal Disabilities Council, and an independent-living center.
e. *Health:* Diabetes Health Education Program, Intertribal FAS/FAE Network, Community Wellness Center, and a Self-Empowerment Program.

The manner in which people progressed with their programs reflected how well they were able to see a clear path from their own personal self-sufficiency to a mobilized effort for the program they wanted to see actualized. There were three observable levels of progress among those developing and implementing the above programs: (1) unclear support and uncertain course of action; (2) clear support and defined course of action; and (3) clear support and implemented action.

(1) UNCLEAR SUPPORT AND UNCERTAIN COURSE OF ACTION. Of the five participants who made preparatory steps towards proceeding with their project beyond their efforts in the workshop, three saw lack of time and support as the major obstacle in completing what they set out to do. Their work, while frequently seen as feasible and exuberantly expressed during the workshop, became less focused over the intervening months. Their efforts stopped at early stages of the project's development; that is, a person might reach a preliminary stage in the program's organization, hold an initial meeting or see if others like the idea, but not go beyond that point. While some of the comments reflect a person's dissatisfaction with him- or herself for losing track of the project, others, who were less empowered, directed the cause for this lack of action outside of themselves. A couple of individuals acknowledged that they had the support of the agency that would be overseeing the project and of the general community, but said that because their new jobs had been consuming their available time, they were unable to continue their work on their projects. Some of these individuals also saw "tribal politics" as a major impediment to achieving their goals. For most of these individuals, their setbacks or lack of progress were attributed to forces outside of themselves that were beyond their control.

(2) CLEAR SUPPORT AND DEFINED COURSE OF ACTION. Nine participants fell into this category. Members of this group were intent on keeping themselves focused on solving the problems in implementing their projects. They were also clear about expressing their needs: "[I] need more grants-writing training," "[help] with dealing with people who say they will help and then back out." And sometimes they simply wanted feedback on their work. One person was implementing her project even while looking for areas in which to expand and fund her program. Another person, interested and motivated to do an intertribal information network on fetal alcohol syndrome/fetal alcohol effect (FAS/FAE), found out during the preliminary stages of organization that before the network could do anything constructive, the group first had to find out what human and material resources were available among the group members.

Each individual was intent on pursuing his or her goals. They appreciated the support of their communities ("everybody is committed to a prevention-type program," "we had a lot of directors from different programs supporting us"), and possibly because of that, were willing to pursue funding outside of the tribe. Seeking outside funding was frequently cited as a more viable option to working through their tribal councils for financial support. They also saw their own personal commitment to the project as critical to its viability: "If I quit and say 'forget it,' you guys can handle it and go home and stay there, it may never take place." Each person focused on the problem and pursued the tasks necessary to keep the plan alive and to write the proposal that could provide the necessary funding.

265

(3) CLEAR SUPPORT AND IMPLEMENTED ACTION. These individuals have been able to put their projects into action within the context they defined. The six participants who did this pursued projects that bore no great similarity to each other but in fact mirrored the diversity of the other projects. This diversity was also seen in what people brought to the workshop. For example, some participants had strong ties to their spiritual beliefs while others had drifted somewhat away from their traditional ways, as was evidenced in such areas as coping with and relieving personal conflict and anger. What distinguished this group was that all of them did projects within the framework of their jobs. They all had the support of their supervisors, and in the few cases, they were able to develop grant proposals as part of their jobs. Similarly, each of these individuals enjoyed the support of their community, and ultimately, the tribal council. A person who had originally wanted to develop a language and culture class for young children to attend while on their school breaks soon turned her attention toward the larger issue of what the community saw as its primary needs. To this end, she successfully developed, executed, and analyzed the results of a community-needs assessment and continues to work to address the community's concerns. Not only does this show transference of action from a specific to a broad scope, it also shows a commitment to transfer the decision-making process to those most personally affected by it. This was also observed in the efforts of another participant who, as a service coordinator, focused her attention on the housing situation in her district. With the help of a mentor she brought together a cadre of volunteer experts and personnel from inside and outside the community to work on a construction-material demonstration project. The tribe is currently discussing the possibility of setting aside a large area of land to locate the new housing.

In a smaller program we see the creation and full funding of a youth resource center. The interest and motivation expressed for the development of this program were evident during the first workshop this participant attended. During this time, she defined her efforts within the context of the goals she was seeking for herself and the community. The young woman who developed the resource center took her own desires, interests, and concerns and used them to attain something for the youth in her community. Drawing on the self-empowerment process and her own spirituality, she saw a similarity of focus and goal: "Even in our own language, that's what's always been said, that it's really up to me, that it's up to me to decide whatever I want." Harnessing this intent, she developed her project and wrote a grant proposal that was funded. The center is a resource hub for the young people in the community and generated several smaller programs, including a dance group, traditional games, and community-service activities.

Having the support of an employer or an organization to develop and complete a project is extremely helpful. Yet, this support does not guarantee the successful development and completion of a project, nor does it qualify as the sole, overriding determinant for the lack of successful development and completion. Other factors reflect what the individual and the community bring to the effort. Whereas the community must see the idea as supportable, the individuals developing the project should: (1) have the ability to use self-empowerment to enhance their self-sufficiency on a scale that is larger than personal interaction; (2) possess a strong internalized perception of support—that is, motivation and commitment to the project; and (3) not perceive obstacles, such as politics or funding, as barriers.

Discussion

This program and the issues raised about self-sufficiency have helped to inform us about how individuals and communities understand and implement change. For the program to support empowerment and self-sufficiency among the participants, it had to provide people with the tools and instructions to move beyond guilt or anger. It also had to provide participants the means to look creatively at their own lives and the lives of their communities to enable them to create programs to enhance the lives of their people.

It would be wrong-headed to develop a program that would put people in constant conflict with existing social and political constraints, so it was important that no agenda was imposed that went beyond the interests or capabilities of the community structure. Yet, it was neither wrong nor disempowering to provide people with the skills to learn how to develop projects and write grants that would enable them to work outside of the political fray. Just as each person took what she or he could from both the empowerment and the project-development components of the program, such a program must not push people into a fixed agenda of preconceived outcomes because success and health can come at all levels of involvement.

Self-sufficiency is not a blanket concept that can be isolated as a strict definition. It draws its expression from the circumstances and situations of the daily life of the people. Some of those experiences are personal and limited, and some of them are expansive and communal. All support family, and draw from the support of family and through community cohesion. Self-sufficiency is part of a sequential series of steps from personal empowerment to community revitalization. Self-empowerment, while personal by definition, was used by these participants as a way to reconnect to the spiritual and cultural ties of their people, while also connecting them to real problems and issues in their communities.

The multiple expression of self-sufficiency evident throughout this analysis emphasizes both the subtlety and complexity by which it was expressed and

realized. The analysis shows that the notion of self-sufficiency is not only difficult to separate from self-empowerment, motivation, and commitment, but is
also actually integrally connected by the person to all three. The people whose
voices were heard in this chapter saw and used self-empowerment as a means
for working with daily-life events. It helped them understand their own reactions and their interactions with others. Yet, even though the explanations and
theory were new, comments and analysis were couched in a familiarity that
facilitated the use of the process. Familiarity and resonance with their own spirituality was helpful to the participants in understanding how the self-empowerment process could be incorporated into their lives without conflicting with
their beliefs. Both the Indian participants and the non-Indian instructor focused
on the person as an intrinsically "whole and complete" beautiful and healthy
being whose source of upset/disharmony came from believing that happiness
lay in outside attainments and possessions. This sense of spiritual oneness and
being centered and in balance became a strong tie between the program and the
people.

While the commitment and motivation were easier to secure at the personal level where the participants were accountable to and for themselves and
their interaction with family members, friends, and co-workers, they were
much more difficult to sustain when program participants had to develop and
implement a project in their communities. At this point it became necessary
for community members to not only share their vision of change, but also to
experience their own sense of power and hope. This was not trivial, because
for people to commit to a plan or an idea for change necessitated that they
reassess their abilities as vehicles for change, a perspective that required a view
of themselves as empowered and as decision-makers. It also required much
more from the person interested in instituting the project. Here motivation
and commitment had to take on a more proactive role in achieving self-sufficiency. As much as personal self-sufficiency required a level of internalized
support based on one's beliefs, so the development of community-level self-
sufficiency heavily relied on the external support of the social system. If there
was resistance to the project—for example, if official tribal approval was not
forthcoming or other people were not taking more active roles—then they
might drop the project or diminish its importance in their lives. This could
occur if having trouble getting funding or having difficulty obtaining a proposal or a request through tribal bureaucracy became translated into a lack of
time to work on the project (diminished motivation and commitment).
Conversely, some participants took the same difficulties and interpreted them
as challenges and pursued other avenues of support (sustained motivation and
commitment). Consensus may play an important role in determining whether
or not a person chooses to pursue completion of his or her project. This kind
of support from the community appears to be important for the translation of

the motivation and commitment of personal self-sufficiency into a community-level project.

There were multiple levels at which the participant could apply the self-empowerment process towards self-sufficiency. On the personal level, individuals did this through their view of their health; how they were able to make choices; and the manner in which the self-sufficiency they achieved was transferred to others. If the progress and understanding of the tools of self-empowerment were incorporated and used in their personal lives, then the individuals were more likely to use the process to bring self-sufficiency to their communities. And yet, this did not occur for all participants who were able to use the self-empowerment process at the personal level. Everyone did not start or make significant progress with his or her project. Therefore, it is necessary to examine some other underpinning cultural, social, and economic factors that influenced this aspect of the program, as well as the program itself, to understand why some participants were able to transfer the knowledge and others did not want to or were unable to do it.

The majority of the comments reflects perceptions people have about their ability to approach the projects from conception to execution. Some, while secure in using the self-empowerment learning process at the personal level, were unable to translate it into self-sufficiency at the community level when they needed to know more about some specific skill, for example, grants writing or how to turn community support into community action. While a few participants requested and received direct assistance from the empowerment-program staff outside of the workshops to implement their goals, others simply made no contact and made no progress in developing their project when they felt that they lacked the necessary knowledge to proceed. Finally, while time was the most frequently cited reason for inaction or stalled action, a few simply noted that they did not know how to move beyond their present point of inaction. There was a desire to work on the project, but an inability to take a direction or to mobilize the necessary people to proceed with the plan. For individuals in this situation, self-sufficiency at the community level was not operating.

The question remains not so much whether people can give an accurate portrayal of their own self-sufficiency, but what has prevented some persons from using their tools of empowerment while others have used them at all levels of interaction. While we cannot disregard other factors in the participants' lives that impact their progress, these other circumstances and events may not be the whole explanation. Part of the answer may lie in whether they were able to initiate and actualize projects within their current employment (Did they work for the tribe? What was their position?), and part may have been the need to achieve consensus before they proceeded with their plan. How other community members perceive the individual may also play a role in the person's ability to obtain support for her or his project. The answer may take any number of forms from personal characteristics to life experiences to length of time living in the community. The problem could even be the project itself: is it perceived by others as benefiting the person directly, socially, politically, or financially?

Obtaining consensus took diverse forms: polling the community in public meetings, conducting informal surveys, and conducting door-to-door formal needs assessments. How people sought consensus was determined by their position in the community: employees of the tribe went to the council or conducted a formalized needs assessment; a member of the disabled community informally surveyed other people with disabilities; and a parent concerned about the youth in the community organized a public meeting. Culture, in particular, played a role in how a program was developed or implemented. A participant from one tribe needed to obtain approval from a broad consensus, whereas another participant only needed the approval of a politically powerful supervisor. Some individuals who found support for their projects in their community but were reluctant to work through tribal government sought financial support from outside sources. Many who applied for funding but were turned down did not give up their interest in obtaining a grant and improving their grant-writing skills. The difference between action and inaction for those who did and those who did not develop or progress with their programs suggests that there is a strong need to address the barriers to translating self-sufficiency from the personal to the community level. In so doing, the apathy and the political and bureaucratic situations present in many of their reservations will be perceived not so much as barriers, but as hurdles to community revitalization.

There is yet another level of self-sufficiency for American Indians that should be addressed: self-determination and sovereignty. Because we were able to see expressions of nondependence at the personal level and its translation over to the community level, we were not surprised to find that these expressions are also part of a larger socioeconomic and political picture. This is best exemplified by the comments of one of the participants in a similar program for youth. This young person talked about her frustration with her tribe and tribal council because of the decision to plan and to build another casino on tribal land: "Why," she wanted to know, "were they building another casino for the entertainment of white people? Why weren't they directing more of their attention towards the needs of the tribal people themselves?" She was not, as one might assume, unaware of the monetary gains the casinos bring. She was instead protesting the role of the tribe as being a source of amusement for non-Indians rather than as a source of strength for Indian people. To use Freire's terms,[18] it was as if she did not want the oppressor to be seen as raising the oppressed. For this individual this process is the antithesis of self-determination; that is, the casinos were not liberating her people from dependence on the dominant society—they were linking them to it.

This protest should not be discounted as a motivating influence. Self-sufficiency as seen through self-determination is an important area for future work. It is implicated in personal awareness, understanding, and interpersonal and community interaction among American Indians. It is ultimately implicated in the power relationships Indian people have with the dominant society.

Notes

1. We gratefully acknowledge the W. K. Kellogg Foundation, whose support made this project possible. We would also like to thank Paul H. Skinner, Ph.D. for his suggestions and encouragement. Finally, we would like to offer our thanks to the many people who participated in this project and whose own experiences and comments have enriched our understanding of how self-sufficiency is developed and realized.

2. H. F. Dobyns, *Their Numbers Became Thinned: Native American Population Dynamics in Eastern North America* (Knoxville: University of Tennessee Press, 1983); D. T. Reff, "The Demographic and Cultural Consequences of Old-World Disease in the Greater Southwest, 1520–1660." Unpublished doctoral dissertation, University of Oklahoma, 1985; M. Trimble, "Epidemiology in the Northern Plains: A Cultural Perspective." Unpublished doctoral dissertation, University of Missouri-Columbia, 1985; J. R. Joe, and R. S. Young, eds., "Introduction" in *Diabetes as a Disease of Civilization* (Berlin: Mouton de Gruyter, 1994).

3. N. Gray, "Addressing Trauma in Substance Abuse Treatment with American Indian Adolescents," *Journal of Substance Abuse Treatment* 15 (1998): 393–99.

4. M. Foucault, *The Birth of the Clinic* (London: Oxford University Press, 1973).

5. M. Foucault, *The Archaeology of Knowledge and the Discourse on Language* (New York: Pantheon Books, 1972).

6. F. Fanon, *The Wretched of the Earth* (New York: Grove Press, 1968).

7. G. C. Anders and S. J. Langdon, "Alaska Native Regional Strategies," *Human Organization* 48 (1989): 162–72; G. C. Anders and K. K. Anders, "Incompatible Goals in Unconventional Organization: The Politics of Alaska Native Corporations," *Organizational Studies* 7 (1986): 213–33.

8. S. Cornell, "Land, Labour and Group Formation: Blacks and Indians in the United States," *Ethnic and Racial Studies* 13 (1990): 368–88; C. M. Snipp, "'Who Are American Indians?' Some Observations about the Perils and Pitfalls of Data for Race and Ethnicity," *Population Research and Policy Review* 5 (1986): 237–52.

9. *Trends in Indian Health, 1996* (Rockville, MD: U.S. Department of Health and Human Services, Public Health Service, Indian Health Service, 1996).

10. R. D. Walker, M. D. Lambert, P. S. Walker, and D. R. Kivlahan, "Treatment Implications of Comorbid Psychopathology in American Indians and Alaska Natives," *Culture, Medicine and Psychiatry* 16 (1993): 555–72.

12. P. H. Skinner, *Alternative Medicine: Healing the Self* (Mt. Clemens, MI: Gold Leaf Press, 1995).

13. P. Freire, *Pedagogy of the Oppressed* (New York: Continuum Press, 1990).

14. L. M. Guiterrez, "Working with Women of Color: An Empowerment Perspective," *Social Work* 35 (1990): 149–53; M. A. Zimmerman, "Psychological Empowerment: Issues and Illustrations," *American Journal of Communal Psychology* 23 (1995): 581–99.

15. J. Rappaport, "The Power of Empowerment Language," *Social Policy* 17 (1985): 15–21.

16. J. R. Joe and R. S. Malach, "Families with Native American Roots," in G. W. Lynch and M. T. Hanson, eds., *Developing Cross-Cultural Competence: A Guide for Working with Young Children and Their Families* (Northvale, NJ: Lawrence Erlbaum Associates, 1993).

17. To insure anonymity, personal identifying criteria were altered or eliminated.

18. Freire, *Pedagogy of the Oppressed*.

INDEX

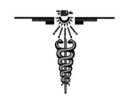

Page numbers in italics indicate tables.

ABOUT THE CONTRIBUTORS

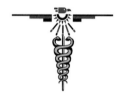

DONNA L. AKERS (Choctaw) is an assistant professor of history at Purdue University.

TODD BENSON wrote his Ph.D. on the history of federal Indian health care policy during the first half of the twentieth century. He is currently associate director of advising at the Stanford School of Medicine.

LINDA BURHANSSTIPANOV (Western Cherokee) has been working in Native American Cancer Prevention and Control since the latter part of the 1980s. She is the executive director of Native American Cancer Research, and Indian-owned and operated non-profit corporation.

JOHN CASKEN is an assistant professor, University of Hawaii at Manoa, School of Public Health/School of Medicine. He has had extensive experience in the recruitment of American Indians and Alaska Natives into higher educational institutions, and teaches in the area of indigenous health care.

EDWARD D. CASTILLO (Cahuilla-Luiseño Mission descendant) is a professor of Native American Studies at Sonoma State University. He is a nationally recognized author and expert on California Indian history.

DOUGLAS FREEMAN, JR. (cover art) is an artist for Gravitywell Productions, a web-based provider of comic books, animated cartoons, and illustrations. He can be reached and his work viewed at <http://www.gravitywell.com>.

JAMES HAMPTON (Choctaw and Chickasaw) is one of two Native American oncologists in the United States. He has been recognized as a community and professional advocate for Native American cancer-prevention and -control efforts for more than 30 years. He is chair of the National Network of Cancer Control Research among American Indian and Alaska Native Populations.

JEANETTE HASSIN, Ph.D. is a medical anthropologist and consultant to the College of Public Health, the Arizona Cessation Training and Evaluation Unit at the University of Arizona. Her major interests are substance abuse and contemporary American Indian health and community issues.

ERIC HENDERSON is a social anthropologist in the Department of Social Sciences, Great Basin College.

FELICIA SCHANCHE HODGE, Dr. P.H., is a Wailaki Indian from Northern California. She is the director of the Center for American Indian Research and Education at the University of California, San Francisco and is professor of nursing at the University of Minnesota. Dr. Hodge has received numerous research grants in areas of cancer prevention and control, smoking cessation, nutrition, diabetes and wellness—all targeting American Indian and Alaska Native populations. She is a member of the University Breast Cancer Research Council, on the board of SACNAS, and a member of the National Cancer Institute Director's Consumer Liaison Group.

TROY JOHNSON is an associate professor of American Indian studies and history at California State University, Long Beach. His publications include *The Occupation of Alcatraz Island: Indian Self-Determination and The Rise of Indian Activism* and *American Indian Activism: Alcatraz to the Longest Walk*.

JEAN A. KELLER is completing her Ph.D. in history at University of California, Riverside.

STEPHEN J. KUNITZ is a professor in the Department of Community and Preventive Medicine at the University of Rochester School of Medicine and Dentistry, Rochester, New York.

JEROME M. LEVI is associate professor of anthropology in the Sociology/ Anthropology Department at Carleton College, Northfield, Minnesota.

JERROLD E. LEVY is a professor emeritus at the University of Arizona, Department of Anthropology.

BROOKE OLSON, a medical anthropologist, teaches at Ithaca College and engages in multicultural health research and consulting. She serves on the Advisory Board of Ithaca's Integrative Community Wellness Center, where she aids in the development of integrative and community-based models of health care and wellness.

NANCY REIFEL (Rosebud Sioux) is a commissioned officer serving in the Dental Branch of the Indian Health Service, Public Health Service. Through an agreement between IHS and the University of California, Los Angeles, she is stationed at the UCLA School of Dentistry.

MARTHA J. TENNEY, MPH, is a program officer for Colorado Action for Healthy People. Her work includes assisting with local needs assessments and health promotion and education.

HOLLY TOMREN graduated Phi Beta Kappa from California State University, Long Beach in 1997 and is a graduate student in American Indian Studies at the University of California, Los Angeles.

CLIFFORD E. TRAFZER (Wyandot) is a professor of history and director of Native American Studies at the University of California, Riverside.

DIANE WEINER is a professional research anthropologist at the American Indian Studies Center, University of California, Los Angeles. Her work focuses on the analysis of chronic illness and health beliefs and behaviors and the development of health-education materials.

ROBERT S. YOUNG, Ph.D. is a research associate at the Native American Research and Training Center, in College of Medicine, the University of Arizona. His major interests are diabetes and substance abuse problems among American Indians.